Mucosal Vaccine Delivery Systems: The Future of Immunization

(Part 2)

Edited by

Shaweta Sharma
School of Medical and Allied Sciences
Galgotias University, Yamuna Expressway
Gautam Buddha Nagar, Uttar Pradesh-201310
India

Aftab Alam
School of Pharmacy Katihar Medical College
Campus Alkarim University Katihar-854106 Katihar
India

&

Akhil Sharma
R.J. College of Pharmacy, Raipur, Gharbara
Tappal, Khair Uttar Pradesh, India

Mucosal Vaccine Delivery Systems: The Future of Immunization *(Part 2)*

Editors: Shaweta Sharma, Aftab Alam, and Akhil Sharma

ISBN (Online): 979-8-89881-024-5

ISBN (Print): 979-8-89881-025-2

ISBN (Paperback): 979-8-89881-026-9

need for a court order if at any point you breach any terms of this License Agreement. In no event will any delay or failure by Bentham Science Publishers in enforcing your compliance with this License Agreement constitute a waiver of any of its rights.

3. You acknowledge that you have read this License Agreement, and agree to be bound by its terms and conditions. To the extent that any other terms and conditions presented on any website of Bentham Science Publishers conflict with, or are inconsistent with, the terms and conditions set out in this License Agreement, you acknowledge that the terms and conditions set out in this License Agreement shall prevail.

Bentham Science Publishers Pte. Ltd.
No. 9 Raffles Place
Office No. 26-01
Singapore 048619
Singapore
Email: subscriptions@benthamscience.net

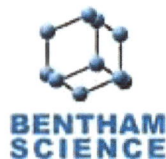

CONTENTS

Koushal Dhamija, Alok Bhardwaj, Sudhir Kumar, Shekhar Sharma and *Rupali Sharma*

FOREWORD

Vaccination has long been a cornerstone of public health, and mucosal vaccine delivery systems represent a transformative step toward safer, more effective immunization strategies. Mucosal Vaccine Delivery Systems: The Future of Immunization – Part II delves into key advancements shaping this field, offering a comprehensive exploration of scientific, regulatory, economic, and clinical perspectives. This volume addresses critical topics, including regulatory considerations, economic implications, and applications in both human and veterinary medicine. Special focus is given to mucosal vaccination's role in combating emerging infectious diseases and cancer immunotherapy, alongside innovations in adjuvants and bioprocessing challenges in large-scale production. By bridging fundamental research with real-world applications, this book serves as an essential resource for researchers, healthcare professionals, and policymakers dedicated to advancing immunization strategies. As mucosal vaccines continue to evolve, their potential to revolutionize global health remains unparalleled.

Shivkanya Fuloria
Pharmaceutical Chemistry Unit
Faculty of Pharmacy, AIMST University
Kedah 08100 Malaysia

PREFACE

The field of mucosal vaccination continues to revolutionize immunization strategies, offering innovative approaches to disease prevention across human and veterinary medicine. As research advances, addressing regulatory, economic, and manufacturing challenges is crucial to ensuring the widespread adoption and success of these vaccines. Mucosal Vaccine Delivery Systems: The Future of Immunization – Part II delves into these critical aspects while exploring groundbreaking applications in emerging diseases and cancer immunotherapy.

This volume begins with an in-depth discussion of regulatory considerations, outlining the frameworks that govern mucosal vaccine approval and distribution. It then examines the economic impacts of mucosal vaccination programs, highlighting cost-effectiveness and public health benefits. The book further explores the role of mucosal vaccines in emerging and pandemic infectious diseases, emphasizing their potential to offer rapid, scalable solutions during global health crises.

Beyond human medicine, mucosal vaccination in veterinary science is addressed, showcasing its significance in controlling zoonotic diseases. Advances in adjuvant technology for mucosal vaccines are explored, focusing on innovations that enhance immune response and vaccine stability. Additionally, challenges in bioprocessing and large-scale production are examined, ensuring that these vaccines can be manufactured efficiently and affordably. Finally, the book highlights the promising role of mucosal vaccines in cancer immunotherapy, paving the way for novel, non-invasive cancer treatments.

By addressing these key topics, this volume serves as a valuable resource for researchers, policymakers, and industry professionals. We hope it inspires further innovation and collaboration to shape the future of mucosal immunization.

Shaweta Sharma
School of Medical and Allied Sciences
Galgotias University, Yamuna Expressway
Gautam Buddha Nagar, Uttar Pradesh-201310
India

Aftab Alam
School of Pharmacy Katihar Medical College
Campus Alkarim University Katihar-854106 Katihar
India

&

Akhil Sharma
R.J. College of Pharmacy, Raipur, Gharbara
Tappal, Khair Uttar Pradesh, India

List of Contributors

Ashish	Mangalmay Pharmacy College, Plot No. 9, Knowledge Park II, Greater Noida, Uttar Pradesh 201306, India
Akhil Sharma	R. J. College of Pharmacy, 2HVJ+567, Raipur, Gharbara, Tappal, Khair, Uttar Pradesh 202165, India
Akanksha Sharma	R. J. College of Pharmacy, 2HVJ+567, Raipur, Gharbara, Tappal, Khair, Uttar Pradesh 202165, India
Alok Bhardwaj	Lloyd Institute of Management & Technology, Plot No.-11, Knowledge Park-II, Greater Noida, Uttar Pradesh-201306, India
Koushal Dhamija	Lloyd Institute of Management & Technology, Plot No.-11, Knowledge Park-II, Greater Noida, Uttar Pradesh-201306, India
Md Nasar Mallick	School of Medical and Allied Sciences, Galgotias University, Yamuna Expressway, Gautam Buddha Nagar, Uttar Pradesh-201310, India
Neeraj Kumar Fuloria	Department of Pharmaceutical Chemistry, Faculty of Pharmacy, AIMST University, Semeling Campus, Jalan Bedong-Semeling, Bedong, Kedah Darul Aman, Malaysia
Rupali Sharma	Amity University Haryana, Manesar, Gurugram, India
Shivkanya Fuloria	Faculty of Pharmacy, AIMST University, Semeling Campus, Bedong, Kedah, Malaysia
Sunita	Metro College of Health Sciences and Research, Greater Noida, India
Shaweta Sharma	School of Medical and Allied Sciences, Galgotias University, Yamuna Expressway, Gautam Buddha Nagar, Uttar Pradesh-201310, India
Shekhar Singh	Babu Banarasi Das Northern India Institute of Technology, Faculty of Pharmacy, Lucknow, Uttar Pradesh, 226028, India
Sudhir Kumar	Faculty of Pharmaceutical Sciences, DAV University, Jalandhar, India
Shekhar Sharma	Lloyd Institute of Management & Technology, Plot No.-11, Knowledge Park-II, Greater Noida, Uttar Pradesh-201306, India

CHAPTER 1

Regulatory Considerations for Mucosal Vaccination

Shivkanya Fuloria[1], Sunita[2], Ashish[3], Shaweta Sharma[4] and Akhil Sharma[5,*]

[1] *Faculty of Pharmacy, AIMST University, Semeling Campus, Bedong, Kedah, Malaysia*

[2] *Metro College of Health Sciences and Research, Greater Noida, India*

[3] *Mangalmay Pharmacy College, Plot No. 9, Knowledge Park II, Greater Noida, Uttar Pradesh 201306, India*

[4] *School of Medical and Allied Sciences, Galgotias University, Yamuna Expressway, Gautam Buddha Nagar, Uttar Pradesh-201310, India*

[5] *R. J. College of Pharmacy, 2HVJ+567, Raipur, Gharbara, Tappal, Khair, Uttar Pradesh 202165, India*

Abstract: Mucosal vaccination has the potential to revolutionize immunization and has several benefits over other conventional parenteral vaccination routes, including enhanced mucosal immune responses and ease of administration. However, the regulatory environment for mucosal vaccines is complex and diverse, necessitating a detailed understanding of the requirements for their development, approval, and deployment. This section offers an in-depth examination of how a regulatory framework is constituted around mucosal vaccinations. This chapter starts with an overview of mucosal vaccination and its importance in the fight against infectious diseases. It proceeds to explore various regulatory policies provided by leading regulatory agencies, which include the Food and Drug Administration (FDA), European Medicines Agency (EMA), and World Health Organization (WHO). It gives a comprehensive look into what makes the control of mucosal vaccines different from others, such as immunological mechanisms, administration routes that are best, formulation stability, and safety assessment. The chapter presents critical insights and best practices for navigating the regulatory landscape effectively through analysis of diverse case studies representing successful regulatory approval processes for mucosal vaccines. Also, it talks about future perspectives on emerging technologies, regulatory adaptations to accommodate evolving scientific advancements, and the necessity for global collaboration to accelerate the development and regulatory approval of mucosal vaccination strategies. The main purpose of synthesizing contemporary regulatory knowledge and giving practical advice in this chapter was to create a useful tool for investigators, producers, and regulatory officials who are working on mucosal vaccines. In the long run, this work will help advance global public health programs.

* **Corresponding author Akhil Sharma:** R. J. College of Pharmacy, 2HVJ+567, Raipur, Gharbara, Tappal, Khair, Uttar Pradesh 202165, India; E-mail: xs2akhil@gmail.com

Shaweta Sharma, Aftab Alam & Akhil Sharma (Eds.)

Keywords: Emerging technologies, European Medicines Agency (EMA), Food and Drug Administration (FDA), Global collaboration, Immunological considerations, Public health initiatives, Safety assessment, World Health Organization (WHO).

INTRODUCTION

Mucosal immunization is a novel form of vaccination that has numerous advantages over traditional injectable vaccines. It induces potent immune responses at the same sites on the mucosa, such as respiratory, gastrointestinal, and genitourinary tracts, where pathogens commonly invade the system. This affords an emergency response to infection-targeting pathogens before they become systematic [1].

An important advantage of mucosal immunization is its potential to result in local and systemic immune responses. Consequently, these immunizations not only prevent initial infections but also confer systemic protection, thus improving the overall efficacy of vaccines. For microbes that can invade both mucosal and systemic tissues, such double immunity guarantees total protection against numerous infectious agents [2].

Furthermore, mucosal vaccines provide additional benefits that can help to increase immunization coverage and public health outcomes. Patients with needle aversion or fear of needles are more likely to be interested in this method of injection without a needle or painful one. As a result, higher rates of vaccination and improved neighborhood security against the spread of infectious diseases may occur. Again, ease of administration and the possibility for self-administration in certain instances make mucosal vaccines the ideal means of reaching remote regions or areas with limited healthcare services [3].

Moreover, the adaptability of mucosal vaccine systems enables the creation of vaccines for an array of pathogens, including parasites, bacteria, and viruses. These vaccines can be given through several noninvasive alternatives, such as oral tablets, nasal sprays, or aerosols, that do away with the use of needles and syringes, hence minimizing needlestick injuries. This also promotes safety in addition to making possible mass immunization campaigns and hastening world-wide immunization initiatives [4].

On the other hand, the use of mucosal vaccination faces a number of challenges that should be considered and studied continuously. Among the major issues researchers in this area have to deal with are working towards overcoming mucosal barriers, formulating vaccines for stability and effectiveness, and ensuring safety and tolerability. In addition, unlike systemic responses, mucosal immune responses might require tailored approaches to vaccine design and evaluation [5].

Mucosal vaccination has great potential for stopping infectious diseases and for improving public health. Because they use mucosal immunity, these vaccines are a new, effective strategy to keep populations immune from many pathogens. To fully benefit from this aspect of health in the world we are facing today, further research on mucosal immunization and development should be conducted [6].

Importance of Regulatory Considerations

Regulatory considerations are paramount in the development, approval, and deployment of any vaccine, including mucosal vaccines.

Safety

Safeguarding public health, regulatory agencies play a crucial role by ensuring that vaccines, which include mucosal vaccines, meet strict safety standards during their development and deployment. Mucosal vaccines often require extensive evaluation to tackle dangers like local irritation or systemic adverse reactions through innovative delivery modalities or formulations. Regulatory oversight is necessary throughout the preclinical and clinical developmental cycle in order to effectively identify and counteract safety issues [7]. In the preclinical stage, regulatory authorities demand a lot of laboratory testing so as to evaluate the safety profiles of various mucosal vaccine candidates. Such works include determining their potential toxicity, immunogenicity, and pharmacokinetics. There are also experiments carried out on animals in order to examine the biological effects of vaccines and confirm if they would lead to an appropriate immune response without causing harm [8].

When mucosal vaccines are advanced to clinical trials, regulatory oversight becomes even more imperative. Phase I trials are aimed at establishing the safety profile of the virus in a small number of people who will get it for experimental purposes; following this, it is given to them in different doses so that they can determine which dose is the best. In phase II, the number of individuals being studied rises so as to evaluate safety and immunogenicity within a bigger cohort, thereby providing more information about risks and benefits [9]. In phase III trials, the regulatory body looks at the safety data collected from a large and diverse population to confirm that the vaccine is safe as well as effective. Adverse events are reported and analyzed in considerable detail in order to identify unexpected reactions or patterns. Besides, regulators evaluate if the vaccine prevents infection or disease by setting efficacy thresholds for product approval purposes.

During the regulatory review process, manufacturers must comply with GMP to maintain uniformity and purity of mucosal vaccines. In order to confirm conformity with set standards, Regulatory agencies inspect manufacturing facilities and scrutinize production processes [10]. This is because it is necessary to continue monitoring the effectiveness and safety of mucosal vaccines in the long term, even after regulatory authorities have approved them. Governments then create means of monitoring adverse events after immunization (AEFI) and carry out pharmacovigilance work designed to detect early warning signs for safety problems. Evaluating the safety of mucosal vaccines and protecting public health is the pivotal role that regulatory agencies play. Their stringent oversight helps to identify and mitigate potential risks, thus ensuring only those vaccines that meet the highest standards of safety are approved for use. By strictly observing these regulatory standards, confidence in mucosal vaccines is enhanced, and this contributes greatly to effective combat against infectious diseases around the world [11].

Efficacy

The efficacy of mucosal vaccines is thoroughly evaluated by regulatory agencies through a careful examination of clinical data, setting strict standards to establish their effectiveness against specific pathogens. A comprehensive analysis is carried out to determine the effects on host immune responses, such as the magnitude, duration, and correlates of protection [12]. Typically, randomized, double-masked studies are conducted in diverse populations as the mainstay of clinical trials, and they are designed to provide substantial evidence concerning vaccine efficacy. The goal of these trials is to assess whether the vaccine can prevent infection, reduce disease severity, or block transmission. Regulatory agencies establish quantifiable standards for HIV endpoints such that vaccines must show a significant drop in targeted diseases' frequencies or severities relative to the placebo or comparator group [13].

Regulatory agencies also evaluate immunological markers and clinical endpoints. Such markers may be particular antibody levels, cellular immunity, or even immune responses along mucosal surfaces. By doing so, the vaccine evaluation process can be simplified and regulatory decision-making expedited [14]. Moreover, the efficacy data is evaluated by regulatory agencies according to the time during which this kind of immunity has been induced. However, long-term follow-up studies are carried out to determine if vaccinated persons still keep their immune responses and if vaccines remain effective over several years or decades.

This information is important for establishing the best patterns of vaccination as well as informing public health policies [15, 16].

There is a need to have adequate data on vaccine efficacy in order for vaccines to be licensed and also to maintain public trust in immunization programs. Regulatory authorities are very careful when examining clinical trial results so that they can ensure that mucosal vaccines meet certain efficacy levels before granting marketing approval. Communication of efficacy data should, therefore, be clear enough for healthcare providers, policymakers, and the public at large, who need to know more about vaccine benefits and encourage their acceptance by all people [17]. The regulatory evaluation of the efficiency of mucosal vaccines is largely based on firm clinical information that covers numerous aspects, including the magnitude of immune responses, duration, and correlates of protection. In order to maintain public health and ensure confidence in immunization programs, government regulators have strict standards for evaluating the effectiveness of vaccines. By putting in place strict parameters, regulatory agencies ensure maximum safety and efficiency, thereby safeguarding public health and instilling confidence in immunization programs [18].

Quality Control

There is a significant role regulatory authorities play in the creation and implementation of quality standards for mucosal vaccine production to ensure they have strict requirements on uniformity, purity, and potency. These standards are essential to maintaining product identity, reducing chances of contamination, and guaranteeing vaccine safety and efficacy [19]. Regulatory agencies, therefore, perform periodic inspections of all vaccine manufacturing plants that cover every stage of production. In order to comply with GMP, they must go through manufacturing procedures, equipment, facilities, and personnel qualifications. The regulations of GMP are exhaustive in terms of the design, monitoring, and control of manufacturing processes, including raw material handling and final product testing [20].

Beginning with the selection and testing of raw materials, manufacturers are required to source high-quality ingredients and conduct rigorous testing to verify their identity, purity, and potency. At every stage of vaccine production, stringent quality control measures are implemented. Any deviations from established specifications, which would lead to product defects or safety issues, are thoroughly investigated [21]. To make vaccines, regulatory bodies scrutinize vital process parameters to ensure uniformity and reproducibility. They watch over things such as formulation, mixing, sterilization, and filling that are necessary for the vaccine quality and its power. By carrying out constant monitoring and validation of the process, any problems can be detected early enough before they affect the safety or effectiveness of vaccines [22].

Quality control tests are conducted at different stages of the manufacturing process to check for product purity, potency, and even stability. These tests might involve an assay of antigen content, potency, sterility/purity, and endotoxin levels, among others. Batch release testing ascertains that each batch of vaccine meets predetermined specifications before it is allowed for distribution [23]. Besides this, regulatory bodies overseeing manufacturing standards also supervise the storage, transportation, and handling systems of vaccines to prevent them from being damaged or tampered with. To keep the vaccines stable and in good condition throughout the process of distribution, it is important to adhere to strict temperature control measures during shipment; proper labeling and secure storage practices should be employed without fail [24]. Stringent quality control measures are of utmost importance to ensure the safety, efficacy, and reliability of mucosal vaccines. Regulatory authorities maintain public confidence in immunization programs and contribute to the prevention and control of infectious diseases by setting up and implementing firm quality standards [25].

Clinical Trial Oversight

Regulatory agencies oversee clinical trials to ensure that they are ethically conducted, that there is safety for patients, and that the integrity of data collected is maintained throughout the development of vaccines such as those for mucosa. Their supervision is very necessary in maintaining scientific excellence and ensuring that only safe and efficient immunizations are released to the public [26]. Study protocols must be scrutinized and endorsed by regulatory agencies before clinical trials can proceed; they critically evaluate trial designs to make sure they are scientifically sound and ethically acceptable. In this regard, participant eligibility criteria, intervention protocols, and outcome measures are thoroughly examined. Regulatory review ensures the protection of the rights and welfare of participants in trials as well as the harmonization of research objectives with ethical considerations and statutory standards [27].

In the course of clinical trials, regulatory agencies oversee trial progress in order to make sure that approved protocols and regulatory standards are followed accordingly, such as by ensuring that participants are recruited well and consented properly. Protocol deviations or ethical breaches do not occur. Trial site monitoring visits, as well as audits, are done regularly to help identify and deal with any problems that might come up throughout the trial [28]. Regulatory agencies also have the responsibility of evaluating and handling adverse events (AEs) reported during clinical trials in addition to trial monitoring. All side effects or safety concerns observed for the patients in a clinical trial should be reported without delay, irrespective of their link to the vaccine being tried out. Regulatory review of adverse event data facilitates early identification of possible safety signals and informs risk reduction strategies to ensure safety for trial participants [29].

Additionally, the regulatory oversight of clinical trial data is vital in evaluating vaccine safety and efficacy before being approved. Regulatory authorities examine clinical trial findings covering effectiveness endpoints, immunogenicity results, and safety profiles to determine the overall benefit-risk profile of the research vaccine. The only vaccines that can get regulatory approval for public use are those that have passed this rigorous evaluation and shown enough efficacy and safety. Clinical trials require regulatory oversight to protect patient safety, maintain scientific integrity, and ensure the credibility of vaccine development. Regulatory agencies influence mucosal vaccine progress, and they promote public health by overseeing trial performance, monitoring adverse events, and examining clinical trial information [30].

Post-marketing Surveillance

Upon authorization and deployment in real life, regulatory agencies are required to engage in post-marketing surveillance so as to monitor the efficiency and safety of vaccines such as mucosal vaccines. Therefore, there is a need for perpetual monitoring to establish negative effects that might occur after vaccination (AEFI) and allow ongoing protection against vaccines that are safe already. Regulatory bodies create mechanisms for healthcare practitioners, vaccine producers, and people in general to submit their reports on AEFIs as a way of ensuring post-marketing surveillance. These systems are commonly referred to as pharmacovigilance programs that facilitate the timely retrieval or collection, examination, and appraisal of adverse event information linked to vaccination. Healthcare providers are urged to report any adverse events regardless of their opinions on whether these were caused by vaccines [31].

To determine any possible safety signals that may suggest unknown risks or patterns of side effects, regulatory bodies scrutinize reported adverse events. In analyzing reported AEFIs, they look at factors such as severity, frequency, and the relation between vaccination and the occurrence of these events. Additionally, regulatory agencies compare observed rates of adverse events with expected background rates to assess whether there is a risk that exceeds what would be expected in the absence of vaccination [32]. Post-marketing surveillance data may be employed to assess the effectiveness of vaccines in real-world populations. Regulatory agencies monitor vaccine coverage rates, disease incidence rates, and vaccine effectiveness studies to evaluate the effect of vaccination programs on disease prevention and control. Such information assists in formulating public health policies and vaccination programs that ensure continuing tangible benefits for individuals who have been vaccinated or specific communities [33].

The results of post-marketing surveillance may lead regulatory authorities to take regulatory measures against noticed dangers or attend to fresh safety concerns. These moves might involve revisions of vaccine labels in order to incorporate current safety information, introduction of further risk management approaches or rare circumstances, and withdrawal from the vaccine market if grave safety issues are discovered [34]. A very important function in the long-term safety and efficacy of vaccines such as mucosal vaccines is ensuring ongoing surveillance by regulatory authorities. This is done by monitoring AEFIs, detecting safety signals, and evaluating vaccine effectiveness in real-life settings, enabling regulators to refine vaccination programs and enhance public health protection as they go along [35].

Labeling and Packaging

These agencies are very careful when reviewing vaccine labels and packaging to confirm that they accurately indicate the product, including its indications, contraindications, dosing schedules, and storage recommendations. Healthcare professionals and recipients of vaccines need to have clear and comprehensive labeling so as to make informed decisions on their use and administer them safely [36]. Vaccine labeling is subject to regulation to ensure that it provides accurate and clear information about the vaccine's intended use. It must specify what the vaccine is licensed for, such as preventing particular contagious diseases or defending people from specific pathogens. Regulatory agencies also call for contraindications to be incorporated into vaccine labels, which are conditions or circumstances in which vaccination should not take place because of possible dangers to the recipient [37].

Another important part of vaccine labeling reviewed by regulatory agencies is the dosing schedules. Labels for vaccines contain information on dosage, route of administration, and timing of doses required to achieve maximum protection from specific diseases. Healthcare providers need this information in order to give the injections as directed by the manufacturer [38]. Also, the labels for vaccines are carefully written to include storage requirements in order to make sure that they stay safe and active. The regulatory authorities establish specific storage conditions like temperature and humidity ranges, which will maintain vaccine efficiency and integrity. Vaccine labels instruct on how vaccines should be stored, handled, and disposed of properly so that product spoilage or contamination is avoided [39].

Moreover, vaccine labels may contain information about possible side effects one might experience after using the vaccine. This is vital as it helps healthcare providers and recipients to weigh the risks and benefits of vaccination, hence making informed decisions about its use [40]. To promote vaccine safety and effectiveness, as well as to guarantee public trust in immunization programs, it is necessary to have proper labeling that is clear and comprehensive. In order to meet established standards of accuracy, clarity, and completion, vaccine labels must be reviewed and approved by regulatory agencies. Regulators contribute to the safe use of vaccines and protect public health through accurate information on labeling [41].

Emergency Use Authorization

When there are public health emergencies such as pandemics or outbreaks of infectious diseases, emergency use authorization (EUA) may be granted by regulatory agencies for the use of vaccines. This EUA allows quicker access to vaccines based on limited clinical data and risk-benefit assessments, weighing the pressing need for intervention against safety and efficacy maintenance. Provisional licenses grant medical practitioners and public health officials the right to instantly utilize vaccines to manage the expansion of ailment and thus minimize its occurrence and death rate. It speeds up compliance with regulations, making it possible to reach lifesaving therapies quickly in times of urgency. Nevertheless, the EUA does not negate safety and effectiveness requirements; instead, it involves an elaborate review of existing data regarding the need to get vaccinated against risks associated with emergencies [42].

Regulatory oversight remains important even though an accelerated EUA process is followed in order to monitor vaccine safety and effectiveness after authorization. Real-world data on vaccine performance, adverse events, and population-level outcomes are continuously being collected and analyzed by regulatory agencies. This surveillance enables the identification of new safety issues or efficacy concerns that may not have been observed during the initial approval stage. Also, the EUA can include other specifications imposed by regulatory bodies, such as extended post-marketing surveillance, increased data collection, and risk management strategies. Such actions are meant to ensure that vaccination remains safe and effective for everyone and outweighs any possible risks involved in it [43]. During an outbreak of a public health emergency, there is a crucial means to bypass regulatory obstacles and provide access to vaccines; this is called Emergency Use Authorization. In such situations, regulatory agencies may approve and deploy vaccines even on the basis of minimal data; however, licensing authorities must still be in place to evaluate product safety and efficacy after authorization, as well as maintain the highest levels of public health safeguards [44].

Global Harmonization

Harmonization of regulations is crucial for international cooperation and easing some processes in vaccine development, assessment, and distribution. Harmonization efforts align regulatory standards, requirements, and processes across regions to foster standardization, compatibility, and reciprocal recognition of regulatory decisions, improving timely access to vaccines globally [45]. Regulatory harmonization has a great advantage: it minimizes duplication and repetition of regulatory requirements. Consequently, when these agencies adopt the same methods, vaccine developers can easily move through the regulatory arena without needing to repeat similar tests or surveys for every country. Thus, this sequential process saves time and resources, speeding up the development and licensing of vaccines.

Further, harmonized regulatory standards help to make the regulatory process more predictable and transparent. For instance, it enhances certainty and confidence in regard to the regulatory pathway for vaccine developers by giving them clear guidelines and expectations. This allows makers to plan better and execute their development programs, leading to faster and more predictable timelines for vaccine approval [46]. In addition, having the same standards makes collaboration easier for international and regulatory agencies. To exchange ideas on vaccine regulation, the best approach is for these organizations to standardize their practices so that they can share scientific knowledge as well as pooled resources efficiently. This joint methodology strengthens regulatory expertise and increases its capacity to protect public health by ensuring vaccine safety, efficacy, and quality.

In addition, the harmonized regulatory standards also encourage mutual recognition of regulatory decisions in various jurisdictions. Should regulators have confidence in one another's systems and practices, they may embrace each other's regulations and determinations, leading to vaccines being available much quicker across several markets. This duplicity reduction through mutual recognition reduces vaccine availability timeframes to the global population [47]. Efforts to harmonize global regulations have been crucial in promoting health by simplifying procedures for developing, assessing, and delivering vaccines. This ensures that regulatory decisions are consistent, interoperable, and mutually recognized, thus leading to harmonized regulatory standards that promote timely access to safe and effective vaccines, thereby preventing and controlling global infectious diseases [48]. Fig. (**1**) summarizes the importance of regulatory considerations in mucosal vaccines.

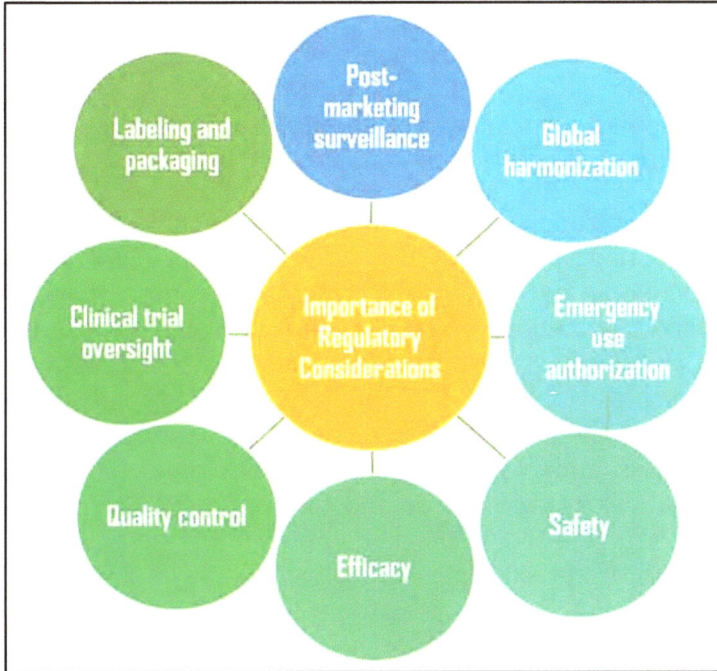

Fig. (1). Importance of regulatory considerations.

OVERVIEW OF REGULATORY BODIES

Regulatory bodies are pivotal institutions charged with overseeing and enforcing laws, regulations, and standards governing various sectors, including healthcare, pharmaceuticals, and biotechnology. When it comes to vaccines, their role is paramount. The Food and Drug Administration (FDA) in the United States, alongside its Center for Biologics Evaluation and Research (CBER), meticulously evaluates vaccines for safety, efficacy, and quality, ensuring they meet rigorous standards before approval. Similarly, the European Medicines Agency (EMA) in the European Union (EU) oversees vaccine regulation through its Committee for Medicinal Products for Human Use (CHMP), providing thorough assessments for marketing authorization across EU member states [49].

Furthermore, Health Canada, as the regulatory body in Canada, rigorously evaluates vaccines for marketing authorization within the country through its Biologics and Genetic Therapies Directorate (BGTD). Additionally, at the global level, the World Health Organization (WHO) provides leadership, guidance, and recommendations on vaccines, including a prequalification process for United Nations agencies to procure them as well as assessments of their safety and efficacy and support of vaccination programs across the globe [50]. In many countries, some NRAs oversee vaccines nationally. They evaluate them, approve them for marketing authorization, inspect manufacturing plants, and monitor their post-marketing safety and effectiveness. Moreover, organizations such as the European Directorate for the Quality of Medicines & Health (EDQM) set standards and provide advice on how to ensure uniformity and consistency in vaccine manufacturing processes and standards [51].

In Japan, the Pharmacopeia and Medics Device Agency (PMDA) plays a very vital role in regulating vaccines by evaluating them for marketing authorization approval and watching over their safety and effectiveness after they have been approved. In the USA, although NIH does not have regulatory authority, it leads vaccine research, funding ventures and academic collaborations as well as industry partnerships to foster vaccine development and invention. These regulatory organizations work in tandem to ensure that vaccines meet the strictest safety, effectiveness, and quality standards, thereby protecting public health and supporting global disease prevention and control campaigns. Thus, they ensure vaccines satisfy stringent requirements before entering the market, which boosts trust among healthcare practitioners as well as people at large while also saving lives [52].

REGULATORY GUIDELINES

FDA (Food and Drug Administration)

The FDA has come under intense scrutiny in recent years as a result of a number of things, which brought to the fore the necessity for more regulation and supervision. A major obstacle is the growth in new technologies and healthcare breakthroughs like gene therapies, personalized medicine, and digital health products. Such developments yield new cures and diagnostic tools but also create intricate compliance concerns about these issues: safety, efficacy, and patient access [53]. Further, the FDA is finding it more difficult to secure imported substances than before due to globalization and the expanding global supply chain. The agency has to deal with different regulatory environments and handle emerging threats such as counterfeit drugs and foodborne illnesses [54].

Apart from these external forces, the FDA has also been hindered by internal factors, including resource constraints and staff insufficiencies in their attempts to perform their duties efficiently. The agency's capability to respond to new risks and introduce new treatments may be hampered by budgetary limitations and administrative barriers. In addition, public health emergencies, including the opioid epidemic and COVID-19, have served to emphasize the significance of the FDA's duty to protect public well-being. As a result of these situations, there is now a clamor for a more flexible and proactive regulatory approach from the FDA to adapt quickly to emerging challenges and fast-track access to vital life-saving treatments [55]. The FDA faces a growing mandate and increasingly complex regulatory landscape, requiring it to adapt and innovate to meet the evolving needs of public health while maintaining rigorous standards of safety and efficacy [56].

Requirements for Clinical Trials

For a drug, biologic, or medical device to be made available to the public, it must undergo clinical trials that comply with the stringent standards set by the FDA. The purpose of these requirements is to ensure that patients' rights are protected, that welfare is taken care of during studies, and that sufficient data is provided for making regulatory decisions [57]. Some components of FDA requirements for clinical trials:

Investigational New Drug (IND) Application

Before conducting clinical trials on a drug being tested, researchers must submit an Investigational New Drug (IND) application to the FDA. This application consists of preclinical data, proposed clinical study protocols, and information about manufacturing processes [58].

Institutional Review Board (IRB) Approval

A team of scientists, ethicists, and community members must review and approve clinical trial protocols. This review ensures that the study is ethical and safeguards participants' rights [59].

Informed Consent

Participants must provide informed consent before enrolling in a clinical trial. This involves comprehensively explaining the trial's purpose, procedures, potential risks and benefits, and participants' rights. Informed consent is an ongoing process throughout the trial [60].

Good Clinical Practice (GCP)

Clinical trials must adhere to GCP guidelines, which outline standards for designing, conducting, recording, and reporting trials. GCP ensures the integrity and credibility of trial data [61].

Safety Monitoring and Reporting

Researchers must monitor subjects for adverse events throughout the trial. Serious events must be reported promptly to the FDA and IRB. Additionally, the FDA receives periodic safety reports throughout the study [62].

Efficacy Assessment

Clinical trials must be planned to show the efficacy of a new medicinal product for its intended use. This often involves randomized controlled trials comparing the test drug with a placebo or standard treatment [63].

Data Collection and Analysis

A detailed plan for data collection, analysis, and statistical methods should be provided prior to the study. This will enable the generation of reliable and strong data from the experiment [64].

Regulatory Submission

Researchers present their findings in an application called a New Drug Application (NDA) or a Biologics License Application (BLA), which they submit to the FDA. Such applications contain numerous data from previous studies and clinical trials indicating that the drug is both safe and effective [65].

Post-Marketing Surveillance

Post-approval safety and real-world effectiveness of a product are monitored by post-marketing surveillance. Adverse events and other relevant data are collected and evaluated continuously [66]. Table **1** summarizes the FDA's safety and efficacy standards for medical products.

Manufacturing Guidelines

The FDA's manufacturing directives are a crucial tool for protecting public health by outlining stringent standards that oversee pharmaceuticals, medical devices, biologics, and other regulated products. As a foundation stone, these criteria ensure product quality, safety, efficacy, *etc.*, and inspire confidence in consumers as well as medical practitioners [73]. The central purpose of this guideline is Good Manufacturing Practices (GMP), which is a quality assurance system that ensures that products are consistently produced and controlled according to quality standards. By following the guidelines for GMP, manufacturers can minimize risks such as product contamination, variabilities, and defects, thereby improving patient safety and safeguarding public health [74].

Table 1. FDA's safety and efficacy standards for medical products.

Safety Standards	Efficacy Standards
Preclinical Testing	**Clinical Trial Design**
- Laboratory and animal studies to assess safety	- Well-designed, randomized controlled trials
- Identify potential toxicities and adverse effects [67]	- Predefined endpoints
Adverse Event Monitoring	- Statistical analysis
- Monitoring participants for adverse events	- Sample size calculation
- Timely reporting to FDA and regulatory authorities [68]	- Subgroup analysis
Risk Management Plans	- Comparative effectiveness studies
- Develop plans to minimize and manage known risks [69]	- Evaluation of comparative efficacy [71, 72]
Post-Marketing Surveillance	
- Continued monitoring of product safety in real-world	
- Reporting and evaluation of adverse events [70]	

The guidelines cover a wide range of manufacturing aspects from installation design maintenance of equipment to record keeping and staff training. Manufacturers are supposed to construct and maintain facilities under strict regulations concerning their layout, construction, and sanitation to ensure safe and efficient production operations. Routine instrument service checks like calibrations are required to yield the best possible performance and dependability, thus reducing the danger of interfering with production and product variability [75]. The manufacturing procedure includes a lot of records and documentation that are very important in showing that the company complies with the requirements set by the relevant regulatory bodies. It is through these records that the manufacturer ensures transparency and accountability to regulatory authorities. These include information about deviations, quality control tests, and detailed manufacturing processes [76].

Furthermore, these principles give prominence to the significance of checking and qualifying manufacturing processes and equipment in order to maintain uniform product quality as well as performance. Manufacturers are able to manage risks linked with product variability and non-conformity through documented evidence of process effectiveness and reliability [77]. The guidelines also cover supply chain management, which necessitates manufacturers to have strong frameworks for assessing and managing their suppliers in order to ensure that raw materials and components are of the right quality and integrity. This proactive approach helps protect against possible threats resulting from disruptions in the supply chain or the use of inferior materials [78].

Innovation and proactive risk prevention are at the heart of Food and Drug Administration manufacturing guidelines for improved productivity and safety. They can minimize public health risks while enhancing product quality, safety, and compliance through the continuous monitoring of performance metrics, data analysis, and taking corrective actions or preventive measures by manufacturers to ensure that the company complies with established regulatory standards. Regulated industries must adhere to the FDA's manufacturing regulations because they guarantee regulatory compliance and that consumer confidence remains high through the foundation of public health. By strictly following these guidelines, manufacturers can maintain global quality, safety, and efficacy standards, thus meeting their goal of providing safe and effective products to patients across the world [78].

EMA (EUROPEAN MEDICINES AGENCY)

The European Medicines Agency (EMA) is responsible for the scientific assessment, control, and safety control of medicines in the European Union (EU) and European Economic Area (EEA). EMA was founded in 1995 to regulate pharmaceuticals and ensure that drugs sold within the EU conform to high standards of quality, safety, and efficacy. The following are the major activities undertaken by EMA.

Scientific Evaluation

The EMA performs scientific evaluations of products for marketing authorization submitted in the EU/EEA. This includes examining information derived from pharmaceutical firms on the quality, safety, and efficacy of the products to decide if they meet regulatory standards [79].

Marketing Authorization

EMA grants marketing authorization for medicines that meet the necessary standards based on scientific evaluation. This authorization enables pharmaceutical companies to market their products within the EU/EEA [80].

Pharmacovigilance

The EMA is responsible for regulating the safety of drugs already on the market. This encompasses collecting and analyzing adverse drug reaction (ADR) reports and other regulatory measures like amending drug labels or imposing safety advisories.

Scientific Advice

During the drug development process, the EMA offers scientific advice to pharmaceutical companies. This will help companies conduct clinical trials, optimize study protocols, and address regulatory requirements, eventually enabling them to develop safe and effective medicines [81].

Guidelines and Standards

To harmonize regulatory requirements across the EU/EEA, EMA develops guidelines and standards. A pharmaceutical company's guide to various aspects of drug development, manufacturing, and regulatory compliance is outlined in these guidelines [82].

Collaboration

The EMA collaborates with national regulatory authorities within the EU/EEA and with international regulatory agencies and organizations to promote regulatory convergence and facilitate global access to safe and effective medicines [83].

Transparency

The EMA promotes transparency by making available information about its regulatory actions, including drug evaluations, regulatory rulings, and safety updates. Such openness helps build public confidence and enables medical practitioners and patients to make informed choices [84]. Table **2** summarizes the comparison between the European Medicines Agency (EMA) and the U.S. Food and Drug Administration (FDA).

Table 2. Comparison of the European Medicines Agency (EMA) and the U.S. Food and Drug Administration (FDA).

Aspect	EMA	FDA
Regulatory Authority	European Union (EU) and European Economic Area (EEA) [85].	United States of America [86].
Scope	Regulates medicines in the EU/EEA [87].	Regulates medicines, food, dietary supplements, medical devices, cosmetics, and tobacco products in the United States [88].
Scientific Evaluation	Conducts scientific assessments of medicines for marketing authorization in the EU/EEA [89].	Conducts scientific evaluations for marketing authorization in the United States [90].
Marketing Authorization	Grants marketing authorization for medicines meeting EU/EEA standards [91].	Grants marketing approval for products meeting FDA standards [92].

(Table 2) cont.....

Aspect	EMA	FDA
Pharmacovigilance	Oversees safety monitoring of medicines post-approval in the EU/EEA [93].	Oversees safety monitoring of drugs and medical products post-approval in the United States [94].
Scientific Advice	Provides scientific advice to pharmaceutical companies during drug development [95].	Provides scientific guidance to companies during drug development [96].
Guidelines and Standards	Develops regulatory guidelines and standards for the EU/EEA market [97].	Develops regulatory guidelines and standards for the United States market [98].
Collaboration	Collaborates with national regulatory authorities in the EU/EEA and international agencies [99].	Collaborates with other federal agencies, international regulatory agencies, and organizations [100].
Transparency	Provides access to information on regulatory activities, assessments, and decisions [101].	Provides access to regulatory information, including product approvals, safety alerts, and enforcement actions [102].

EUROPEAN REGULATORY FRAMEWORK

To ensure safe, effective, and high-quality medicinal products in the European Union (EU) and European Economic Area (EEA), Europe has put in place an elaborate system of medicines regulation. Key players handle various legislative, regulatory, and procedural elements that make up the framework. Fig. (**2**) provides a summary of how medicine is regulated in Europe.

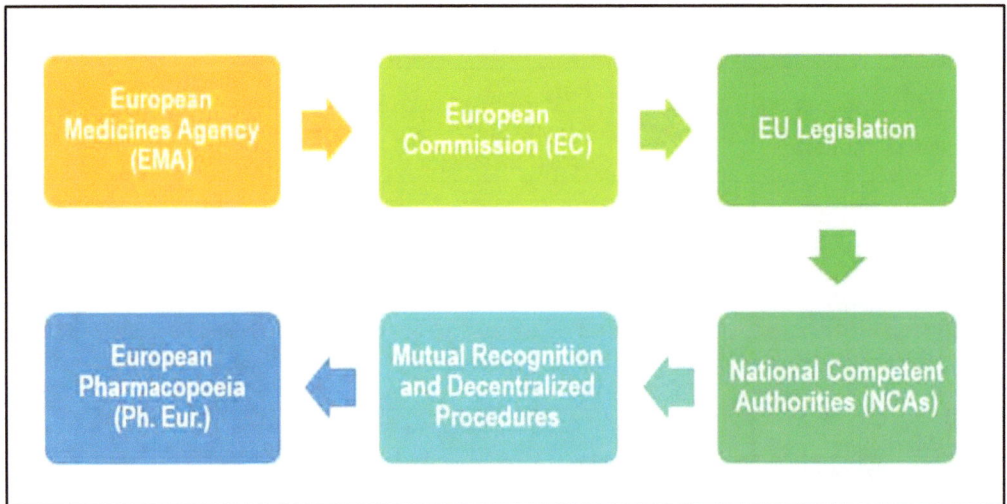

Fig. (2). European regulatory framework.

Approval Processes

The European Medicines Agency (EMA) supervises the authorization of medicinal products proposed for marketing within the European Union (EU) as well as the European Economic Area (EEA). Authorization processes involve several major steps, such as preauthorization procedures and postapproval activities. The approval processes managed by the EMA are as follows:

Pre-Marketing Authorization Procedures

Centralized Procedure

The primary way to get marketing approval in the EU/EEA for some medicines is through the centrality process. A solitary application is sent to EMA for appraisal and endorsement. The EMA arranges the logical evaluation of the drug product by way of its Committee for Medicinal Products for Human Use (CHMP) or Committee for Medicinal Products for Veterinary Use (CVMP), as applicable (human or veterinary). Following authorization by the European Commission, this marketing authorization can be used inside all member countries within the EU/EEA [103].

Decentralized Procedure

Pharmaceutical companies can use the decentralized procedure to seek marketing authorization simultaneously in several EU/EEA member states on the basis of a single application. In this process, there is a reference member state (RMS) where an applicant submits the marketing authorization application initially, and concerned member states (CMS) evaluate it later. The RMS coordinates the assessment with contributions from the CMS members. On satisfactory completion of the assessment, the RMS grants marketing authorization that is valid in all participating states [104].

Mutual Recognition Procedure

The mutual recognition procedure is broadly similar to the decentralized procedure but applies to medicinal products that have already been authorized in one EU/EEA member state. To market the product in other member states, a pharmaceutical firm can make an application for recognition on a mutual basis through their national regulatory authorities. The regulatory authorities evaluate this application based on the existing marketing authorization, and they may grant marketing authorization in their respective jurisdictions [105].

National Procedure

Some circumstances may require individual EU/EEA states to go through the national approval process before deciding whether to approve a medicine. This is usually for products that do not fall under the centralized, decentralized, or mutual recognition procedures [106].

Post-Authorization Activities

Pharmacovigilance

Pharmaceutical companies are required to conduct pharmacovigilance activities after marketing authorization to monitor the safety of their medicinal products. This involves collecting and analyzing adverse drug reaction (ADR) reports and implementing risk minimization measures where needed. The EMA collaborates with national competent authorities (NCAs) to oversee pharmacovigilance activities [107].

Variations and Renewals

Pharmaceutical companies may submit marketing authorization variations to request changes in the authorized products, for instance, updating product information or manufacturing processes. Moreover, a renewal of marketing authorizations is done periodically to ascertain continuous conformity with regulatory prerequisites [108].

Post-Marketing Studies

Approval of medicinal products by the European Medicines Agency (EMA) may necessitate post-authorization safety studies or post-marketing studies in order to examine the effectiveness, safety, or efficacy of such drugs [109].

WHO (WORLD HEALTH ORGANIZATION)

The most important position in global health governance is occupied by the World Health Organization (WHO), which serves as the foremost international authority that addresses public health issues. Established in 1948, WHO's mandate includes a broad range of functions that seek to protect and enhance the health of populations globally. Through its stewardship, WHO influences the global health agenda and leads efforts to tackle prioritized health issues, including infectious diseases, non-communicable diseases, and healthcare disparities [110, 111].

To ensure that nations follow scientific guidelines and health care practices, the WHO has three main objectives. WHO assists many countries in improving their health systems, enhancing disease surveillance, and developing public health infrastructure through its expertise [112]. In moments of emergencies, the WHO plays a leading part in organizing worldwide responses to health crises like pandemics and natural calamities. The provision of funding, alignment of common goals among stakeholders, and timely relaying of data help the WHO reduce health shocks that result in loss of life [113].

Furthermore, WHO acts as a facilitator for global health research, promoting creativity and transfer of information in the medical world. WHO collaborates with academic institutions and other research organizations to ensure that studies carried out are translated into policies and actions. The role played by the World Health Organization (WHO) is critical in influencing the global health agenda, fostering social justice in health, and working towards the achievement of the best attainable state of health for all people [114, 115].

Global Regulatory Standards

The WHO stands as the key to the development and spread of global norms for control across grounds of public health. The mandate includes making rules and benchmarks to achieve safety, efficacy, and quality in products and services that relate to health on a worldwide scale. WHO plays an essential role in coordinating regulatory activities among state members and international partners, promoting cross-border cooperation, harmonizing regulatory practices, and ensuring equitable access to vital healthcare interventions [116, 117].

The World Health Organization (WHO) takes the lead in strengthening regulatory systems, which entails establishing norms and standards for evaluating, licensing, and post-market surveillance of medicines in countries. Its prequalification program evaluates key medicines' quality, safety, and efficacy while improving procurement processes and solidifying the integrity of supply chains. WHO's oversight equally applies to vaccines, through which it develops stringent criteria for safeguarding their quality, safety, and efficacy to ensure that they remain available and reliable for immunization programs globally [117]. WHO, in partnership with the Food and Agriculture Organization (FAO), works towards the Codex Alimentarius Commission, which is responsible for setting international food safety standards that protect consumer health and ensure fair trading practices. In addition, WHO provides policies on nutrition as a response to malnutrition and diet-related diseases by supporting measures that depend on scientific evidence with the aim of improving dietary behaviors and overcoming nutritional gaps [118].

WHO provides technical support to countries for the regulation and monitoring of medical devices and technologies. The aim is to improve the dependability and efficiency of medical devices by encouraging adherence to quality management systems as well as international standards, ultimately protecting patient health [119]. Moreover, the WHO's establishment of a framework convention on tobacco control has been exemplary in its global cooperation towards slowing down the spread of tobacco across the globe. The WHO is challenging for settings that are driven by evidence-based policies and interventions so as to reduce tobacco consumption, prevent diseases associated with tobacco use, and protect public health from the risks caused by smoking [120].

Guidelines for Vaccine Development

In the development of vaccines, WHO acts as a leading institution that provides comprehensive guidance on the entire process from its start to when they are distributed. These guidelines are important in ensuring that vaccines are safe, effective, and of good quality, which ensures that Public health is globally protected. WHO provides important recommendations from the preclinical phase, which help in the selection of vaccine candidates and carrying out preliminary laboratory tests to determine their immunological and safety profiles [121, 122]. As vaccines move towards clinical trials, the WHO guidelines provide a set of strict rules that describe trial design, participant selection, and data analysis to guarantee strong evidence is obtained on safety and efficacy.

WHO is closely cooperating with national regulators to facilitate the review and approval process by the regulatory authorities themselves, making use of its prequalification program to gauge whether vaccines comply with global norms. Guidelines for post-marketing surveillance are important for monitoring the safety and efficacy of vaccines in reality so as to promptly detect and respond to any adverse events that may arise. Moreover, the WHO provides vaccine deployment strategic guidance that includes prioritization approaches and monitoring tools to enhance the benefits of immunization programs. To sum up, as a starting point for stakeholders, WHO's exhaustive guidelines on vaccine development are maps that help such individuals navigate through difficult terrains related to research on vaccine production or distribution process that will lead to an enhancement in well-being and durability globally [123].

Collaborative Efforts

This WHO is renowned for its collaboration across a broad range of public health areas, building partnerships, and fostering cooperation in response to global health challenges. By way of an extended network of member countries, international organizations, civil society, academia, and private sector involvement, the WHO combines knowledge and resources to fulfill its mission of ensuring better health [124].

Multilateral Partnerships

In addition, WHO partners closely with other UN agencies like UNICEF, UNFPA, and UNAIDS to coordinate efforts in addressing issues of maternal and child health, family planning, HIV/AIDS prevention and treatment, and humanitarian aid. These partnerships take advantage of each organization's respective advantages to provide holistic healthcare services for people at high risk worldwide [125].

Bilateral Cooperation

WHO forms bilateral partnerships with individual countries to offer technical support, capacity-building assistance, and collaborative research initiatives tailored to specific health contexts and priorities. The main aim of these partnerships is to facilitate knowledge exchange, technology transfer, and mutual learning, which can foster sustainable health development at both national and regional levels [125].

Public-Private Partnerships

The WHO collaborates with the private sector, including pharmaceutical companies, medical device manufacturers, and technology firms, to drive innovation, expand access to essential health products and services, and strengthen health systems. The WHO works with industry partners such as the Access to COVID-19 Tools (ACT) Accelerator to hasten the development, production, and equitable distribution of COVID-19 vaccines, therapeutics, and diagnostics [126].

Academic and Research Collaborations

WHO partners with academic institutions, research organizations, and scientific networks to generate evidence, build research capacity, and develop guidelines in priority areas of public health. These collaborations enhance scientific knowledge, inform policy decisions, and improve health outcomes through evidence-based interventions and innovations [127].

Civil Society Engagement

WHO also supports civil society organizations, community groups, and NGOs to increase their voices, mobilize grassroots actions, and promote health equity and social justice. These alliances sustain the importance of WHO's programs being informed by community perspectives and needs, thus enhancing inclusive and participatory health policies and programs [128].

CHALLENGES IN MUCOSAL VACCINATION REGULATION

It is necessary to consider the unique challenges involved in regulating mucosal vaccines and how they can be addressed. These challenges cover various aspects such as immunological considerations, administration routes, stability and shelf life, safety concerns, and method standardization.

Immunological Considerations

Mucosal surfaces differ from systemic vaccination routes in terms of their immunological features. In evaluating the efficacy and immunogenicity of mucosal vaccines, regulators should consider diversity and healthiness in the mucosal immune response, including MALT activation, mucosal antibody production, and mechanisms of mucosal tolerance [129].

Route of Administration

There are vaccines given on the mucosal surfaces. The advantages include being free from injections, superior mucosal immunity responses, and probable protection in distant mucosal areas. Choose route administration cunningly—for instance, oral, intranasal, or intravaginal—considering such aspects as vaccine stability, target population, and desired immune responses. The regulators need to assess the safety and efficiency of each route of administration while ensuring consistent delivery across different populations.

Stability and Shelf-life

Since mucosal vaccines come into contact with different environmental conditions and mucosal secretions during administration, they encounter some difficulties related to stability and shelf-life. Some of the factors that can affect vaccine effectiveness include temperature sensitivity, water exposure, and enzymatic breakdown. As a result, regulators have to ensure that their stability testing protocols are stringent enough and that storage is stipulated throughout the manufacturing process, distribution chain, and immunization [130].

Safety Concerns

The safety of mucosal vaccination is cause for concern as it may lead to local or systemic reactions, irritation of the mucosal lining, or impairment of the barrier integrity. Regulators need to evaluate the safety profile of mucosal adjuvants, delivery systems, and vaccine constituents to reduce risks and enhance immune responses. Continuous vigilance and monitoring are crucial to quickly detect and respond to any potential safety issues that might arise post-licensure.

Standardization of Methods

Different methods for vaccinating mucosa exist, such as formulation, device delivery, dosing schedule, and mucosal sampling techniques. Standardizing vaccine development, manufacturing, quality control, and evaluation methodologies is necessary for achieving uniformity, comparability, and reproducibility of different kinds of mucosal vaccines. The regulators are responsible for harmonizing regulatory requirements and guidelines to support the development and authorization of mucosal vaccines [131]. Challenges in mucosal vaccination regulation are summarized in Fig. (**3**).

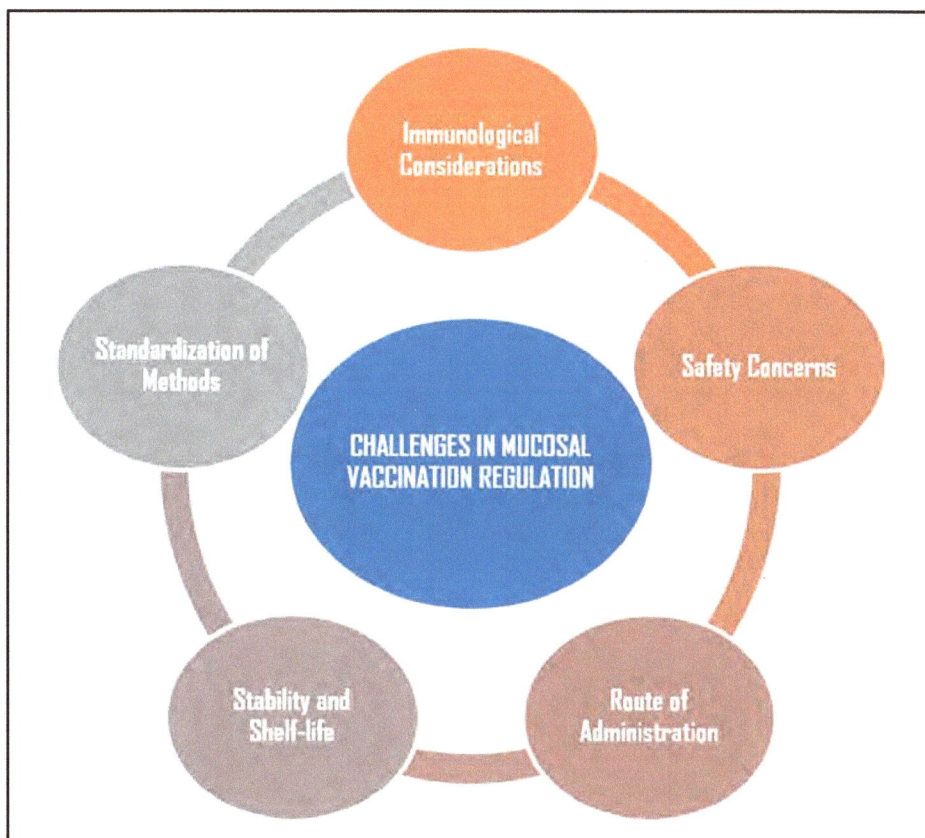

Fig. (3). Challenges in mucosal vaccination regulation.

EXAMPLES OF SUCCESSFUL REGULATORY APPROVAL

Examples of successful regulatory approvals for mucosal vaccines across different administration routes:

Nasal Spray Vaccines

FluMist® Quadrivalent (Live Attenuated Influenza Vaccine)

FluMist® is the nasal spray flu vaccine produced by AstraZeneca. It was first approved by regulatory agencies like the US FDA and the European Medicine Agency (EMA). It helps to stimulate mucosal immune responses in the respiratory tract to provide protection against seasonal influenza viruses. In eligible patients aged 2 to 49, FluMist® may be used [132, 133].

Oral Vaccines

Rotarix® (Rotavirus Vaccine, Live, Oral)

Rotarix® is an oral rotavirus vaccine that GlaxoSmithKline (GSK) designed to prevent infantile gastroenteritis caused by this condition. It has received worldwide approval from regulatory bodies such as the FDA and EMA. Rotarix® contains weakened, living strains of rotaviruses and is given orally in two doses starting at 6 weeks of age in infants. In terms of severe rotavirus diarrhea case reduction, the vaccine has shown effectiveness in reducing hospitalizations related to it [134, 135].

Inhaled Vaccines

FluMist® Quadrivalent (Live Attenuated Influenza Vaccine)

Apart from being a nasal spray, FluMist® is also a successful example of an inhaled vaccine. It is approved for intranasal administration and has been widely used for seasonal flu vaccination in populations eligible for it. The vaccine has shown the ability to produce both systemic and mucosal immune responses, thus presenting another choice against injectable influenza vaccines [136, 137].

FUTURE PERSPECTIVES

Advancements in technology can totally change sectors and communities, ranging from artificial intelligence and quantum computing to biotechnology and renewable energy. By solving complex problems, these developments promise unimaginable chances for creativity and expansion [138].

This requires that regulatory adaptations be made to facilitate responsible and ethical deployment of new technologies. Balancing innovation and protection from risks such as algorithmic biases, privacy breaches, and cyber threats will be a tightrope walk for governments and regulatory bodies. In this age of globalization, there is an increasing need for global collaboration to deal with common challenges like climate change, pandemics, and economic inequality. International cooperation will facilitate the sharing of resources, knowledge, and ideas to address multifaceted cross-border problems [139].

This is a future world where our success will depend on our ability to seize the potential of nascent technologies while observing regulatory requirements and improving collaboration across borders. Our adoption of these principles will ensure a sustainable future that incorporates everyone [140].

CONCLUSION

In summary, as we go forward into the future, the importance of moving through the new technology landscape, regulatory adaptations, and global cooperation cannot be overemphasized. These pillars underpin our collective progress, each contributing to our common fate. Essential points summarizing recognize the transformative potential that exists within emerging technologies across sectors such as artificial intelligence and biotechnology, with breakthroughs promising to change industries and societies completely. However, this optimism cannot overlook the urgent demand for regulatory changes that will ensure the responsible and ethical utilization of these technologies and in line with public opinion. A compliance regime is pivotal in this direction; it has several purposes, such as reducing risks associated with technological advances and ensuring that they do not promote discriminatory practices or inequalities within society. The future direction is outlined by the glow from the horizon through which the need for worldwide cooperation can be seen. Today, problems that we face are not limited to certain geographical regions. Still, they go beyond such divisions, hence the need to approach them in a unified manner by making use of knowledge, materials, and creativity collectively. In addition, fostering collaborations among countries, disciplines, and cultures allows for more effective global solutions while addressing complex challenges such as climate change, pandemics, economic disparity, *etc*. While traversing this impermanent terrain, the decisions we make now will resonate for many years later. Should we decide to promote openness in the market while ensuring adherence to regulatory frameworks and enhancing global solidarity, then we can shape a fair future that is not only sustainable but also prosperous for our successive generations. In the midst of transformation, let us mold a tomorrow that respects the inherent honor and abilities of each person, thereby preserving our global environment's health.

ACKNOWLEDGEMENTS

Authors are highly thankful to their Universities/Colleges for providing library facilities for the literature survey.

REFERENCES

[1]   Huang M, Zhang M, Zhu H, Du X, Wang J. Mucosal vaccine delivery: A focus on the breakthrough of specific barriers. Acta Pharmaceutica Sinica B. Chinese Academy of Medical Sciences; 2022; 12, 3456–74.

[2]   Dotiwala F, Upadhyay AK. Next Generation Mucosal Vaccine Strategy for Respiratory Pathogens. Vaccines. Multidisciplinary Digital Publishing Institute (MDPI), 2023; 11.
[http://dx.doi.org/10.3390/vaccines11101585]

[3]   Huang M, Zhang M, Zhu H, Du X, Wang J. Mucosal vaccine delivery: A focus on the breakthrough of specific barriers. Acta Pharmaceutica Sinica B. Chinese Academy of Medical Sciences; 2022; 12, 3456–74.

[4]   Azegami T, Kiyono H. The Mucosal Immune System for Vaccine Development Aayam Lamichhane. 2014. Available from: https://www.elsevier.com/open-access/userlicense/1.0/

[5]   Hameed SA, Paul S, Dellosa GKY, Jaraquemada D, Bello MB. Towards the future exploration of mucosal mRNA vaccines against emerging viral diseases; lessons from existing next-generation mucosal vaccine strategies. npj Vaccines. Nature Research; 2022; 7.

[6]   Chatterjee SK, Saha S, Munoz MNM. Activation of mucosal immunity and novel prophylactic and therapeutic strategy in combating COVID-19. Exploration of Immunology. Open Exploration Publishing Inc; 2021; 1, 374–97.

[7]   Anggraeni R, Ana ID, Wihadmadyatami H. Development of mucosal vaccine delivery: an overview on the mucosal vaccines and their adjuvants. Clinical and Experimental Vaccine Research. Korean Vaccine Society; 2022; 11, 235–48.

[8]   Otczyk DC, Cripps AW. Mucosal immunization: A realistic alternative. Hum Vaccin 2010; 6(12): 978-1006.
[http://dx.doi.org/10.4161/hv.6.12.13142] [PMID: 21150284]

[9]   Holmgren J, Czerkinsky C. Mucosal immunity and vaccines. Nat Med 2005; 11(S4) (Suppl.): S45-53.
[http://dx.doi.org/10.1038/nm1213] [PMID: 15812489]

[10]   Scheuplein RJ, Shoaf SE, Brown RN. Role of pharmacokinetics in safety evaluation and regulatory considerations. Annu Rev Pharmacol Toxicol 1990; 30(1): 197-218.
[http://dx.doi.org/10.1146/annurev.pa.30.040190.001213] [PMID: 2188568]

[11]   Myhr AI. DNA vaccines: Regulatory considerations and safety aspects. Curr Issues Mol Biol 2017; 22: 79-88.
[http://dx.doi.org/10.21775/cimb.022.079] [PMID: 27705898]

[12]   Eichler HG, Bloechl-Daum B, Abadie E, Barnett D, König F, Pearson S. (). 2010. Available from: www.nature.com/reviews/drugdisc

[13]   Reed SD, Anstrom KJ, Seils DM, Califf RM, Schulman KA. Use of larger versus smaller drug-safety databases before regulatory approval: the trade-offs. Health Aff (Millwood) 2008; 27(5) (Suppl. 1): w360-70.
[http://dx.doi.org/10.1377/hlthaff.27.5.w360] [PMID: 18682441]

[14]   Krause PR, Roberts J. Scientific and regulatory considerations for efficacy studies of cytomegalovirus vaccines. J Infect Dis 2020; 221 (Suppl. 1): S103-8.
[http://dx.doi.org/10.1093/infdis/jiz523] [PMID: 32134485]

[15]   Eichler HG, Abadie E, Breckenridge A, Flamion B, Gustafsson LL, Leufkens H, Rowland M, Schneider CK, Bloechl-Daum B. Bridging the efficacy–effectiveness gap: a regulator's perspective on addressing variability of drug response. Nat rev Drug discov 2011; 10(7): 495-506.

[16]   Fonseca-Santos B, Corrêa MA, Chorilli M. Sustainability, natural and organic cosmetics: consumer, products, efficacy, toxicological and regulatory considerations. Braz J Pharm Sci 2015; 51(1): 17-26.
[http://dx.doi.org/10.1590/S1984-82502015000100002]

[17]   Myhr AI. DNA vaccines: Regulatory considerations and safety aspects. Curr Issues Mol Biol 2017; 22: 79-88.
[http://dx.doi.org/10.21775/cimb.022.079] [PMID: 27705898]

[18]   Bent S. Herbal medicine in the United States: review of efficacy, safety, and regulation: grand rounds at University of California, San Francisco Medical Center. J Gen Intern Med 2008; 23(6): 854-9.
[http://dx.doi.org/10.1007/s11606-008-0632-y] [PMID: 18415652]

[19]   Okpala COR, Korzeniowska M. Understanding the Relevance of Quality Management in Agro-food Product Industry: From Ethical Considerations to Assuring Food Hygiene Quality Safety Standards and Its Associated Processes. Food Reviews International. Taylor and Francis Ltd.; 2023; 39, 1879–952.

[20]   Paul MJ, LeDuc SD, Lassiter MG, Moorhead LC, Noyes PD, Leibowitz SG. Wildfire Induces Changes in Receiving Waters: A Review With Considerations for Water Quality Management. Water Resources Research. John Wiley and Sons Inc; 2022; 58.

[21]   Ongley ED. Water quality management: design, financing and sustainability considerations-II. 2000; 1

[22]   Gervais A, Dirksen EHC, Pohl T, *et al.* Compliance and regulatory considerations for the implementation of the multi-attribute-method by mass spectrometry in a quality control laboratory. Eur J Pharm Biopharm 2023; 191: 57-67.
[http://dx.doi.org/10.1016/j.ejpb.2023.08.008] [PMID: 37582411]

[23]   Béghin L, Castera M, Manios Y, *et al.* Quality assurance of ethical issues and regulatory aspects relating to good clinical practices in the HELENA Cross-Sectional Study. Int J Obes 2008; 32(S5) (Suppl. 5): S12-8.
[http://dx.doi.org/10.1038/ijo.2008.179] [PMID: 19011647]

[24]   Chu CT. A pivotal role for PINK1 and autophagy in mitochondrial quality control: implications for Parkinson disease. Hum Mol Genet 2010; 19(R1): R28-37.
[http://dx.doi.org/10.1093/hmg/ddq143] [PMID: 20385539]

[25]   Misra G. Books Quality Control and Regulatory Aspects for Biologicals: Regulations and Best Practices. 2024. Available from: https://books.google.co.in/books?id=sR35EAAAQBAJ&dq=Importance+of+Regulatory+Considerations:+Quality+control&lr=&source=gbs_navlinks_s

[26]   Massella M, Dri DA, Gramaglia D. Regulatory Considerations on the use of Machine Learning based tools in Clinical Trials. Health Technol (Berl) 2022; 12(6): 1085-96.
[http://dx.doi.org/10.1007/s12553-022-00708-0] [PMID: 36373014]

[27]   Ellenberg SSmith, Fleming TR, DeMets DL. Data monitoring committees in clinical trials: a practical perspective. J. Wiley & Sons; 2002; 191.

[28]   McNair L. Ethical and regulatory oversight of clinical research: The role of the Institutional Review Board. Vol. 247, Experimental Biology and Medicine. SAGE Publications Inc., 2022; 561–6.

[29]   Davis JR, Institute of Medicine (U.S.). Roundtable on Research and Development of Drugs B. Assuring data quality and validity in clinical trials for regulatory decision making: workshop report: Roundtable on Research and Development of Drugs, Biologics, and Medical Devices. National Academy Press; 1999; 76.

[30]   Califf RM, Sugarman J. Exploring the ethical and regulatory issues in pragmatic clinical trials. Clin Trials 2015; 12(5): 436-41.
[http://dx.doi.org/10.1177/1740774515598334] [PMID: 26374676]

[31]   Zhengwu L. Technical challenges in designing post-marketing eCRFs to address clinical safety and pharmacovigilance needs - ScienceDirect. 2010.

[32]   Alomar M, Tawfiq AM, Hassan N, Palaian S. Post-marketing surveillance of suspected adverse drug reactions through spontaneous reporting: current status, challenges and the future. Therapeutic Advances in Drug Safety. SAGE Publications Ltd; 2020; 11.

[33] Fritsche E, Elsallab M, Schaden M, Hey SP, Abou-El-Enein M. Post-marketing safety and efficacy surveillance of cell and gene therapies in the EU: A critical review. Cell Gene Ther Insights 2019; 5(11): 1505-21.
[http://dx.doi.org/10.18609/cgti.2019.156]

[34] Gad SC. Books Safety Pharmacology in Pharmaceutical Development: Approval and Post Marketing Surveillance, Second Edition Selected pages Importance of Regula. 2012. Available from: https://books.google.co.in/books?id=AHA2g-qq6WwC&dq=Importance+of+Regulatory+Considerations:+Post-marketing+surveillance&lr=&source=gbs

[35] Aronson JK. Post-marketing drug withdrawals: pharmacovigilance success, regulatory problems Arrêts de commercialisation des médicaments post-autorisation: succès de la pharmacovigilance, problèmes réglementaires 2017.

[36] Schifferstein HNJ, de Boer A, Lemke M. Conveying information through food packaging: A literature review comparing legislation with consumer perception. Journal of Functional Foods. Elsevier Ltd; 2021; 86.

[37] Mackey TK, Liang BA, Novotny TE. Evolution of tobacco labeling and packaging: international legal considerations and health governance. Am J Public Health 2013; 103(4): e39-43.
[http://dx.doi.org/10.2105/AJPH.2012.301029] [PMID: 23409884]

[38] Pascall MA, DeAngelo K, Richards J, Arensberg MB. Role and Importance of Functional Food Packaging in Specialized Products for Vulnerable Populations: Implications for Innovation and Policy Development for Sustainability. Foods 2022; 11(19): 3043.
[http://dx.doi.org/10.3390/foods11193043] [PMID: 36230119]

[39] Boz Z, Korhonen V, Sand CK. Consumer considerations for the implementation of sustainable packaging: A review. Sustainability (Switzerland). 2020 Mar 1;12(6).
[http://dx.doi.org/10.3390/su12062192]

[40] Institute of Medicine (U.S.). Committee on Examination of Front-of-Package Nutrition Rating Systems and Symbols., Wartella Ellen, Institute of Medicine (U.S.). Food and Nutrition Board. Front-of-Package Nutrition Rating Systems and Symbols: Promoting Healthier Choices. National Academies Press; 2012; 163.

[41] Restuccia D, Spizzirri UG, Parisi OI, *et al.* New EU regulation aspects and global market of active and intelligent packaging for food industry applications. Food Control 2010; 21(11): 1425-35.
[http://dx.doi.org/10.1016/j.foodcont.2010.04.028]

[42] Patel NG, Kesselheim AS, Darrow JJ. Trust and Regulation: Assuring Scientific Independence in the FDA's Emergency Use Authorization Process. J Health Polit Policy Law 2023; 48(5): 799-820.
[http://dx.doi.org/10.1215/03616878-10637726] [PMID: 36995365]

[43] Kent-Jensen L, Quinney SJ. Emergency Use Authorizations in the Time of Coronavirus Emergency Use Authorizations in the Time of Coronavirus Recommended Citation. Utah Law Rev 2022; 2022: 2022-413.
[http://dx.doi.org/10.26054/0d-5nj3-gp2r]

[44] Badnjević A, Pokvić LG, Džemić Z, Bečić F. Risks of emergency use authorizations for medical products during outbreak situations: A COVID-19 case study. BioMedical Engineering Online. BioMed Central Ltd 2020; p. 19.

[45] Lindström-Gommers L, Mullin T. International conference on harmonization: Recent reforms as a driver of global regulatory harmonization and innovation in medical products. Clinical Pharmacology and Therapeutics. Nature Publishing Group; 2019; 105, 926–31.

[46] Kephalopoulos S, De Bruin YB, Arvanitis A, Hakkinen P, Jantunen M. Issues in consumer exposure modeling: Towards harmonization on a global scale. J Expo Sci Environ Epidemiol 2007; 17(S1) (Suppl. 1): S90-S100.

[http://dx.doi.org/10.1038/sj.jes.7500605] [PMID: 17668010]

[47]   Wolf DC, Aggarwal M, Battalora M, *et al.* Implementing a globally harmonized risk assessment-based approach for regulatory decision-making of crop protection products. Pest Manag Sci 2020; 76(10): 3311-5.
[http://dx.doi.org/10.1002/ps.5793] [PMID: 32077588]

[48]   Simmons BA. The international politics of harmonization: The case of capital market regulation. Int Organ 2001; 55(3): 589-620.
[http://dx.doi.org/10.1162/00208180152507560]

[49]   Oberweis CV, Marchal JA, López-Ruiz E, Gálvez-Martín P. A worldwide overview of regulatory frameworks for tissue-based products. Tissue Engineering - Part B: Reviews. Mary Ann Liebert Inc.; 2020; 26, 181–96.
[http://dx.doi.org/10.1089/ten.teb.2019.0315]

[50]   Godlove N. Regulatory Overview of Virtual Currency. Oklahoma Journal of Law and Technology 2014; 10.

[51]   Ndomondo-Sigonda M, Mahlangu G, Agama-Anyetei M, Cooke E. A new approach to an old problem: Overview of the East African Community's Medicines Regulatory Harmonization initiative. PLoS Medicine. Public Library of Science; 2020; 17.

[52]   OECD Publishing. Regulatory Impact Analysis Best Practices in OECD Countries_ Best Practices OECD - Google Books. 1997.

[53]   latest from JAMA Oncology, including those for text and data mining, AI training, and similar technologies.2024. Available from: https://jamanetwork.com/journals/jamaoncology/article-abstract/2250350

[54]   Mukherjee S. The United States Food and Drug Administration (FDA) regulatory response to combat neglected tropical diseases (NTDs): A review. PLoS Neglected Tropical Diseases. Public Library of Science; 2023; 17.

[55]   Hackett JL, Gutman SI. Introduction to the food and Drug Administration (FDA) regulatory process. Vol. 4. J Proteome Res 2005; 4(4): 1110-3.
[http://dx.doi.org/10.1021/pr050059a] [PMID: 16083260]

[56]   Ross S. Functional foods: the Food and Drug Administration perspective. Am J Clin Nutr 2000; 71(6): 1735S-8S.

[57]   Razavi M, Glasziou P, Klocksieben FA, Ioannidis JPA, Chalmers I, Djulbegovic B. US Food and Drug Administration Approvals of Drugs and Devices Based on Nonrandomized Clinical Trials: A Systematic Review and Meta-analysis. JAMA Network Open. American Medical Association; 2019; 2.
[http://dx.doi.org/10.1001/jamanetworkopen.2019.11111]

[58]   Zhao Q, Han Z, Wang J, Han Z. Development and investigational new drug application of mesenchymal stem/stromal cells products in China. Stem Cells Translational Medicine. John Wiley and Sons Ltd; 2021; 10, S18–30.

[59]   Musoba GD, Jacob SA, Robinson LJ. The Institutional Review Board (IRB) and faculty: Does the IRB challenge faculty professionalism in the social sciences? Qual Rep 2014; 19(51): 1-14.

[60]   Beauchamp T, Faden R, Barry R. The Linacre Quarterly. The Linacre Quarterly. 1987; 54. Available from:
https://epublications.marquette.edu/lnqAvailableat:https://epublications.marquette.edu/lnq/vol54/iss2/15

[61]   Verma K. Base of a Research: Good Clinical Practice in Clinical Trials. J Clin Trials 2013; 3(1)
[http://dx.doi.org/10.4172/2167-0870.1000128]

[62]   Califf RM, Sugarman J. Exploring the ethical and regulatory issues in pragmatic clinical trials. Clin

Trials 2015; 12(5): 436-41.
[http://dx.doi.org/10.1177/1740774515598334] [PMID: 26374676]

[63] Colopy MW, Gordon R, Ahmad F, Wang WW, Duke SP, Ball G. Statistical Practices of Safety Monitoring: An Industry Survey. Ther Innov Regul Sci 2019; 53(3): 293-300.
[http://dx.doi.org/10.1177/2168479018779973] [PMID: 29991276]

[64] Kairuz T, Crump K, John O'brien A. Perspectives on qualitative research. Part 2: Useful tools for data collection and analysis. Article in Pharmaceutical Journal. 2007. Available from: https://www.researchgate.net/publication/43499524

[65] Macdonald JC, Isom DC, Evans DD, Page KJ. Digital Innovation in Medicinal Product Regulatory Submission, Review, and Approvals to Create a Dynamic Regulatory Ecosystem—Are We Ready for a Revolution? Front Med (Lausanne) 2021; 8: 660808.
[http://dx.doi.org/10.3389/fmed.2021.660808] [PMID: 34109196]

[66] Dart RC. Monitoring risk: Post-marketing surveillance and signal detection. Drug Alcohol Depend. 2009; 105(SUPPL. 1).

[67] Dhruva SS, Darrow JJ, Kesselheim AS, Redberg RF. Experts' Views on FDA Regulatory Standards for Drug and High-Risk Medical Devices: Implications for Patient Care. J Gen Intern Med 2022; 37(16): 4176-82.
[http://dx.doi.org/10.1007/s11606-021-07316-0] [PMID: 35138547]

[68] Lievevrouw E, Marelli L, Van Hoyweghen I. The FDA's standard-making process for medical digital health technologies: co-producing technological and organizational innovation. Biosocieties 2022; 17(3): 549-76.
[http://dx.doi.org/10.1057/s41292-021-00232-w] [PMID: 34002115]

[69] Van Norman GA. Drugs, Devices, and the FDA: Part 2. JACC Basic Transl Sci 2016; 1(4): 277-87.
[http://dx.doi.org/10.1016/j.jacbts.2016.03.009] [PMID: 30167516]

[70] Specialist AKS, Policy IH. FDA Regulation of Medical Devices. 2023.

[71] Policy P. Read the clinical trial. Get the latest from JAMA Internal Medicine including those for text and data mining, AI training, and similar technologies 2024. Available from: https://jamanetwork.com/journals/jamainternalmedicine/article-abstract/1910557

[72] Kramer DB, Tan YT, Sato C, Kesselheim AS. Ensuring Medical Device Effectiveness and Safety: A Cross-National Comparison of Approaches to Regulation 2014.

[73] Cox Gad S. Pharmaceutical manufacturing handbook regulations and quality 2008.

[74] Di Prima M, Coburn J, Hwang D, Kelly J, Khairuzzaman A, Ricles L. Additively manufactured medical products – the FDA perspective. 3D Print Med. 2016; (1).

[75] Gupta NV, Padickakunnel GS. Modern FDA Guidance and comparative overview of FDA and EMA on process validation. Article in International Journal of Pharmacy and Pharmaceutical Sciences. 2014. Available from: https://www.researchgate.net/publication/263657534

[76] Ravi G, Vishal Gupta N, Ravi G. Citations 3 reads 6,718. Vol. 5, Article in International Journal of PharmTech Research. 2013. Available from https://www.researchgate.net/publication/263657531

[77] Urbaniak M, Zimon D, Madzik P, Šírová E. Risk factors in the assessment of suppliers Plos one 2022; 17(8): e0272157.

[78] Lincoln JE. Overview of the us fda gmps: Good manufacturing practice (gmp)/quality system (qs) regulation (21 CFR part 820). J Valid Technol 2012; 18(3): 17.

[79] Townend D, van de Pas R, Bongers L, Haque S, Wouters B, Pilot E, Stahl N, Schroder-Back P, Shaw D, Krafft T. What is the Role of the European Union in the COVID-19 Pandemic?. Med & L 2020; 39: 249.

[80] Di Prima M, Coburn J, Hwang D, Kelly J, Khairuzzaman A, Ricles L. Additively manufactured

medical products – the FDA perspective. 3D Print Med. 2016; 2(1).

[81]   Mantus D, Pisano DJ. Books FDA Regulatory Affairs: Third Edition. 2014. Available from: https://books.google.co.in/books?id=6O71EAAAQBAJ&dq=FDA:+Manufacturing+Guidelines&lr=& source=gbs_navlinks_s
[http://dx.doi.org/10.1201/b16471]

[82]   José (Pepe) Rodríguez-Pérez. Bridging_the_efficacy_effectiveness_gap. 2014.

[83]   Dal-Ré R, Kesselheim AS, Bourgeois FT. Increasing Access to FDA Inspection Reports on Irregularities and Misconduct in Clinical Trials. JAMA - Journal of the American Medical Association. American Medical Association; 2020; 323, 1903–4.
[http://dx.doi.org/10.1001/jama.2020.1631]

[84]   Arcidiacono JA, Bauer SR, Kaplan DS, Allocca CM, Sarkar S, Lin-Gibson S. FDA and NIST Collaboration on Standards Development Activities Supporting Innovation and Translation of Regenerative Medicine Products. 2018.
[http://dx.doi.org/10.1016/j.jcyt.2018.03.039]

[85]   Anderson M, Forman R, Mossialos E. Navigating the role of the EU Health Emergency Preparedness and Response Authority (HERA) in Europe and beyond. The Lancet Regional Health - Europe. Elsevier Ltd; 2021; 9.

[86]   Iandomenico Majone G. Eui Working Papers In Political and Social Sciences Eui Working Paper SPS No. 90/6 Cross-National Sources of Regulatory Policy-Making in Europe and the United States. 1990.

[87]   Ziller J. The european union and the territorial scope of european territories. 2007.

[88]   Hastedt JE, Bäckman P, Clark AR, *et al.* Scope and relevance of a pulmonary biopharmaceutical classification system AAPS/FDA/USP Workshop March 16-17th, 2015 in Baltimore, MD. AAPS Open 2016; 2(1): 1.
[http://dx.doi.org/10.1186/s41120-015-0002-x]

[89]   Haan den K, Bs H, der Zandt van. EUROPEAN UNION SYSTEM FOR TEE EVALUATION OF SUBStances. Vol. 34, Chemosphere. Elsevier AU rights-cd; 1997.

[90]   Cormier JW. Advancing FDA's Regulatory Science through Weight of Evidence Advancing FDA's Regulatory Science through Weight of Evidence Evaluations Evaluations. Vol. 28, Journal of Contemporary Health Law & Policy. 1985. Available from: https://scholarship.law.edu/jchlp/vol28/iss1/2

[91]   Narla SK. Marketing authorization of human medicinal products to European Union/European Economic Area. Int J Pharm Sci Rev Res. 2011; 10(1): 1-8.

[92]   Muchmore AI. Penn State Law eLibrary Penn State Law eLibrary Journal Articles Faculty Works 2022. 2022. Available from: https://elibrary.law.psu.edu/fac_works

[93]   Felix T, Jordan JB, Akers C, Patel B, Drago D. Current state of biologic pharmacovigilance in the European Union: improvements are needed. Expert Opinion on Drug Safety. Taylor and Francis Ltd; 2019; 18, 231–40.

[94]   Harpaz R, DuMouchel W, LePendu P, Bauer-Mehren A, Ryan P, Shah NH. Performance of pharmacovigilance signal-detection algorithms for the FDA adverse event reporting system. Clin Pharmacol Ther 2013; 93(6): 539-46.
[http://dx.doi.org/10.1038/clpt.2013.24] [PMID: 23571771]

[95]   Young M, Flink T, Dall E. Science Diplomacy in the Making: Case-based insights from the S4D4C project Preface The editors. 2020. Available from: www.S4D4C.eu

[96]   McIntyre TD, Pappas M, DiBiasi JJ. How FDA Advisory Committee Members Prepare and What Influences Them. Ther Innov Regul Sci 2013; 47(1): 32-40.
[http://dx.doi.org/10.1177/0092861512458096] [PMID: 30227490]

[97]   Legido-Quigley H, Panteli D, Brusamento S, *et al.* Clinical guidelines in the European Union:

Mapping the regulatory basis, development, quality control, implementation and evaluation across member states. Health Policy 2012; 107(2-3): 146-56.
[http://dx.doi.org/10.1016/j.healthpol.2012.08.004] [PMID: 22939646]

[98] Kaza M, Karaźniewicz-Łada M, Kosicka K, Siemiątkowska A, Rudzki PJ. Bioanalytical method validation: new FDA guidance vs. EMA guideline. Better or worse? J Pharm Biomed Anal 2019; 165: 381-5.
[http://dx.doi.org/10.1016/j.jpba.2018.12.030] [PMID: 30590335]

[99] Cunningham JA, Link AN. Fostering university-industry R&D collaborations in European Union countries. Int Entrep Manage J 2015; 11(4): 849-60. http://link.springer.com/article/
[http://dx.doi.org/10.1007/s11365-014-0317-4]

[100] Ackley D, Birkebak J, Blumel J, *et al.* FDA and industry collaboration: Identifying opportunities to further reduce reliance on nonhuman primates for nonclinical safety evaluations. Regul Toxicol Pharmacol 2023; 138: 105327.
[http://dx.doi.org/10.1016/j.yrtph.2022.105327] [PMID: 36586472]

[101] Hillebrandt M. Transparency as a platform for institutional politics: The case of the council of the European Union. Politics Gov 2017; 5(3): 62-74.
[http://dx.doi.org/10.17645/pag.v5i3.975]

[102] Wood SF, Perosino KL. Increasing TransParency at the fda: The impact of the fda amendments act of 2007. Vol. 123, Public Health Reports. 2007. Available from: http://www.fda

[103] Padel S. Economic Analysis of Certification Systems in Organic Food and Farming The european regulatory framework and its implementation in influencing organic inspection and certification systems in the eu deliverable 11. 2010. Available from: http://www.certcost.org

[104] Musazzi UM, Marini V, Casiraghi A, Minghetti P. Is the European regulatory framework sufficient to assure the safety of citizens using health products containing nanomaterials? Drug Discovery Today. Elsevier Ltd; 2017; 22 870–82.
[http://dx.doi.org/10.1016/j.drudis.2017.01.016]

[105] Verbeken G, Pirnay JP, De Vos D, *et al.* Optimizing the European regulatory framework for sustainable bacteriophage therapy in human medicine. Arch Immunol Ther Exp (Warsz) 2012; 60(3): 161-72.
[http://dx.doi.org/10.1007/s00005-012-0175-0] [PMID: 22527355]

[106] Carvalho M, Sepodes B, Martins AP. Regulatory and scientific advancements in gene therapy: State-of-the-art clinical applications and of the supporting European regulatory framework. Frontiers in Medicine. Frontiers Media S.A. 2017; 4.

[107] Vettorazzi A, de Cerain AL, Sanz-Serrano J, Gil AG, Azqueta A. European regulatory framework and safety assessment of food-related bioactive compounds. Nutrients. MDPI AG 2020; 12.

[108] Kerscher S, Arboleya P. The key role of aggregators in the energy transition under the latest European regulatory framework. 2022.
[http://dx.doi.org/10.1016/j.ijepes.2021.107361]

[109] Herrero-Martinez E, Hussain N, Roux NL, *et al.* Dynamic Regulatory Assessment: evolving the European Regulatory Framework for the Benefit of Patients and Public Health—an EFPIA View. Clin Ther 2022; 44(1): 132-8.
[http://dx.doi.org/10.1016/j.clinthera.2021.11.001] [PMID: 34848082]

[110] The first ten years of the World Health Organization. 1958.

[111] World Health Organization. The second ten years of the World Health Organization. World Health Organ 1968; 1958-67. https://iris.who.int/handle/10665/39254

[112] Ahonen EQ, Benavides FG, Benach J. Immigrant populations, work and health—a systematic literature review. Scand J Work Environ & Health 2007; 1: 96-104.

[113] World Health Organization. The World Health Report 2005: Make every mother and child count. World Health Organ 2005; 23.

[114] McCarthy M. A brief history of the World Health Organization. Lancet 2002; 360(9340): 1111-2. [http://dx.doi.org/10.1016/S0140-6736(02)11244-X] [PMID: 12387972]

[115] World Health Organization. The World Health Report 2001_ Mental Health _ New Understanding, New Hope - World Health Organization - Google Books. 2001.

[116] Cassese S. Global standards for national administrative procedure. 2006. Available from: http://law.duke.edu/journals/lcp

[117] Young AR. Europe as a global regulator? The limits of EU influence in international food safety standards. J Eur Public Policy 2014; 21(6): 904-22. [http://dx.doi.org/10.1080/13501763.2014.910871]

[118] Magaldi De Sousa M. New Thinking and the New G20 Series. 2015.

[119] Wielsch D. Global Law's Toolbox: Private Regulation by Standards. Am J Comp Law 2012; 60(4): 1075-104. [http://dx.doi.org/10.5131/AJCL.2012.0012]

[120] Kane EJ (Edward J. Relevance and Need for International Regulatory Standards. Brookings-Wharton Papers on Financial Services. 2001; 2001(1): 87–115.

[121] Dretler AW, Rouphael NG, Stephens DS. Progress toward the global control of Neisseria meningitidis: 21st century vaccines, current guidelines, and challenges for future vaccine development. Human Vaccines and Immunotherapeutics. Taylor and Francis Inc.; 2018; 14, 1146–60.

[122] Kaufmann SHE, Juliana McElrath M, Lewis DJM, Del Giudice G. Challenges and responses in human vaccine development. Current Opinion in Immunology. Elsevier Ltd; 2014; 28, 18–26 [http://dx.doi.org/10.1016/j.coi.2014.01.009]

[123] Brisse M, Vrba SM, Kirk N, Liang Y, Ly H. Emerging Concepts and Technologies in Vaccine Development. Frontiers in Immunology. Frontiers Media S.A. 2020; 11.

[124] Zwaan CM, Kolb EA, Reinhardt D, Abrahamsson J, Adachi S, Aplenc R, et al. Collaborative efforts driving progress in pediatric acute myeloid leukemia. Journal of Clinical Oncology. American Society of Clinical Oncology; 2015; 33, 2949–62. [http://dx.doi.org/10.1200/JCO.2015.62.8289]

[125] Martens J 1962. Multistakeholder partnerships - future models of multilaterism? 2007.

[126] Broadbent J, Laughlin R. Public private partnerships: an introduction. Account Audit Account J 2003; 16(3): 332-41. [http://dx.doi.org/10.1108/09513570310482282]

[127] Sargent LD, Waters LE. Careers and academic research collaborations: An inductive process framework for understanding successful collaborations. J Vocat Behav 2004; 64(2): 308-19. [http://dx.doi.org/10.1016/j.jvb.2002.11.001]

[128] Rasmussen A, Reher S. Civil Society Engagement and Policy Representation in Europe. Comp Polit Stud 2019; 52(11): 1648-76. [http://dx.doi.org/10.1177/0010414019830724]

[129] Zhang X, Zhang J, Chen S, He Q, Bai Y, Liu J, *et al.* Progress and challenges in the clinical evaluation of immune responses to respiratory mucosal vaccines. 2024. [http://dx.doi.org/10.1080/14760584.2024.2326094]

[130] Venu G, Dutta S, Panwar K, Sarkar R, Sinha E, Arun A, *et al.* Mucosal vaccines: Strategies and challenges: A brief overview. The Pharma Innovation Journal. 2023; 12(6): 4980–90. Available from: www.thepharmajournal.com

[131] Shewen PE, Carrasco-Medina L, McBey BA, Hodgins DC. Challenges in mucosal vaccination of

cattle. Vet Immunol Immunopathol 2009; 128(1-3): 192-8.
[http://dx.doi.org/10.1016/j.vetimm.2008.10.297] [PMID: 19046777]

[132] Luczo JM, Bousse T, Johnson SK, *et al.* Intranasal powder live attenuated influenza vaccine is thermostable, immunogenic, and protective against homologous challenge in ferrets. NPJ Vaccines 2021; 6(1): 59.
[http://dx.doi.org/10.1038/s41541-021-00320-9] [PMID: 33883559]

[133] Gasparini C, Acunzo M, Biuso A, *et al.* Nasal spray live attenuated influenza vaccine: the first experience in Italy in children and adolescents during the 2020–21 season. Ital J Pediatr 2021; 47(1): 225.
[http://dx.doi.org/10.1186/s13052-021-01172-8] [PMID: 34774062]

[134] Folorunso OS, Sebolai OM. Overview of the development, impacts, and challenges of live-attenuated oral rotavirus vaccines. Vaccines. MDPI AG 2020; 8: pp. 1-64.

[135] Kirkwood CD, Ma LF, Carey ME, Steele AD. The rotavirus vaccine development pipeline. Vaccine 2019; 37(50): 7328-35.
[http://dx.doi.org/10.1016/j.vaccine.2017.03.076] [PMID: 28396207]

[136] Nigwekar PV, Kumar A, Padbidri VV, Choudhury A, Chaudhari AB, Kulkarni PS. Safety of Russian-Backbone Trivalent, Live Attenuated Seasonal Influenza Vaccine in Healthy Subjects: Open-Label, Non-randomized Phase 4 Study. Drug Saf 2018; 41(2): 171-7.
[http://dx.doi.org/10.1007/s40264-017-0605-3] [PMID: 29027148]

[137] Trombetta CM, Gianchecchi E, Montomoli E. Influenza vaccines: Evaluation of the safety profile. Human Vaccines and Immunotherapeutics. Taylor and Francis Inc.; 2018; 14, 657–70.

[138] Baker JR Jr, Farazuddin M, Wong PT, O'Konek JJ. The unfulfilled potential of mucosal immunization. J Allergy Clin Immunol 2022; 150(1): 1-11.
[http://dx.doi.org/10.1016/j.jaci.2022.05.002] [PMID: 35569567]

[139] Rhee JH. Current and new approaches for mucosal vaccine delivery. Mucosal Vaccines: Innovation for Preventing Infectious Diseases. Elsevier 2019; pp. 325-56.

[140] Hameed SA, Paul S, Dellosa GKY, Jaraquemada D, Bello MB. Towards the future exploration of mucosal mRNA vaccines against emerging viral diseases; lessons from existing next-generation mucosal vaccine strategies., npj Vaccines. Nature Research; 2022; 7.

CHAPTER 2

Economic Impacts of Mucosal Vaccination Programs

Neeraj Kumar Fuloria[1], Akhil Sharma[2], Sunita[3], Akanksha Sharma[2] and **Shaweta Sharma[4,*]**

[1] *Department of Pharmaceutical Chemistry, Faculty of Pharmacy, AIMST University, Semeling Campus, Jalan Bedong-Semeling, Bedong, Kedah Darul Aman, Malaysia*

[2] *R. J. College of Pharmacy, 2HVJ+567, Raipur, Gharbara, Tappal, Khair, Uttar Pradesh 202165, India*

[3] *Metro College of Health Sciences and Research, Greater Noida, India*

[4] *School of Medical and Allied Sciences, Galgotias University, Yamuna Expressway, Gautam Buddha Nagar, Uttar Pradesh-201310, India*

Abstract: Mucosal vaccination is a new method of immunization with the potential to revolutionize strategies in the prevention of diseases. Although more attention has been paid to its ability to generate strong immunity, its economic implications have not been adequately discussed. This abstract gives an inclusive summary of the economic effects of disease prevention programs with their possible advantages and drawbacks. There are various advantages of mucosal vaccination compared to traditional injection approaches, including improved immunity at the mucosal level, lesser rates of transmission, and faster acquisition of herd immunity. Consequently, all these benefits lead to substantial economic gains across different sectors. In the health system, a considerable amount of money can be saved if there are fewer ill people due to reduced disease burden, which would lower the costs of treatment and strain on healthcare infrastructure. Mucosal vaccination, apart from better healthcare, can have various economic implications on society and industries. A healthy labor force translates to higher productivity levels, reduced absenteeism rates as well as improved living standards for people and their families. In addition, the production and distribution of mucosal vaccines promote pharmaceutical growth as well as biotechnological sectors by encouraging research and development activities while expanding vaccine manufacturing capacities. However, the advantages of mucosal immunization initiatives in economic terms must be counterbalanced with their challenges. Some of the major things to consider in this case are high development and deployment costs, accessibility and distribution issues as well as public perception and acceptance. However, such problems are surmountable as the use of mucosal vaccination has been shown to be cost-effective and economically beneficial in the future. Eventually, vaccination programs targeting the mucosal surfaces provide a potential solution for

* **Corresponding author Shaweta Sharma:** School of Medical and Allied Sciences, Galgotias University, Yamuna Expressway, Gautam Buddha Nagar, Uttar Pradesh-201310, India;
E-mail: shawetasharma@galgotiasuniversity.edu.in

not only effective healthcare delivery but also considerable economic growth. Policymakers, healthcare providers, and industries should understand the economic consequences of vaccination through the mucosal route and should work together to overcome hindrances that might come their way in order to prevent disease and make the economy prosperous.

Keywords: Biotech sensors, Economic impact, Disease,, Healthcare, Industry, Immunization, Mucosal vaccination, Prevention, Treatment, Transmission, Vaccination programs.

INTRODUCTION

Mucosal vaccination is a new approach to immunization that focuses on the mucosal surfaces of the body, mainly in the respiratory, gastrointestinal, and genitourinary systems, instead of following traditional injection procedures. Mucosal vaccines do not act like regular vaccines that stimulate a systemic immune response through intramuscular or subcutaneous injection; rather, they elicit both mucosal and systemic immunity. Mucosal surfaces are the main entry points for many pathogens, such as respiratory viruses, sexually transmitted infections, and gastrointestinal pathogens [1].

By precisely aiming at such sites, mucosal immunization intensifies the body's ability to prevent infections better and control disease transmission. Most importantly, though, mucosal vaccines can also induce mucosal IgA antibodies that serve as a first line of defense against invading pathogens at portals of entry, thus partly filling the gap between systemic immune responses induced by conventional vaccines. These two aspects of immunity work together to not only improve protection against infection but also lead to herd immunity, reducing the overall incidence of a particular disease within a population [2].

Preventing infectious diseases from spreading and reducing disease rates is the way vaccination programs contribute to public health. Vaccination, in history, has been one of the most cost-effective interventions in public health, leading to the elimination or near eradication of a number of fatal diseases such as smallpox, polio, and measles, among others. Not only have vaccines saved millions of lives, but they have also had significant economic benefits through saving costs for healthcare, increasing productivity, and avoiding economic impacts triggered by outbreaks of disease [3].

Vaccination programs have a direct effect on individual health; they also contribute to better social equity, minimize healthcare discrepancies, and improve global health security. Besides that, immunization is a critical part of sustainable development as it facilitates economic growth, promotes the attainment of education, and enhances social integration among people. That is why investment in vaccination programs can be considered an allocation of resources that can bring about substantial public health results alongside economic prosperity [4].

The economic impacts of mucosal vaccination programs go beyond public health and affect various sectors of the economy and society. From a health perspective, mucosal immunization can potentially result in significant cost savings by reducing the burden of infectious diseases. Prevention of illness and complications due to mucosal vaccines can reduce healthcare costs associated with treatment, hospitalizations, and long-term care, thus relieving healthcare systems and resources [5].

Moreover, immunizing staff against contagious illnesses makes them stronger and more prepared to contribute towards economic expansion. Furthermore, societies as a whole profit economically from mucosal vaccinations since healthier communities mean higher productivity levels as well as lower rates of absenteeism coupled with enhanced living standards. Industries, including biotechnology and pharmaceuticals, may benefit from mucosal vaccination initiatives in a variety of ways that can lead to innovation, research, and development. There are always new markets to be created when making or using vaccines through the mucosa, which also prompt investments into this type of infrastructure while at the same time fostering partnerships among different governments as well as with businesses across various industries [6].

Mucosal vaccination also promotes global health security by reducing the likelihood of pandemics and epidemics, which can cause severe economic damage on national or global scale. Therefore, multiple economic effects of mucosal vaccination programs exist, including those that reduce healthcare costs, improve societies, and foster sustainable development, global health equity, and the overall growth of various economies.

ECONOMIC IMPACTS ON HEALTHCARE SYSTEM

The economic impacts of mucosal vaccination programs on the healthcare system are presented in Fig. (**1**) and discussed below.

Cost Savings

Mucosal vaccination programs are cost-effective for healthcare systems by alleviating the burden of infectious diseases. These programs decrease the demand for treatment, hospitalization, and medication by preventing infections or lowering their severity. Consequently, fewer individuals become sick, thus cutting down on health spending linked to infectious disease management. In particular, reduced rates of in-patient care for avoidable infections significantly affect hospitalization costs, which account for a significant proportion of healthcare expenditure [8].

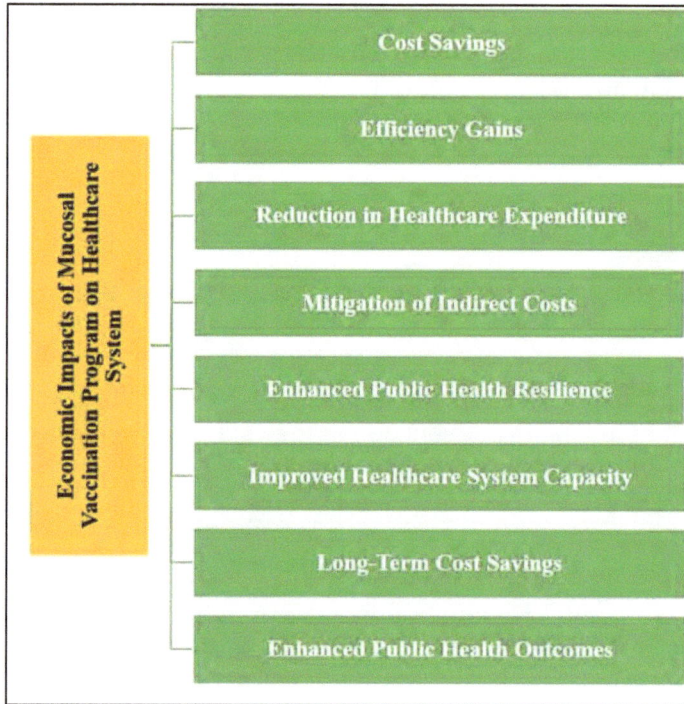

Fig. (1). Economic impacts of the mucosal vaccination program on the healthcare system.

Besides, it eases the burden on healthcare resources through mucosal immunization, which leads to a better distribution of medical staff, facilities, and tools. In conclusion, mucosal vaccination is a cost-saving measure in healthcare systems that helps free up resources that can be used in other important areas, hence improving healthcare quality as well as access for communities [9, 10].

Efficiency Gains

When people are vaccinated through the mucosal route, there is increased effectiveness in healthcare delivery because infections can be stopped before they start or their severity reduced. Fewer patients with preventable infectious diseases mean that health providers can use resources more efficiently, concentrating on life-saving interventions rather than addressing outbreaks. Consequently, such an approach will help cut down queues for treatment as well as consultations and diagnostic procedures so that patients get immediate assistance and attention [11].

In addition, healthcare services are also eased by a lighter load of diseases that cause infections. With the resources previously used in managing infections, care becomes more accessible through channeling them into the expansion of services and implementing outreach initiatives. Hence, through mucosal vaccination programs, there is better overall quality and response of the health systems, which improves the health outcomes for individuals and society at large [12].

Reduction in Healthcare Expenditure

The implementation of mucosal vaccination strategies results in a decrease in healthcare costs by curbing the demand for medical care. Such programs reduce the severity of infections, prevent them and, therefore, minimize the need for medical interventions to manage infectious diseases. Fewer people visit physicians, thus decreasing the number who are likely to fall ill due to preventable causes. This means that there will be fewer laboratory assays as well as imaging procedures such as X-rays, which will be needed since the prevalence rate has fallen [13].

Mucosal vaccination also reduces the need for intravenous fluids and other supportive care measures, such as respiratory support, thereby averting severe disease and its complications. As such, this makes the healthcare system eventually reduce its spending, thus allowing effective use of available resources and possibly more monies that can be set aside for health investments in other health priorities. Mucosal vaccination programs help in reducing healthcare expenditure hence making healthcare services sustainable and affordable [14].

Mitigation of Indirect Costs

Mucosal vaccination programs have a critical role in containing the collateral expenses of infectious diseases. These diseases lead to losses in economic activities, such as absenteeism at workplaces or schools, among other medical charges. Mucosal vaccines indirectly help ease these costs by preventing infections and also reducing disease spread. Reduced attendance of employees or students due to lowered sickness rates will ensure that productivity levels do not decline, leading to a stable economy [15].

In addition, fewer people are in need of support from caregivers when they fall ill or have complications. The existence of mucosal vaccination programs to curb infectious diseases leads to a healthier workforce and community, which enhances social and economic participation. Lastly, the overall health of society and resilience towards economic uncertainties is improved through the reduction of indirect costs by practicing mucosal vaccinations, which may affect many other sectors in an economy positively [16].

Enhanced Public Health Resilience

The resilience of public health is supported by programs on mucosal immunizations, which help in repelling new infectious diseases. They focus on the sites where pathogens enter the body to stop infections and promote community resistance to widespread transmission. It further contributes to lowering the risk of epidemic outbreaks by minimizing risks of policy reactions like isolation, seal-off, or travel bans during such times. This reduces economic damages due to disease prevalence, thus ensuring that society remains unaffected amidst such eventualities [17].

Mucosal vaccination improves the healthcare system's ability to handle health crises by preventing the spread of infectious diseases in advance. Furthermore, this reduces the cost of responding to epidemics and enhances public trust in health interventions. Therefore, mucosal vaccination strengthens community preparedness for health shocks, thus aiding society in adjusting to and surmounting new challenges that arise due to changed health circumstances [18].

Improved Healthcare System Capacity

Enhanced healthcare system capacity through the reduced number and severity of infectious diseases is one of the key roles played by mucosal vaccination. Consequently, these systems can ably manage many patients, which leads to timely healthcare for all people both those with non-communicable diseases or emergencies. This, therefore, reduces pressure on hospitals, clinics, and health personnel since fewer people are affected by infectious diseases that could have been prevented through immunization. The result will be a decreased burden of infectious diseases on healthcare facilities, allowing for better response to patient load and to ensure access for all patients, including those with non-communicable conditions or emergency problems, in time so as to get medical care [19].

Additionally, there is a greater capacity for healthcare providers to optimize resource allocation through concentrating on quality care delivery and prevention of disease transmission. Mucosal vaccination programs enhance overall health system responsiveness, allowing them to effectively meet the demands of their population while ensuring that they are still compliant with the quality measures and safety of patients [20].

Long-Term Cost Savings

Long-term savings could be achieved by the healthcare system through mucosal vaccination programs that prevent future outbreaks and eliminate expensive interventions. Mucosal vaccines, which are administered at the site of pathogenic entry, can, therefore, protect and safeguard communities from pathogen transmission, thereby avoiding treatment costs incurred due to widespread epidemic infections. Furthermore, mucosal vaccination also supports long-term prevalence reduction for infectious diseases, which would, in turn, save on costs as fewer cases may present to hospitals or seek medical attention [21].

In addition, the proactive character of mucosal vaccination also prevents other measures that must be taken in response to an infection, such as quarantine or mass vaccinations, which can consume a lot of resources and cause economic difficulties. Investing in programs for this type of immunization is a wise choice financially because it leads to great gains in health preservation over many years and saves money for the future sustainability of the economy [22].

Enhanced Public Health Outcomes

Boosting public health is one of the main reasons for mucosal vaccination programs. Such programs prevent diseases and reduce their severity as well. They do this by immunizing people against pathogens where they get into the body. Therefore, such initiatives minimize the chances of catching infections, which leads to lower morbidity and mortality rates within a society. In addition, when fewer people fall sick or develop serious problems due to preventable illnesses, it results in better general well-being of the population, thereby creating healthier communities that are able to withstand any form of adversity [23].

In addition, mucosal vaccination programs also help to alleviate the strain on healthcare systems by preventing diseases and reducing their transmission. This allows for better use of resources, which can then be redirected to meet other healthcare demands effectively. Consequently, access to care is increased while service quality is enhanced, leading to healthier people of all ages. Ultimately, these positive results in terms of public health achieved through mucosal vaccination programs play a vital role in ensuring sustainable development, thereby creating a stronger tomorrow that is full of good health for everyone [24].

ECONOMIC IMPACTS ON SOCIETY

The economic effects of mucosal vaccination programs on society go beyond healthcare and include all areas of socio-economic welfare. The economic impacts of these programs on society are discussed below and summarized in Fig. (**2**).

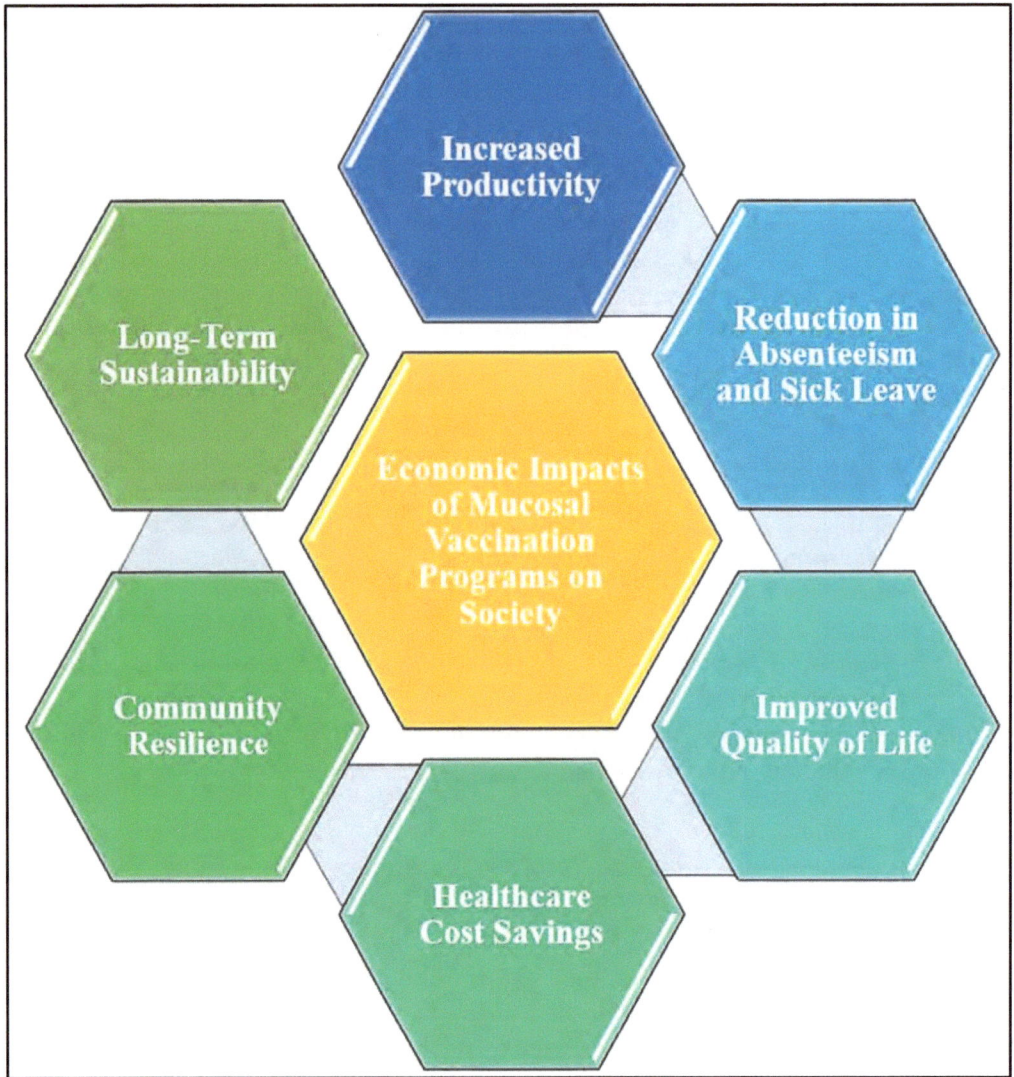

Fig. (2). Economic impacts of mucosal vaccination programs on society.

Increased Productivity

To ensure a stronger workforce and prevent infectious diseases from spreading effectively, it is important to have vaccination programs for mucus. This will help reduce the number of people who contract common infections such as flu, pneumonia, and gastroenteritis by immunizing them against these diseases at entry points, such as the respiratory system or digestive tract. Consequently, workers are less likely to get sick, which means they take fewer days off from work, thus leading to higher productivity levels at work places [25].

Fewer operational interruptions and workflow disturbances are experienced by businesses when their employees are healthy and at work. There is a decrease in instances of employees being absent because of sickness, and these personnel can keep up the required performance levels throughout. It is not just individual companies' effectiveness that benefits from this increased productivity; it also enhances national economic development and competitiveness.

Additionally, a healthier workforce creates a good working atmosphere, which is known for its enthusiastic spirit, reduced rates of employees leaving their jobs, and higher levels of commitment among them. Companies also save money on healthcare when they do not have to treat illnesses in staff or find temporary workers as replacements. Ultimately, the effect that these immunization initiatives have on productivity due to mucosal surface infection prevention will extend beyond individual businesses but rather wider socio-economic gains for all communities [26].

Reduction in Absenteeism and Sick Leave

Mucosal vaccination is important as it helps to reduce absenteeism from work or school by preventing the spread of contagious diseases. The programs achieve this by immunizing people against common pathogens, including flu viruses and respiratory viruses, among others that cause gastrointestinal infections, thereby lowering the rate at which people get sick in a given community. Consequently, fewer individuals fall sick to the extent that they need to stay away from their normal duties, thus cutting down on absentees [27].

Employers save money in many different directions when absenteeism is reduced. This means that they do not have to spend as much on temporary staff to fill in for absent people, and it also leads to lower healthcare costs since there are not as many sick workers. Furthermore, businesses enjoy increased productivity and smoother functioning because employees show up for work and do what they are supposed to do [28].

Correspondingly, educational institutions take advantage of decreased student absenteeism. They can keep up with their schoolwork and succeed academically if they do not miss many days because of sicknesses. This produces better educational results and more elevated levels of involvement among the pupils, which makes them stick around for longer. The mucosal vaccination initiative decreases sick leave and absenteeism, thus making workers more effective at work while helping them achieve better educational outcomes, which may be seen as another step towards prosperity in any given society [29].

Improved Quality of Life

Enhancing the well-being of people and societies is the main effect of mucosal vaccination programs as they help in prevention and decrease in severity of illnesses. The systems reduce instances of ill health by preventing attacks from common pathogens like pneumonia, influenza, and those causing gastroenteritis, among others, which may lead to chronic illness or death. Consequently, this results in less number of sick days thereby improving physical fitness levels [30].

In addition to having physical benefits, mucosal vaccination campaigns may also relieve emotional and financial problems frequently accompanying diseases. The families and the caretakers of the patients are able to feel less worried or tense because they have fewer interruptions in their daily lives looking after someone who is ill. Furthermore, this saves them from spending too much money on hospital bills; it also allows them to spend less time away from work and pay lower healthcare prices, thereby giving them a chance to meet other basic requirements.

Additionally, such programs improve general health and happiness. Fewer illnesses mean that people recover faster and are not bedridden for long periods. Consequently, they can interact more with others and participate in social events, which consequently leads them to live happier lives. Furthermore, the benefits of mucosal vaccination programs touch on a wider scope than just personal wellness; they extend to overall public welfare, thus fostering stronger communities characterized by increased levels of joy and resilience [31].

Healthcare Cost Savings

Saving costs for healthcare systems is the main function of mucosal vaccination initiatives. This objective is achieved through the effective prevention of disease transmission and reduction of the medical interventions needed. These programs lower the occurrence and seriousness of infectious illnesses by vaccinating people against common pathogens like influenza, respiratory viruses, and gastrointestinal infections, among others, within regions. Therefore healthcare utilization will decrease, including doctor visits, admissions into hospitals, diagnostic examinations, and treatment [32].

The medical systems can use their money best in the world after they save a lot by objecting themselves to the mucous coat vaccine program. This means that the health providers will not have to spend more on treating these infections but instead put those funds into other important sectors like preventive services, controlling chronic illnesses and improving facilities related to healthcare care provision; taking this into consideration, the overall performance will increase, access levels shall rise, and all communities' healthcare requirements must be met under such circumstances [33].

Additionally, mucosal vaccination programs help maintain long-term cost control and sustainability in healthcare spending through the promotion of community health and prevention of disease outbreaks. If healthcare systems put more money into preventative care, they can reduce the economic burden from treating preventable diseases, which would then optimize healthcare resources benefiting all of society. Ultimately, the wide-reaching consequences on affordability, accessibility, and efficacy within different areas of health provision that are brought about by saving costs through this method have been found to ensure improved individual and community health outcomes at large [33].

Community Resilience

To prevent outbreaks of diseases and minimize the economic impact of health emergencies, we must be ready all the time. Every society can keep itself safe by ensuring that it is able to neutralize viruses that invade the body through inhalation or ingestion. This is achieved through immunization programs that target mucosal tissues where pathogens first enter the body. In this way, infections are controlled within communities, thereby preventing massive disease outbreaks and global pandemics that strain healthcare systems and paralyze societies [34].

Mucosal vaccination programs help maintain community spirit and togetherness by reducing disease transmission. When people are strong and less vulnerable to diseases, it becomes easier for societies to keep their balance even when faced with difficulties. Thus, people begin trusting each other more and showing support, which allows them to solve problems jointly as a team.

Also, the overall resilience of communities is supported by mucosal vaccination programs that lessen the socioeconomic toll of health crises. By preventing widespread sickness and poverty caused by preventable illnesses, societies are more prepared to cope with and bounce back from disruptions in their daily routines and sources of income. This robustness enhances social cohesion, allowing neighborhoods to adjust and prosper under difficult circumstances such as these, which will eventually result in a stable, healthy life for everyone [35].

Long-Term Sustainability

Investing in mucosal vaccination programs is a good idea to make sure that socio-economic sustainability remains for many years. Preventing diseases from spreading and promoting public health are the main reasons these strategies were set up. This leads to increased productivity among workers due to reduced illness, which results in low workforce morbidity rates as well as mortality levels, hence saving on medical bills throughout the years. When people do not get sick often, hospitals save money, too because they will not spend much treating preventable diseases, thus freeing up resources for other important needs like managing chronic conditions or improving facilities at hospitals, among others [36].

Moreover, mucosal vaccination initiatives help maintain economic steadiness and affluence through promoting efficiency in a dynamic society. When fewer people fall sick, necessitating school or work absenteeism, productivity goes up, thus spurring economic advancement and competitiveness. Apart from this, such programs reduce socio-economic disruptions caused by health emergencies like pandemics; they also allow communities to better withstand and recover from disasters. In the end, such resilience builds cohesion among different groups within a community, leading to stability, which in turn enhances prosperity over time [37].

Basically, the immediate public health benefits and also sustainable economic growth are the two main advantages of investing in mucosal vaccination programs. These projects contribute to stability and prosperity through long-term economic sustainability by bettering results in public health, cutting down on healthcare expenses as well, and creating a robust society that can withstand shocks, which therefore guarantees a promising tomorrow for all our children's children [38].

Mucosal vaccines are a boon to the economy in general. Because they improve productivity and lower healthcare expenses and at the same time enhance the quality of life and community resilience, these initiatives are vital for the welfare of both persons and societies because they deal with both health-related issues as well as those concerning socio-economic aspects, thus fostering individual success within a nation alongside communal development too [37].

ECONOMIC IMPACTS ON INDUSTRIES

Mucosal vaccination programs' economic effects are not limited to healthcare and the community only but also to all sectors that have unique impacts on them. The economic impacts of mucosal vaccination programs on industries are described below and summarized in Fig. (3).

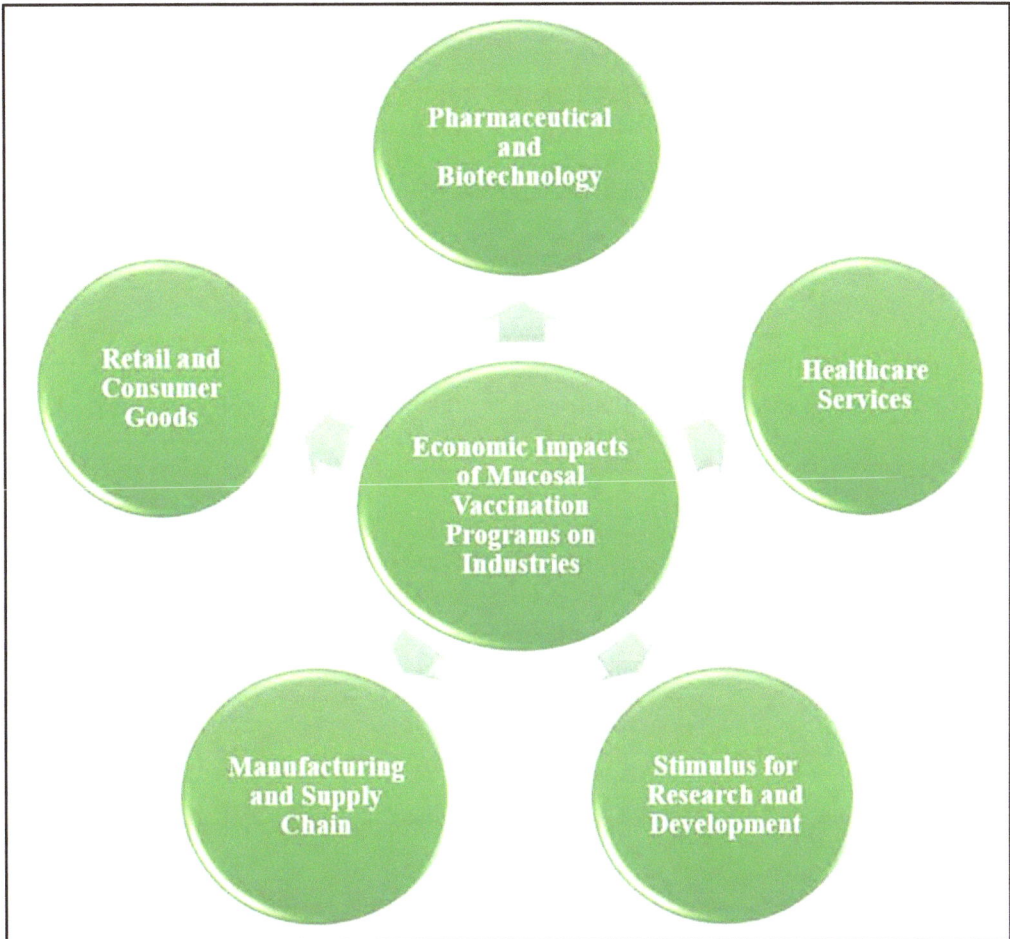

Fig. (3). Economic impacts of mucosal vaccination programs on industries.

Pharmaceutical and Biotechnology

Mucosal vaccination programs create the requirement for vaccines and associated technologies, which in turn stimulate advancements and investments in pharmaceuticals and biotechnology. These initiatives are aimed at preventing infectious diseases on mucosal surfaces like respiratory or gastrointestinal systems; thus, such ventures need specific vaccine types designed to provoke efficient immune responses at these sites through appropriate delivery systems that would work best for them [39].

Meeting the demand is what companies that develop, produce, and distribute vaccines are doing. These organizations invest in research and development for new mucosal vaccinations, which can provide strong protection against many different types of infections over a long period. For example, this involves trying out various vaccine formats like viral vectors, nanoparticles, or adjuvants designed specifically for use through the mucous membranes [40].

In addition, an increase in the number of mucosal vaccination initiatives presents a chance for drug and biotech firms to make more money. Governments and healthcare institutions are now giving preventive healthcare much emphasis; hence, there is a need for vaccines against pathogens that infect through the mucosal surfaces, which has resulted in higher incomes as well as wider markets for producers of vaccines. The pharmaceutical industry experiences growth and development due to these programs, thus enabling them to take advantage of new prospects brought about by worldwide demand for immunizations [40 - 42].

Healthcare Services

Healthcare services are greatly affected by mucosal vaccination programs as they significantly reduce the need for treatments, hospital stays, and emergency care. The fact that these initiatives stop preventable contagious diseases from spreading implies that fewer people will have to seek medical help for conditions associated with illness. Despite the fact that it may cause health providers to lose money in the form of the reduced number of patients coming in or being admitted, this has huge advantages in the end [43].

In the long run, healthcare systems save money and improve efficiency through mucosal vaccination programs. This frees up resources that would have been used in treating preventable diseases and redirects them to other needs like chronic illness management, prevention services, or building health facilities, among others, thereby enabling them to provide better services as well as ensuring a wider range of people are reached with health care in different parts of any given society [44].

In addition, healthcare providers can work more effectively with less time, lower occupancy, and better resource management because of fewer infectious diseases. Such changes not only enhance patient satisfaction and results but also ensure the durability and flexibility of health care over a long period. Even though it might look like mucosal vaccination programs reduce the income generated by healthcare givers during their initial stages, in the end, they save money through cost-cutting measures as well as reallocating inefficiencies towards meeting new demands within community-based systems where this is needed most [45].

Stimulus for Research and Development

Mucosal vaccination contributes to much research and development (R&D) in various sectors by acting as a strong catalyst, which in turn fosters innovation and cooperation among them, including biomedical engineering immunology, among others. Such initiatives are behind attempts to improve immunization through the design of vaccines, their delivery systems, or adjuvants aimed at provoking stronger mucosal immunity that protects against infections more effectively [46].

Biomedical engineering focuses on finding new vaccine types that can be used in the delivery of mucous membranes. This involves creating micro- and nano-sized transporters that can target mucosal surfaces and facilitate efficient delivery of antigens. By using advances in materials science and nanotechnology, researchers hope to improve vaccine stability, immunogenicity, and durability [47].

Immunologists and microbiologists research the basis of mucosal immunity. They strive to understand how germs, mucosal tissues, and the host immune system interact with each other. This knowledge also helps in creating vaccines for use on mucosal surfaces against certain pathogens and environments by provoking immune protection where the disease enters [48].

Also, programs for vaccinating mucosal membranes encourage partnerships among universities, businesses, and public authorities, which then leads to multidisciplinary research and development (R&D) projects that seek to promote the technologies behind mucosal vaccines. The sharing of information between private and public sectors, pooling of resources, and regulatory assistance speed up the process through which findings from scientific investigations are transformed into practical measures for improving community health at large [49].

Such additional funding and investment into R&D initiatives for the making of new mucosal vaccines will only serve to speed up advancements in science within this area. This encompasses help given towards preclinical research, clinical trials, scaling up manufacturing, and solving logistical and regulatory hurdles tied to creating/using such vaccines in the mucosa [50].

This will stimulate research and development programs in different industries, leading to scientific discoveries, technological advancements, and translational medicine endeavors that aim at improving global health issues. Such initiatives foster cooperation and investment in mucosal vaccine technology, thereby helping to create effective vaccines that can be administered easily to people to prevent infections and provide public health protection [51].

Manufacturing and Supply Chain

Mucosal vaccination programs are important for supply chain management and manufacturing because they reduce employee absenteeism and increase consumer trust. Preventing diseases can mean less sick leave is taken by factory staff; therefore, more work gets done, which leads to less disturbance in the production timetable, so there is a flow throughout all aspects of manufacturing. This creates better efficiency and higher yields within the industry as a whole [52].

In addition, the widespread enhancement of public healthcare due to mucosal vaccination initiatives encourages optimism among buyers, leading to increased expenditures. With people feeling more secure while participating in business transactions, there is a greater need for different types of products and services. Such intense consumer pressure prompts development along the entire supply chain, from providers of unprocessed materials to wholesalers and retailers [53].

Moreover, the savings in healthcare costs due to fewer disease transfers release cash that individuals can spend on wants and non-basic needs, thus increasing spending on non-essential items. This encourages economic activity at all stages of production, thereby promoting general economic development and well-being. In addition, mucosal vaccination initiatives help manufacturing and supply chain businesses through employee well-being support, consumer trust building, and the requirement for more goods/services, which drive up their output levels, hence leading them towards becoming stronger economically resilient entities [54].

Retail and Consumer Goods

Mucosal vaccination initiatives augment consumer confidence and expenditure, thus having a considerable positive effect on the consumer goods industry. With growing protection from avoidable infections, people have become more active in socializing and making money, shopping being among the economic undertakings they engage in most. Consequently, this leads to increased numbers of customers coming into contact with different types of retailers, such as online shops or traditional physical outlets, thereby boosting sales volumes made through them [55].

Furthermore, companies in the retail and consumer goods sector can take advantage of rising customer trust by launching novel commodities and amenities that address evolving health and safety concerns. For instance, they can focus more on cleanliness or hygiene while promoting such health-oriented items as vitamins, supplements, and personal protective equipment (PPEs). Establishments should tap into what consumers consider important as this will help boost demand even more, thereby increasing their earnings [56].

Also, when the economy starts to bounce back and people begin spending again, stores might see a comeback in sales of luxury items or services. This lets companies try new things and meet the different needs of customers because they are changing what they like over time. This can attract more buyers to them, which will help keep their business growing for longer in this industry [57].

Immunization through the mucosal surface has economic implications that cut across different businesses, markets, and consumer activities. These programs are important for sustainable development in all sectors since they help improve public health by controlling diseases as well as promoting economic recovery [56].

COST-EFFECTIVENESS OF MUCOSAL VACCINATION

The economic viability of mucosal injection depends on how well the long-term costs are balanced with the initial investment in setting up and sustaining such schemes. Below, we discuss how mucosal vaccination programs demonstrate value for money in public health spending.

Long-term Cost Savings vs. Initial Investment

Efforts towards mucosal immunization are calculated moves that may have substantial financial pay-offs. Indeed, these programs might seem expensive to develop, implement, or expand since they require a lot of money, but in the end, they save more than they consume. Even though much capital may be needed during creation, such investments pay back through economies achieved from better health results among people, which leads to less spending on medical care services and contributes to overall social welfare improvements, too [58].

Mucosal vaccination programs require investment in research and clinical trials aimed at identifying antigens, perfecting vaccine formulas, and determining their safety and efficacy. Usually, this stage collaborates with academia, industry, and government agencies, alongside regulatory measures that guarantee that mucosal vaccines are up to standard. Moreover, it is essential to invest in distribution infrastructure as well as public health campaigns to promote the uptake and adherence of vaccines among the intended recipients [59].

Nonetheless, the long-term benefits of mucosal vaccination schemes are more than worth the cost of setting them up; therefore, they should be used as a cheap method to improve public health and prevent disease transmission. One major advantage of these vaccines is that they can stop infections at their entry points, which in turn also lowers healthcare system loads, besides reducing costs incurred through disease management, hospitalizations, and medical interventions.

Mucosal immunization breaks the chain of infection by acting on pathogens before they cause diseases, thus leading to decreased morbidity rates and less need for healthcare services over time [60].

Additionally, programs for vaccinating mucous membranes can save society a lot of money. This is because they reduce the economic effects of infectious diseases through productivity loss, caregiver burden, and absenteeism. Indirect costs to the community include caregiver burden and loss of wages, among others, which have lasting impacts on the economy, such as reduced workforce productivity. This disease also prevents getting sick, so it saves on healthcare expenses, too, because people do not need hospital stays or days off from work to look after someone else [61].

In addition, mucosal vaccination programs have a greater effect on the economy and society at large than just saving money. Society becomes more resilient and enjoys higher living standards when diseases are stopped from spreading while good health is promoted among the people. This implies that such initiatives promote the prosperity of the entire community, both economically and socially. With good health comes increased productivity, which in turn fuels economic growth through increased individual participation in different sectors [62].

Although the mucosal vaccination projects may need large amounts of money at first, it is an undeniable fact that they are cost-effective in the long run. When it comes to infectious diseases, prevention is better than cure; therefore, mucosal vaccines reduce healthcare costs, lower economic losses due to sicknesses, and improve the overall welfare of communities. Therefore, investment in such programs is wise because it ensures sustainability while benefiting many people through improved health status as well as reduced medical bills, thus making them stronger against different threats [63, 64].

Value for Money in Public Health Spending

Mucosal vaccination programs are best suited to optimizing public health spending due to their cost-effectiveness. Such immunization schemes concentrate on prevention rather than cure, which in turn helps to maximize health outcomes while minimizing costs over time. Instead of waiting for diseases to happen, they direct resources into proactive measures that can effectively contain the transmission of infectious agents at their entry points [65].

The preventive character of mucosal vaccines guarantees the efficiency of resource allocation; this averts dealing with outbreak aftermaths. This anticipatory method is very effective, particularly in infectious diseases, where prompt intervention can substantially decrease healthcare expenses as well as morbidity and mortality related to managing advanced stages of sicknesses. Consequently, mucosal immunization programs interrupt transmission cycles, hence stopping infections from spreading among communities through vaccination against common pathogens on respiratory or gastrointestinal surfaces [66].

The money spent on treating diseases and fixing their economic consequences is high in contrast with the low budgets put into vaccination programs through mucosal routes, which give more returns by way of bettering health, lowering healthcare costs, and improving general welfare. Direct medical costs, like hospitalization fees, medications, *etc.*, are cut down when illness is prevented through vaccination. Still, it also reduces indirect expenditures such as lost productivity hours due to absenteeism from work, among other things, including caregiver burden [67].

Also, programs for mucosal vaccination offer many societal advantages beyond the savings on healthcare. These programs foster productivity, engagement, and resilience among healthy populations, which in turn catalyzes economic growth, social harmony, and community welfare. By stopping disease spread and boosting overall health status, they set off an optimistic chain reaction whose benefits accrue to individuals, families, and entire societies [68].

Moreover, the efficiency of mucosal vaccination campaigns is indicated by their ability to avoid future healthcare spending and economic losses due to outbreaks of contagious diseases. Today's investment in prevention means less expensive interventions in the future, thereby saving health systems and ensuring the sustainability of economies in the long run [69].

Investing in vaccination through mucosa is a very good investment for public health that gives excellent value for money. The best way to achieve higher health outcomes and lower healthcare costs as well as increase social welfare is by prioritizing prevention, which also builds strong communities against future challenges while improving both physical and mental wellbeing, thereby increasing productivity besides mitigating vulnerability, hence promoting overall development; thus investing on preventive healthcare methods such as vaccines should not be seen just as economic sense but more importantly an ethical duty towards safeguarding the present and future generations welfare [70, 71].

SUCCESSFUL MUCOSAL VACCINATION PROGRAMS WORLDWIDE

Mucosal vaccination programs have impressively prevented infectious diseases and improved public health. Table **1** outlines some successful programs worldwide.

Table 1. Successful mucosal vaccination programs worldwide.

Country/Region	Mucosal Vaccines	Targeted Diseases	Key Achievements
United States	FluMist (intranasal influenza vaccine)	Influenza	Decreased incidence of flu among children [72]
Europe	Rotarix and RotaTeq (oral rotavirus vaccines)	Rotavirus	Significant decrease in rotavirus-related morbidity and mortality [73]
India	Polio drops (oral polio vaccine)	Polio	Eradication of wild poliovirus [74]
Brazil	Oral Cholera Vaccine (OCV)	Cholera	Control of cholera outbreaks [75]
China	Nasal Spray Influenza Vaccine	Influenza	Effective prevention of seasonal flu [76]
Australia	FluMist Quadrivalent	Influenza	High vaccine effectiveness against influenza [77]

ECONOMIC OUTCOMES IN SPECIFIC REGIONS OR COUNTRIES

Factors such as vaccine coverage, disease burden, healthcare infrastructure, and socio-economic conditions can lead to different economic outcomes from implementing specific mucosal immunization programs. The economic impacts of mucosal vaccination programs in three specific regions or countries, India, Brazil, and the United States, are discussed below.

India

India has done a good job in conducting various successful programs of mucosal vaccination, the most prominent one being the Oral Polio Vaccine campaign. The effect of this undertaking on the nation's economy is immense. To start with, removing polio from the country has resulted in substantial savings in healthcare spending. By preventing polio-caused paralysis and the lifelong disabilities that come with it, India saved itself from having to bear the cost of providing life-long medical treatment for such people, which also requires continuous rehabilitation [78].

India's economy has also been boosted by the achievement of its polio immunization efforts. This is because it has improved productivity at work and reduced absenteeism due to sickness. When fewer people are affected by polio, there is a good effect on job numbers and wealth created. Moreover, the worldwide eradication of this disease in India has made it more favorable to both tourists and investors, thus leading to economic growth as well as development [79].

Brazil

In Brazil, the utilization of mucosal immunizations has produced considerable economic results. They have been able to prevent outbreaks of cholera, which means they do not have to spend money on managing public health emergencies or responding to diseases like this one. In addition, saving lives from cholera also saves healthcare dollars because fewer people need medical treatment, so there's less need for hospitals, doctors, *etc* [80].

In addition, Brazil's successful cholera vaccination program has also brought about other positive impacts on society, which include improved food security, better water and sanitation facilities, and an increase in tourism income. By protecting public health and ensuring safety standards are met, this country has provided a good atmosphere for growth and wealth creation [81, 82].

United States

Among the mucosal vaccination efforts in America, FluMist has had significant economic consequences, mainly on healthcare. FluMist has cut down the cost of treating seasonal flu by decreasing its occurrence and severity, thus reducing other medical expenses such as hospital stays, medication use, or outpatient visits. Medical care providers and payers are relieved from financial strain due to fewer cases of influenza-related complications or admissions into hospitals [83].

Furthermore, the success of FluMist and other vaccinations that are given through the nose helps to make people work harder by decreasing the amount of time they have to take off work when they get sick with the flu. If a business has healthy workers, it can improve their job satisfaction and lower how many people want to leave, which will increase their overall productivity and help them grow economically as a company and also as an economy in general. Mucosal vaccination programs have considerable financial implications at local or national levels; these include healthcare cost savings, increased workforce productivity, and better economic growth rates. These programs prevent infections and safeguard public health, thus ensuring a brighter tomorrow for all societies across the globe [84, 85].

POLICY IMPLICATIONS

The successful implementation of mucosal vaccination programs hinges on several key policy implications, each playing a crucial role in fostering their adoption and integration into national and global health agendas:

Importance of Government Support and Investment

Governments should support and invest in mucosal vaccination programs. These steps can improve the chances of fighting infectious diseases and improve people's health on a large scale [86].

To begin with, funding from the authorities is imperative as regards vaccine research and related matters such as growing manufacturing capabilities to produce enough vaccines for all. When put in research, it allows us to discover new vaccines, optimize their formulations, or evaluate their safety and efficacy. On the other hand, support from governments also makes provision for setting up solid regulatory systems that are aimed at guaranteeing that mucosal vaccines meet required standards before being integrated into the health programs of nations [87].

Governments also need to distribute mucosal vaccines fairly by sharing all supplies among populations. This requires them to spend money on cold chain infrastructure and transport networks and educate healthcare staff who can help deliver immunizations in remote areas that lack such services. If governments give more resources priority to vaccination distribution, it will mean that even people from marginalized communities, including children or older people, will get life-saving vaccines [88].

Additionally, the role of government is very important in putting into action successful vaccination efforts and dealing with vaccine hesitancy through public education and awareness programs. To promote the acceptance of vaccines and debunk fallacies related to immunization, governments can use their power and authority. They should also involve communities, healthcare workers, and other relevant groups in order to win their trust, which will result in more people receiving this type of immunization, thereby increasing its coverage rate at mucosal levels [89].

Ultimately, investments made in mucosal vaccination programs at the end of the day result in better health outcomes, lower healthcare costs, and improved societal well-being. Mucosal vaccines prevent infections while at the same time lowering pressure on healthcare systems, thus fostering economic growth, productivity, and sustainability. Governments have a key role to play through their support for these initiatives, which they view as wise investments in public health as well as national development [90].

Role of Regulatory Agencies in Facilitating Adoption

Through rigorous evaluation and approval processes, regulatory agencies are important for ensuring the safety, efficiency, and excellence of vaccines that work through the mucous membranes. These organizations function as gatekeepers by evaluating scientific evidence in support of vaccine licenses and giving confidence to healthcare workers, policymakers, and the public about the safety and efficacy of such vaccines [91].

The regulatory agency's initial duties are to set clear rules and benchmarks for the production, testing, and licensing of vaccines intended for mucosal administration. The guidelines provide the conditions necessary for preclinical studies, clinical trials, manufacturing practices, and quality control measures that a vaccine must meet before it is approved as safe and effective for use in humans or animals. Such frameworks should be transparently established on the basis of evidence so that manufacturers know what is expected of them while also allowing the development and evaluation of these types of immunizations to take place more easily [92].

Global acceptance and use of mucosal vaccines require that regulatory requirements be harmonized across countries and regions. Regulatory agencies can speed up the approval of such vaccines by aligning their standards with those of other agencies, thus preventing duplication of work and allowing faster access to new vaccine technology. This kind of harmonization ensures uniformity in regulators' decision-making, which increases trust in them and makes it possible for people all over the world to get critical immunizations on time [93].

Post-licensure safety and continuous efficacy of mucosal vaccines require non-stop checking and watchfulness by regulatory bodies. They carry out post-marketing surveillance, pharmacovigilance, and adverse event monitoring in a bid to detect and act upon any possible safety issues or side effects linked with mucosal vaccines. Concerned authorities can discover new hazards that may arise from the use of these vaccines only when they keep track of their efficiency beyond clinical trial settings; further, they can also find ways to mitigate such risks, thereby ensuring continuing reliance on this mode of vaccination among healthcare workers and members of the public alike [94].

The importance of regulatory agencies in promoting the use of mucosal vaccines cannot be underestimated. This is done by subjecting the vaccines to strict inspection and approval processes to ascertain their safety, effectiveness, and quality. They also help in setting standards, streamlining regulatory requirements as well and performing continual monitoring and surveillance activities that will facilitate successful development, authorization, and continuous assessment of these preventive treatments hence protecting the community against diseases worldwide [95].

Integration into National and Global Health Agendas

Global and national health programs must include vaccines administered on mucus lining for the greatest effect on disease prevention and control strategies. Governments and international healthcare organizations can solve public health problems more effectively and promote fairness in access to immunization that saves lives by giving priority to mucosal vaccines [96].

When it comes to national scope, the integration of mucosal vaccination programs into usual immunization schedules is essential for meeting target populations, including high-risk groups and vulnerable communities. The inclusion of vaccines that target influenza, rotavirus, and polio, among others, should be given priority by national immunization programs so as to offer complete protection against preventable diseases. Countries can promote universal coverage and fair distribution of vaccines if they incorporate them into regular vaccination timetables, thereby lessening the impact of such diseases on health at all levels of society [97].

Moreover, the incorporation of mucosal immunization with other public health approaches makes them more effective and sustainable. These vaccines are crucial in readiness for pandemics when they occur, as well as in responding to outbreaks and promoting health equity through protection from infectious diseases. Adopting these programs on a global scale within already existing structures or systems used in healthcare provision by different countries can help build resilience against future epidemics by preventing their occurrence while limiting their effects where they happen, at the same time ensuring fairness among all communities in terms of wellbeing [98].

On the worldwide stage, international health establishments like the World Health Organization (WHO) and Gavi, as well as the Vaccine Alliance, have an important role to play: they advocate for the worldwide usage of mucosal vaccines. These organizations do a number of things; they mobilize resources, provide technical assistance, and coordinate international efforts to solve problems related to global health, including vaccine-preventable diseases. In promoting global immunization strategies that include mucosal vaccines as one of their components, WHO, together with Gavi, thus enables such countries access to vaccines necessary for saving lives, thereby contributing towards the achievement of Universal Health Coverage (UHC) and Sustainable Development Goals (SDGs) in low income or middle-income settings [99].

It is important to note that mucosal vaccination programs need to be incorporated into national and global health plans for them to have a maximum effect on disease prevention and control strategies. Making the inclusion of mucosal vaccines a priority will strengthen immunization programs in countries and global health organizations, enhance pandemic readiness, promote equity in health among populations, and ultimately save lives and improve public health outcomes worldwide [100, 101].

FUTURE ECONOMIC IMPACT OF MUCOSAL VACCINATION PROGRAMS

Mucosal vaccination programs will have a transformative effect in future economic terms, supported by several notable aspects. First and foremost, mucosal vaccines have been shown to be cost-effective and lead to long-term savings. Mucosal vaccine campaigns decrease the financial burden on healthcare systems by stopping infections at their sources, thereby reducing costs incurred in treating diseases, hospitalization rates, and medical interventions. In addition, it causes a reduction in social costs through reduced productivity and absenteeism as well as caregiver burden, leading to further economic gains over time. Therefore, there is potential for growing emphasis on mucosal vaccination programs as a rational and feasible strategy that promotes public health while inhibiting disease transmission based on cost-effectiveness analysis in the near future among policymakers and healthcare stakeholders [102].

Moreover, constant technological growth and creativity in developing vaccines and delivery systems will have a huge effect on the economy of mucosal vaccination programs. Moreover, there is potential for new mucosal vaccines that are safe, more effective, and with a high immunogenicity profile in relation to different types of infectious diseases due to sustained research and development. The projection, therefore, is that innovative vaccine delivery technologies like needle-free delivery systems and microencapsulation techniques will improve the workability and expand the scope for mucosal vaccination, thereby helping to increase their economic potential as well as reach [103].

Furthermore, mucosal vaccination programs are increasingly seen as important tools for global health security and pandemic preparedness measures' resilience in the world with subsequent discussions on their economic implications. Even as the world continues to face COVID-19 along with increasing infectious disease threats, there is an increased realization that prevention, such as through mucosal vaccines, is necessary in dealing with future pandemics. They help strengthen the immune system's defense mechanisms at various body surfaces, thereby shielding against numerous pathogens, decreasing the chances of widespread infections, and reducing the need for reactive steps that lead to economic disruptions [104].

Mucosal vaccination programs may have a considerable future economic impact due to their cost-effectiveness, technological advancements, and contributions to global health security and preparedness. By using these tendencies and elements, mucosal vaccination programs can potentially result in significant economic gains for various healthcare systems, societies, and economies worldwide, contributing to better public health outcomes and sustainable development [105].

CHALLENGES AND CONSIDERATIONS

Efforts to vaccinate through the mucosa, which may be the key to preventing infectious diseases and promoting public health, must grapple with some noteworthy challenges and considerations that need to be sorted out. The high costs associated with developing and deploying such vaccines are a major barrier. The research, development, and manufacturing of these vaccines are expensive in terms of preclinical and clinical studies, optimization of vaccine formulations, and safety trials [106].

Moreover, the specialized technologies and production processes required for mucosal vaccine manufacturing often result in higher production costs compared to traditional injectable vaccines. Deployment costs further compound the challenge, as mucosal vaccination programs necessitate investment in distribution infrastructure, cold chain storage, and healthcare workforce training. Additionally, the logistical complexities associated with maintaining vaccine stability and effectiveness during transportation and administration pose significant barriers to accessibility and distribution, particularly in resource-limited settings and remote or underserved areas [107].

Meeting these challenges entails mobilizing adequate resources for the development, manufacturing, and distribution of mucosal vaccines. Public-private partnerships, creative financing mechanisms, and technology transfer programs could enable low-cost vaccine manufacturing and supply and increase accessibility to populations on a global scale. Nevertheless, there is a need to adopt equity in access to mucosal vaccination by enhancing the vaccination distribution infrastructure, expanding cold chain capacity, and introducing innovative delivery systems like mobile vaccination clinics and community outreach programs [108].

Another equally important step is overcoming social and cultural obstacles to vaccine acceptance and utilization, which requires effective communication, education, and engagement strategies aimed at building public trust and confidence in mucosal vaccines. Health authorities can encourage broad acceptance and uptake of mucosal immunization programs by dispelling safety and efficacy misconceptions and engaging with communities, healthcare providers, and stakeholders [109].

Mucosal vaccination must be part of national and global health initiatives to ensure maximality in disease prevention and control intervention. This means that the immunization program at the country level should prioritize mucosal vaccines in their routine immunization schedules with a focus on communities that are most vulnerable and populations exposed to the highest risks so as to cover all preventable diseases in our society. Additionally, such programs should be integrated into other health promotion interventions aimed at pandemic preparedness, outbreak response, and health equity initiatives, among others, for faster and more durable protection from infectious diseases [110].

The presence of global health organizations such as the World Health Organization (WHO), Gavi, and the Vaccine Alliance on the world stage is critical in promoting the use of mucosal vaccines. These organizations facilitate the availability of essential vaccines to poor countries by pooling resources, rendering technical support, and coordinating international actions. This helps ensure that universal health coverage is achieved while simultaneously meeting sustainable development goals for low- and middle-income states.

Challenges and considerations related to mucosal vaccine programs necessitate a multi-sectoral collaboration, innovative thinking, and continuous funding in research, infrastructure, and community engagement. If the barriers to vaccine development, accessibility, and acceptance can be overcome, then mucosal vaccination programs could reach their full potential in preventing infectious diseases and improving public health outcomes for populations globally [111, 112].

CONCLUSION

In conclusion, mucosal vaccination programs give low-cost answers to infectious disease prevention and health expense reduction while improving the lives of people. Alongside this, they help unburden health systems from pathogenic invasion, hence leading to huge savings on curative treatments as well as other medical approaches. Further, they also bring about long-term economic gains by reducing indirect costs such as caregiver burden and productivity loss that arise due to disease infection. Moreover, mucosal vaccination initiatives help make healthcare more efficient, enhance healthcare system capacity, and increase public health resilience. They also enable better allocation of resources, shortened waiting times for patients, and improved accessibility to care. In addition, these programs fortify public health resilience through preventive response to emerging infectious disease threats, minimizing the need for reactive measures that disturb economies. To optimize their financial value and enhance health outcomes, ongoing investment in mucosal vaccination initiatives is vital. The full potential of these progressive interventions can be realized by leveraging technological breakthroughs, enhancing vaccine availability and uptake, and including mucosal vaccination in national and international health plans. This essentially means that public health would be better off, thus ensuring a healthier and more adaptable future for all for a long time to come.

ACKNOWLEDGEMENTS

Authors are highly thankful to their Universities/Colleges for providing library facilities for the literature survey.

REFERENCES

[1]   Tsai CJY, Loh JMS, Fujihashi K, Kiyono H. Mucosal vaccination: onward and upward. Expert Review of Vaccines. Taylor and Francis Ltd.; 2023; 22, 885–99.

[2]   Shakya AK, Chowdhury MYE, Tao W, Gill HS. Mucosal vaccine delivery: Current state and a pediatric perspective. J Control Release 2016; 240: 394-413.
[http://dx.doi.org/10.1016/j.jconrel.2016.02.014] [PMID: 26860287]

[3]   Tsai CJY, Loh JMS, Fujihashi K, Kiyono H. Mucosal vaccination: onward and upward. Expert Review of Vaccines. Taylor and Francis Ltd.; 2023; 22, 885–99.

[4]   Lee J, Khang D. Mucosal delivery of nano vaccine strategy against COVID-19 and its variants. Acta Pharmaceutica Sinica B. Chinese Academy of Medical Sciences; 2023; 13, 2897–925.

[5]   Song Y, Mehl F, Zeichner SL. Vaccine Strategies to Elicit Mucosal Immunity. Vaccines. Multidisciplinary Digital Publishing Institute (MDPI); 2024; 12.
[http://dx.doi.org/10.3390/vaccines12020191]

[6]   Feng F, Wen Z, Chen J, Yuan Y, Wang C, Sun C. Strategies to Develop a Mucosa-Targeting Vaccine against Emerging Infectious Diseases. Viruses 2022; 14(3): 520.
[http://dx.doi.org/10.3390/v14030520] [PMID: 35336927]

[7]   Hellfritzsch M, Scherließ R. Mucosal vaccination *via* the respiratory tract. Pharmaceutics. MDPI AG 2019; 11.

[8]   Kovaiou R. D. Age-related changes in immunity_ implications for vaccination in older people _ Expert Reviews in Molecular Medicine _ Cambridge Core. 2007.

[9]   Tortorella GL, Fogliatto FS, Espôsto KF, *et al.* Healthcare costs' reduction through the integration of Healthcare 4.0 technologies in developing economies. Total Qual Manage Bus Excell 2022; 33(3-4): 467-87.
[http://dx.doi.org/10.1080/14783363.2020.1861934]

[10]   García-Sanz-Calcedo J, Al-Kassir A, Yusaf T. Economic and environmental impact of energy saving in healthcare buildings. Applied Sciences (Switzerland). 2018; 8(3).
[http://dx.doi.org/10.3390/app8030440]

[11]   Dhaoui I. Healthcare system efficiency and its determinants: A two-stage Data Envelopment Analysis (DEA) from MENA countries. Giza: Economic Research Forum (ERF) 2019.

[12]   Barroy H, Cylus J, Patcharanarumol W, Novignon J, Evetovits T, Gupta S. Do efficiency gains really

translate into more budget for health? An assessment framework and country applications. Health Policy and Planning. Oxford University Press; 2021; 36, 1307–15.
[http://dx.doi.org/10.1093/heapol/czab040]

[13] Raghupathi V, Raghupathi W. Healthcare Expenditure and Economic Performance: Insights From the United States Data. Front Public Health 2020; 8: 156.
[http://dx.doi.org/10.3389/fpubh.2020.00156] [PMID: 32478027]

[14] Keegan C, Thomas S, Normand C, Portela C. Measuring recession severity and its impact on healthcare expenditure. Int J Health Care Finance Econ 2013; 13(2): 139-55.
[http://dx.doi.org/10.1007/s10754-012-9121-2] [PMID: 23417124]

[15] Elsevier ~-~, Koopmanschap MA, Rutten FFH, Martin Van Ineveld B, Van Roijen L. The friction cost method for measuring indirect costs of disease. 14. J Health Econ 1995.

[16] Razzaq S, Zahidie A, Fatmi Z. Estimating the pre- and post-diagnosis costs of tuberculosis for adults in Pakistan: household economic impact and costs mitigating strategies. Glob Health Res Policy 2022; 7(1): 22.
[http://dx.doi.org/10.1186/s41256-022-00259-x] [PMID: 35858877]

[17] Logar I, van den Bergh JCJM. Methods to Assess Costs of Drought Damages and Policies for Drought Mitigation and Adaptation: Review and Recommendations. Water Resour Manage 2013; 27(6): 1707-20.
[http://dx.doi.org/10.1007/s11269-012-0119-9]

[18] Walton AA, Marr J, Cahillane MJ, Bush K. Building community resilience to disasters: A review of interventions to improve and measure public health outcomes in the northeastern United States. Sustainability (Switzerland). 2021; 13(21).

[19] Bossert TJ, Mitchell AD, Janjua MA. Improving health system performance in a decentralized health system: Capacity building in Pakistan. Health Syst Reform 2015; 1(4): 276-84.
[http://dx.doi.org/10.1080/23288604.2015.1056330] [PMID: 31519095]

[20] Swanson R, Atun R, Best A, *et al.* Strengthening health systems in low-income countries by enhancing organizational capacities and improving institutions. Global Health 2015; 11(1): 5.
[http://dx.doi.org/10.1186/s12992-015-0090-3] [PMID: 25890069]

[21] Rü S, Keck B, Hartmeier C, Maetzel A, Bucher HC. Long-Term Antibiotic Cost Savings from a Comprehensive Intervention Program in a Medical Department of a University-Affiliated Teaching Hospital. 2004. Available from: https://academic.oup.com/cid/article/38/3/348/290954

[22] Jans S, Westra X, Crone M. Elske van den Akker-van Marle M, Rijnders M. Long-term cost savings with Centering-based group antenatal care. Midwifery 2023; 126.

[23] Meier PS, Warde A, Holmes J. All drinking is not equal: how a social practice theory lens could enhance public health research on alcohol and other health behaviours. Addiction 2018; 113(2): 206-13.
[http://dx.doi.org/10.1111/add.13895] [PMID: 28695705]

[24] Tolulope Olorunsogo , Oloruntoba Babawarun , Olorunsogo T, Babawarun O. Leveraging big data and analytics for enhanced public health decision-making: A global review. GSC Advanced Research and Reviews 2024; 18(2): 450-6.
[http://dx.doi.org/10.30574/gscarr.2024.18.2.0078]

[25] Carleton TA, Hsiang SM. Social and economic impacts of climate. Science. American Association for the Advancement of Science; 2016; 353.
[http://dx.doi.org/10.1126/science.aad9837]

[26] Lindberg K. Economic Impacts. 2001. Available from: https://cabidigitallibrary.org

[27] Nunes AP, Richmond MK, Pampel FC, Wood RC. The Effect of Employee Assistance Services on Reductions in Employee Absenteeism. J Bus Psychol 2018; 33(6): 699-709.
[http://dx.doi.org/10.1007/s10869-017-9518-5]

[28]   van Rhenen W, Blonk RWB, Schaufeli WB, van Dijk FJH. Can sickness absence be reduced by stress reduction programs: on the effectiveness of two approaches. Int Arch Occup Environ Health 2007; 80(6): 505-15.
[http://dx.doi.org/10.1007/s00420-006-0157-9] [PMID: 17093962]

[29]   Pauly MV, Nicholson S, Xu J, *et al.* A general model of the impact of absenteeism on employers and employees. Health Econ 2002; 11(3): 221-31.
[http://dx.doi.org/10.1002/hec.648] [PMID: 11921319]

[30]   Carlson LE, Bultz BD. Health and Quality of Life Outcomes Benefits of psychosocial oncology care: Improved quality of life and medical cost offset. 2003. Available from: http://www.hqlo.com/content/1/1/8

[31]   Cohen-Cymberknoh M, Shoseyov D, Kerem E. Managing cystic fibrosis: strategies that increase life expectancy and improve quality of life. Am J Respir Crit Care Med 2011; 183(11): 1463-71.
[http://dx.doi.org/10.1164/rccm.201009-1478CI] [PMID: 21330455]

[32]   Walsh T, Barr PJ, Thompson R, Ozanne E, O'Neill C, Elwyn G. Undetermined impact of patient decision support interventions on healthcare costs and savings: Systematic review. BMJ (Online). 2014; 348.

[33]   Ahn S, Smith ML, Altpeter M, Post L, Ory MG. Healthcare cost savings estimator tool for chronic disease self-management program: a new tool for program administrators and decision makers. Front Public Health 2015; 3: 42.
[http://dx.doi.org/10.3389/fpubh.2015.00042] [PMID: 25964946]

[34]   Sharifi A. A critical review of selected tools for assessing community resilience. Ecol Indic 2016; 69: 629-47.
[http://dx.doi.org/10.1016/j.ecolind.2016.05.023]

[35]   Kirmayer LJ, Whitley R. Community Resilience: Models, Metaphors and Measures. J Aborig Health 2009.

[36]   Chang V, Mills H, Newhouse S. From Open Source to long-term sustainability: Review of Business Models and Case studies. 2007.

[37]   Lin LH, Wang PL, Rumble D, Lippmann-Pipke J, Boice E, Pratt LM, *et al.* Long-term sustainability of a high energy, low diversity crustal biome. 2006.
[http://dx.doi.org/10.1126/science.1127376]

[38]   Fleiszer AR, Semenic SE, Ritchie JA, Richer MC, Denis JL. An organizational perspective on the long-term sustainability of a nursing best practice guidelines program: a case study. BMC Health Serv Res 2015; 15(1): 535.
[http://dx.doi.org/10.1186/s12913-015-1192-6] [PMID: 26634343]

[39]   Wu F, Munkvold GP. Mycotoxins in ethanol co-products: modeling economic impacts on the livestock industry and management strategies. J Agric Food Chem 2008; 56(11): 3900-11.
[http://dx.doi.org/10.1021/jf072697e] [PMID: 18444660]

[40]   Soetaert W, Vandamme E. The impact of industrial biotechnology. Biotechnol J 2006; 1(7-8): 756-69.
[http://dx.doi.org/10.1002/biot.200600066] [PMID: 16897819]

[41]   Scollo M, Lal A. Review of the quality of studies on the economic effects of smoke-free policies on the hospitality industry. 12, Tobacco Control. 2003. Available from: www.pmoptions.com

[42]   Berman EM. The economic impact of industry-funded university R&D. 1989.

[43]   Valderas JM, Starfield B, Sibbald B, Salisbury C, Roland M. Defining comorbidity: implications for understanding health and health services. Ann Fam Med 2009; 7(4): 357-63.
[http://dx.doi.org/10.1370/afm.983] [PMID: 19597174]

[44]   Robert G, Cornwell J, Locock L, Purushotham A, Sturmey G, Gager M. Patients and staff as codesigners of healthcare services. BMJ (Online). 2015; 350:1.

[http://dx.doi.org/10.1136/bmj.g7714]

[45]   Ballegaard SA, Hansen TR, Kyng M. Healthcare in everyday life - designing healthcare services for daily life. In: Conference on Human Factors in Computing Systems - Proceedings. 2008; 1807–16.

[46]   Tidwell DL, Fitzgerald LMay, Heston ML, American Educational Research Association. Self-Study of Teacher Education Practices Special Interest Group. Journeys of hope: risking self-study in a diverse world: 2004, Herstmonceux Castle, East Sussex, England. University of Northern Iowa; 2004; 280.

[47]   Prajogo DI, Ahmed PK. Relationships between innovation stimulus, innovation capacity, and innovation performance. 2006.
[http://dx.doi.org/10.1111/j.1467-9310.2006.00450.x]

[48]   Dymond S, Rehfeldt RA, Schenk J. Nonautomated procedures in derived stimulus relations research: a methodological note. 55. Psychol Rec 2005; 55(3): 461-81.
[http://dx.doi.org/10.1007/BF03395521]

[49]   Bach-y-Rita P, Kaczmarek KA, Tyler ME, Garcia-Lara J. Form perception with a 49-point electrotactile stimulus array on the tongue: a technical note. J Rehabil Res Dev 1998; 35(4): 427-30.
[PMID: 10220221]

[50]   Maydak M. Stimulus_classes_in_matching_to_sample_a. 1995.

[51]   Higbee T, Carr JE, Harrison CD. Further evaluation of the multiple-stimulus preference assessment. Res Dev Disabil 2000; 21(1): 61-73.
[http://dx.doi.org/10.1016/S0891-4222(99)00030-X] [PMID: 10750166]

[52]   Kunovjanek M, Knofius N, Reiner G. Additive manufacturing and supply chains – a systematic review. Prod Plann Contr 2022; 33(13): 1231-51.
[http://dx.doi.org/10.1080/09537287.2020.1857874]

[53]   Radej B, Drnovšek J, Begeš G. An overview and evaluation of quality-improvement methods from the manufacturing and supply-chain perspective. Advances in Production Engineering And Management. Production Engineering Institute; 2017; 12, 388–400.
[http://dx.doi.org/10.14743/apem2017.4.266]

[54]   Bharadwaj S, Bharadwaj A, Bendoly E. The performance effects of complementarities between information systems, marketing, manufacturing, and supply chain processes. Inf Syst Res 2007; 18(4): 437-53.
[http://dx.doi.org/10.1287/isre.1070.0148]

[55]   Wang ZX, Wu JM, Zhou CJ, Li Q. Identifying the factors of China's seasonal retail sales of consumer goods using a data grouping approach-based GRA method Emerald logo. 2024; Available from: https://www.emerald.com/insight/content/doi/10.1108/GS-11-2019-0055/full/html

[56]   Ladd GW, Suvannunt V. A Model of Consumer Goods Characteristics. Am J Agric Econ 1976; 58(3): 504-10.
[http://dx.doi.org/10.2307/1239267]

[57]   Legner C, Schemm J. Toward the inter-organizational product information supply chain - Evidence from the retail and consumer goods industries. J Assoc Inf Syst 2008; 9(3–4): 119-50.

[58]   Pantano E, Priporas CV. The effect of mobile retailing on consumers' purchasing experiences: A dynamic perspective. Comput Human Behav 2016; 61: 548-55.
[http://dx.doi.org/10.1016/j.chb.2016.03.071]

[59]   Stobart J. A history of shopping: the missing link between retail and consumer revolutions. Journal of Historical Research in Marketing 2010; 2(3): 342-9.
[http://dx.doi.org/10.1108/17557501011067860]

[60]   Stevanato N, Lombardi F, Guidicini G, *et al.* Long-term sizing of rural microgrids: Accounting for load evolution through multi-step investment plan and stochastic optimization. Energy Sustain Dev 2020; 58: 16-29.

[http://dx.doi.org/10.1016/j.esd.2020.07.002]

[61]   Bütün H, Kantor I, Maréchal F. An optimization approach for long-term industrial investment planning. Energies 2019; 12(21): 4076.
[http://dx.doi.org/10.3390/en12214076]

[62]   Tidwell DL, Fitzgerald LMay, Heston ML, American Educational Research Association. Self-Study of Teacher Education Practices Special Interest Group. Journeys of hope: risking self-study in a diverse world: 2004, Herstmonceux Castle, East Sussex, England. University of Northern Iowa; 2004; 280.

[63]   Nef DP, Gotor E, Wiederkehr Guerra G, Zumwald M, Kettle CJ. Initial Investment in Diversity Is the Efficient Thing to Do for Resilient Forest Landscape Restoration. Front For Glob Change 2021; 3: 615682.
[http://dx.doi.org/10.3389/ffgc.2020.615682]

[64]   Unützer J, Katon WJ, Fan MY, *et al.* Long-term cost effects of collaborative care for late-life depression. Am J Manag Care 2008; 14(2): 95-100.
[PMID: 18269305]

[65]   Lee JS, Mogasale V, Kim S, *et al.* The potential global cost-effectiveness of prospective Strep A vaccines and associated implementation efforts. NPJ Vaccines 2023; 8(1): 128.
[http://dx.doi.org/10.1038/s41541-023-00718-7] [PMID: 37626118]

[66]   Rodríguez González-Moro JM, Menéndez R, Campins M, *et al.* Cost Effectiveness of the 13-Valent Pneumococcal Conjugate Vaccination Program in Chronic Obstructive Pulmonary Disease Patients Aged 50+ Years in Spain. Clin Drug Investig 2016; 36(1): 41-53.
[http://dx.doi.org/10.1007/s40261-015-0345-z] [PMID: 26547199]

[67]   Klok RM, Lindkvist RM, Ekelund M, Farkouh RA, Strutton DR. Cost-effectiveness of a 10- versus 13-valent pneumococcal conjugate vaccine in Denmark and Sweden. Clin Ther 2013; 35(2): 119-34.
[http://dx.doi.org/10.1016/j.clinthera.2012.12.006] [PMID: 23312274]

[68]   Ellen Wolff. Cost-effectiveness of vaccination and the value of prevention. 2020.

[69]   Haeussler K, Marcellusi A, Mennini FS, *et al.* Cost-Effectiveness Analysis of Universal Human Papillomavirus Vaccination Using a Dynamic Bayesian Methodology: The BEST II Study. Value Health 2015; 18(8): 956-68.
[http://dx.doi.org/10.1016/j.jval.2015.08.010] [PMID: 26686779]

[70]   Wolff E, Elfström KM, Haugen Cange H, *et al.* Cost-effectiveness of sex-neutral HPV-vaccination in Sweden, accounting for herd-immunity and sexual behaviour. Vaccine 2018; 36(34): 5160-5.
[http://dx.doi.org/10.1016/j.vaccine.2018.07.018] [PMID: 30017146]

[71]   Scholz S, Schwarz M, Beck E, *et al.* Public Health Impact and Cost-Effectiveness Analysis of Routine Infant 4CMenB Vaccination in Germany to Prevent Serogroup B Invasive Meningococcal Disease. Infect Dis Ther 2022; 11(1): 367-87.
[http://dx.doi.org/10.1007/s40121-021-00573-w] [PMID: 34877641]

[72]   Nochi T, Takagi H, Yuki Y, Yang L, Masumura T, Mejima M, *et al.* Rice-based mucosal vaccine as a global strategy for cold-chain-and needle-free vaccination. 2007. Available from: www.pnas.orgcgidoi10.1073pnas.0703766104

[73]   Adams A. Progress, challenges and opportunities in fish vaccine development. Fish Shellfish Immunol 2019; 90: 210-4.
[http://dx.doi.org/10.1016/j.fsi.2019.04.066] [PMID: 31039441]

[74]   Grassly NC, Jafari H, Bahl S, *et al.* Mucosal immunity after vaccination with monovalent and trivalent oral poliovirus vaccine in India. J Infect Dis 2009; 200(5): 794-801.
[http://dx.doi.org/10.1086/605330] [PMID: 19624278]

[75]   Barreto ML, Teixeira MG, Fundação);, Cruz O, De Janeiro R, Barreto ML, *et al.* Health in Brazil 3 Successes and failures in the control of infectious diseases in Brazil: social and environmental context, policies, interventions, and research needs. Lancet. 2011;377:1877–89. Available from:

http://dtr2004.saude.gov.br/

[76]   Woodrow KA, Bennett KM, Lo DD. Mucosal vaccine design and delivery. Annu Rev Biomed Eng 2012; 14(1): 17-46.
[http://dx.doi.org/10.1146/annurev-bioeng-071811-150054] [PMID: 22524387]

[77]   Skwarczynski M, Toth I. Non-invasive mucosal vaccine delivery: advantages, challenges and the future. Expert Opinion on Drug Delivery. Taylor and Francis Ltd; 2020; 17, 435–7.

[78]   Sachs JD, Bajpai N, Ramiah A. Understanding Regional Economic Growth in India Working Papers. 2002.

[79]   Ohlan R. Pattern of Regional Disparities in Socio-economic Development in India: District Level Analysis. Soc Indic Res 2013; 114(3): 841-73.
[http://dx.doi.org/10.1007/s11205-012-0176-8]

[80]   Cavalcanti TV, Magalhães AM, Tavares JA. Institutions and economic development in Brazil. Q Rev Econ Finance 2008; 48(2): 412-32.
[http://dx.doi.org/10.1016/j.qref.2006.12.019]

[81]   Haddad EA, Domingues EP, Perobelli FS, Haddad EA. Regional effects of economic integration: the case of Brazil. J Policy Model 2002; 24(5): 453-82.
[http://dx.doi.org/10.1016/S0161-8938(02)00125-4]

[82]   Vincens N, Stafström M. Income inequality, economic growth and stroke mortality in Brazil: Longitudinal and regional analysis 2002-2009. Vol. 10, PLoS ONE. Public Library of Science; 2015.

[83]   Béduwé Catherine, Planas Jordi, European Centre for the Development of Vocational Training. EDEX: educational expansion and labor market: a comparative study of five European countries - France, Germany, Italy, Spain, and the United Kingdom - with special reference to the United States. Office for Official Publications of the European Communities; 2003. 191.

[84]   Supplemental Material for Divided We Stand: Three Psychological Regions of the United States and Their Political, Economic, Social, and Health Correlates. J Pers Soc Psychol 2013.

[85]   Wolff EN, Baumol WJ, Saini AN. A comparative analysis of education costs and outcomes: The United States vs. other OECD countries. Econ Educ Rev 2014; 39: 1-21.
[http://dx.doi.org/10.1016/j.econedurev.2013.12.002]

[86]   Mason CM, Harrison RT. Business angel investment activity in the financial crisis: UK evidence and policy implications. Environ Plann C Gov Policy 2015; 33(1): 43-60.
[http://dx.doi.org/10.1068/c12324b]

[87]   Brewer TL. His publications have appeared in the. Journal of Money, Credit and Banking, and Journal of Comparative Economics. 1992. Available from: www.jstor.org

[88]   Banga R. Impact of government policies and investment agreements on FDI inflows Standard-Nutzungsbedingungen: Impact of government policies and investment agreements on fdi inflows. 2003. Available from: https://hdl.handle.net/10419/189636

[89]   Daniel K, Hirshleifer D, Teoh SH. Investor psychology in capital markets: evidence and policy implications. J Monet Econ 2002; 49(1): 139-209.
[http://dx.doi.org/10.1016/S0304-3932(01)00091-5]

[90]   Dirk Willem. te Velde, Dirk Willem. 2003. Available from https://hdl.handle.net/10419/72818

[91]   Wang G. Renewable and Sustainable Energy Reviews. 2021. Available from: https://doi.org/./j.rser

[92]   Murillo MV. Political Competition and Policy Adoption: Market Reforms in Latin American Public Utilities. 2007. Available from: www.indotel.org.do

[93]   Catan G, Espanha R, Mendes RV, Toren O, Chinitz D. Health information technology implementation - impacts and policy considerations: a comparison between Israel and Portugal. Isr J Health Policy Res 2015; 4(1): 41.

[http://dx.doi.org/10.1186/s13584-015-0040-9] [PMID: 26269740]

[94] Thorne RJ, Hovi IB, Figenbaum E, Pinchasik DR, Amundsen AH, Hagman R. Facilitating adoption of electric buses through policy: Learnings from a trial in Norway. Energy Policy 2021; 155: 112310.
[http://dx.doi.org/10.1016/j.enpol.2021.112310]

[95] Paul H, Jonathan Z. Flexible specialization versus post-Fordism: theory, evidence and policy implications. Econ Soc 1991; 20(1): 1-56.

[96] Paranjape SM, Franz DR. Implementing the global health security agenda: lessons from global health and security programs. Health Secur 2015; 13(1): 9-19.
[http://dx.doi.org/10.1089/hs.2014.0047] [PMID: 25812424]

[97] Cieza A, Kamenov K, Sanchez MG, Chatterji S, Balasegaram M, Lincetto O, *et al*. Burden of disability in children and adolescents must be integrated into the global health agenda. The BMJ. BMJ Publishing Group; 2021; 372.

[98] Bali S, Taaffe J. The sustainable development goals and the global health security agenda: exploring synergies for a sustainable and resilient world. J Public Health Policy 2017; 38: 257-68.

[99] Agyepong IA, M'Cormack-Hale FAO, Brown Amoakoh H, Derkyi-Kwarteng ANC, Darkwa TE, Odiko-Ollennu W. Synergies and fragmentation in country level policy and program agenda setting, formulation and implementation for Global Health agendas: a case study of health security, universal health coverage, and health promotion in Ghana and Sierra Leone. BMC Health Serv Res 2021; 21(1): 476.
[http://dx.doi.org/10.1186/s12913-021-06500-6] [PMID: 34016117]

[100] Tadesse AW, Gurmu KK, Kebede ST, Habtemariam MK. Analyzing efforts to synergize the global health agenda of universal health coverage, health security and health promotion: a case-study from Ethiopia. Global Health 2021; 17(1): 53.
[http://dx.doi.org/10.1186/s12992-021-00702-7] [PMID: 33902625]

[101] Myhre S, Habtemariam MK, Heymann DL, Ottersen T, Stoltenberg C, Ventura D de FL, *et al*. Bridging global health actors and agendas: the role of national public health institutes. Journal of Public Health Policy. Palgrave Macmillan; 2022; 43, 251–65.
[http://dx.doi.org/10.1057/s41271-022-00342-0]

[102] Fernandes EG, Rodrigues CC, Sartori AM, De Soárez PC, Novaes HM. Economic evaluation of adolescents and adults' pertussis vaccination: A systematic review of current strategies. Hum Vaccines & Immunother 2019; 15(1): 14-27.

[103] Fernandes EG, Rodrigues CCM, Sartori AMC, De Soárez PC, Novaes HMD. Economic evaluation of adolescents and adults' pertussis vaccination: A systematic review of current strategies. Human Vaccines and Immunotherapeutics. Taylor and Francis Inc.; 2019; 15, 14–27.

[104] Brotherton JML, Gertig DM. Primary prophylactic human papillomavirus vaccination programs: future perspective on global impact. Expert Rev Anti Infect Ther 2011; 9(8): 627-39.
[http://dx.doi.org/10.1586/eri.11.78] [PMID: 21819329]

[105] Sánchez-Ramón S, Diego R, Dieli-Crimi R, Subiza JL. Extending the clinical horizons of mucosal bacterial vaccines: current evidence and future prospects. Curr Drug Targets 2014; 15(12): 1132-43.
[http://dx.doi.org/10.2174/1389450115666141020160705] [PMID: 25330031]

[106] Ebrahimi N, Yousefi Z, Khosravi G, Malayeri FE, Golabi M, Askarzadeh M, *et al*. Human papillomavirus vaccination in low- and middle-income countries: progression, barriers, and future prospective. Frontiers in Immunology. Frontiers Media S.A. 2023; 14.

[107] Possas C, de Souza Antunes AM, de Oliveira AM, *et al*. Vaccine Innovation for Pandemic Preparedness: Patent Landscape, Global Sustainability, and Circular Bioeconomy in Post-COVID-19 era. Circ Econ Sustain 2021; 1(4): 1439-61.
[http://dx.doi.org/10.1007/s43615-021-00051-y] [PMID: 34888570]

[108] Li M, Wang Y, Sun Y, Cui H, Zhu SJ, Qiu HJ. Mucosal vaccines: Strategies and challenges.

Immunology Letters. Elsevier B.V. 2020; 217: pp. 116-25.

[109]   Poland GA, Jacobson RM, Ovsyannikova IG. Trends affecting the future of vaccine development and delivery: The role of demographics, regulatory science, the anti-vaccine movement, and vaccinomics. Vaccine 2009; 27(25-26): 3240-4.
[http://dx.doi.org/10.1016/j.vaccine.2009.01.069] [PMID: 19200833]

[110]   Pattyn J, Hendrickx G, Vorsters A, Van Damme P, Hepatitis B. Vaccines. J Infect Dis 2021; 224(12) (Suppl. 4): S343-51.
[http://dx.doi.org/10.1093/infdis/jiaa668] [PMID: 34590138]

[111]   Mattison CP, Cardemil CV, Hall AJ. Progress on norovirus vaccine research: public health considerations and future directions. 2018.

[112]   Wood DJ, Sutter RW, Dowdle & WR. Round Table Stopping poliovirus vaccination after eradication: issues and challenges. 2000.

CHAPTER 3

Mucosal Vaccination for Emerging and Pandemic Infectious Diseases

Md Nasar Mallick[1], Akhil Sharma[2], Akanksha Sharma[2], Sunita[3] and Shaweta Sharma[1,*]

[1] *School of Medical and Allied Sciences, Galgotias University, Yamuna Expressway, Gautam Buddha Nagar, Uttar Pradesh-201310, India*

[2] *R. J. College of Pharmacy, 2HVJ+567, Raipur, Gharbara, Tappal, Khair, Uttar Pradesh 202165, India*

[3] *Metro College of Health Sciences and Research, Greater Noida, India*

Abstract: Mucosal vaccination is a revolutionary method for controlling epidemic and pandemic infectious ailments. The technique has an exclusive feature that makes it produce very strong immune responses to pathogens at the entry point. This section gives detailed information on mucosal immunity and its importance in protection against different diseases. It starts by probing into how mucosal immune responses work before presenting arguments that support mucosal vaccination choices over other options. In addition, the chapter provides a contrast between traditional systemic inoculation ways. It shows the superiority and wider range of action of mucosal vaccines when compared with traditional systemic vaccination routes. Detailed scrutiny of manifold mucosal vaccine delivery systems comprising oral, nasal, and pulmonary routes discloses various ways to overcome mucosal barriers and improve the uptake and efficiency of vaccines. The chapter presents success stories of preventing infectious diseases, including influenza, rotavirus, and cholera, through mucosal vaccination, as seen in preclinical and clinical studies. It also identifies complexities within the regulatory environment for a better understanding of those unique obstacles, which ought to be considered when seeking approval for a new type of vaccine, like one that is administered through mucosal routes. The chapter underscores the real-world impact of mucosal vaccination on the disease burden and the shaping of public health outcomes with insightful case studies. However, despite considerable progress made in this field, it is still confronted by various difficulties in the selection of antigens and optimization of formulations, as well as scaling up production. This paper also describes essential scientific tracks for future research along with some technological advancements that are considered to overcome these impediments and open a gateway for a new generation of mucosal vaccines. In summary, this chapter emphasizes the long-term investments and partnerships that are needed to optimize

* **Corresponding author Shaweta Sharma:** School of Medical and Allied Sciences, Galgotias University, Yamuna Expressway, Gautam Buddha Nagar, Uttar Pradesh-201310, India; E-mail: shawetasharma@galgotiasuniversity.edu.in

mucosal vaccination as a major approach to addressing emerging and pandemic infectious diseases. This way, we can build up our ability to protect ourselves by encouraging prevention measures at the mucosal level.

Keywords: Emerging diseases, Mucosal immunity, Pandemic, Regulatory approval, Vaccine delivery systems, Vaccination.

INTRODUCTION

A specialized immunization technique known as mucosal vaccination entails giving vaccines directly into the body's mucosal surfaces, like respiratory, gastrointestinal, and genitourinary tracts. Its main objective is to promote a protective immunity against infectious diseases. Mucosal vaccination differs from the traditional systemic routes of vaccination that often consist of putting vaccines in the bloodstream or muscle tissues since it uses unique traits of mucosal tissues to stimulate immune responses through the spots where pathogens enter [1].

In mucosal vaccination, the vaccine's antigens are brought to the mucosal surfaces *via* several ways, like the oral, nasal, pulmonary, rectal, vaginal, and ocular route of administration. When these antigens reach the surface of the mucus membrane, for example, certain types of immune cells, such as dendritic cells, macrophages, and lymphocytes, play a role in capturing and initiating immune response towards them [2].

One of the most important characteristics of mucosal vaccination is its capacity to elicit both local and systemic immune responses. Mucosal vaccines used for this purpose so often result in the production of secretory immunoglobulin A (sIgA) antibodies, which provide a first line of defense against pathogens at mucosal surfaces through means such as neutralization and prevention of their passage into the body. Moreover, mucosal vaccination also activates systemic immune responses that produce circulating antibodies and activate T cells responsible for long-term immune protection against pathogens that breach the mucosal barrier into the blood stream [3].

Mucosal vaccination has various advantages over traditional systemic vaccination approaches. First, it mimics the natural infection path of several pathogens, leading to the elicitation of immune responses at the site where most likely they would be entering into the body. This is capable of bringing about an increase in mucosal and systemic immunity compared to systemic vaccination. Secondly, mucosal vaccinations can also cause immune reactions at numerous mucosal locations, hence providing a wide range of protection against different types of pathogens. Thirdly, most mucosal vaccines do not require needles and are administered without much strain, making them suitable for mass immunization programs as well as limited-resource settings [4].

Thus, because the vaccines are administered at the mucosal surface of the body, they have several benefits and limitations that need to be considered, such as bypassing immune responses. Nonetheless, the challenges can be overcome by the continued search for answers and swinging of mucosal immunization back into its potentially powerful applications in fighting infectious diseases, from pandemics to emerging ones [5, 6].

Importance in Combating Emerging and Pandemic Infectious Diseases

As a global strategy for the prevention of emerging and pandemic infectious diseases, mucosal vaccination is increasingly important. This is because it can utilize multiple defense tactics at mucosal surfaces, which are the main entry points for various types of pathogens. Mucosal vaccination prevents systemic distribution by directly activating the immune system near the site of infection. This enables the immune response to attack pathogens at their entry point and stops them from spreading further into the body. In addition to stopping infections from developing, this approach also reduces the likelihood of passing on diseases, thus blocking their wide-scale diffusion, which could lead to pandemics [7].

Apart from reacting fast, mucosal vaccination also provides a wide range of guards against different kinds of pathogens. Unlike traditional systematic vaccines that aim at one type of bacterium or virus, this category can activate various defenders, such as sIgA antibodies, mucosal T cells, and innate immune mediators. These many weapons not only destroy the intruders but also make the body resist closely related strains or completely different bugs, thereby increasing its resistance to constantly changing infectious hazards [8].

The strategic advantage of mucosal vaccination, in addition to this, is its ability to prevent mass transmission in crowded areas or impoverished regions. In fact, it can reduce the shedding of pathogens and their spread by breaking the continuous sequence between outbreaks that may otherwise lead to global pandemics. Also, these features make it ideal for large-scale immunization campaigns because there are no needles involved, which makes logistics simpler and faster while ensuring wide-reaching protection necessary during such explosive outbreaks with potential catastrophic health implications [9].

Even though mucosal vaccination has this unmatched beneficial side, it still has its share of difficulties. It is very challenging to design and optimize formulations for mucosal vaccines, which include selecting an antigen, incorporating an adjuvant, and developing a delivery system. Also, the regulatory pathways designed for approving such vaccines demand strict scrutiny on safety assessment as well as evaluation for effectiveness with respect to quality assurance during manufacturing, among other things, which further complicates their development [10].

The significance of mucosal vaccination in the fight against new and global diseases cannot be overstated. This is because it can trigger an immediate and wide-ranging immune reaction at points where pathogens first enter the body, besides being able to prevent transmission and allow for quick deployment, thus making it a necessary tool for protecting public health during times when worldwide health risks are increasing rapidly. Nevertheless, to achieve this aim, there has to be continued investment into research, development, and regulatory processes that will keep mucosal vaccination on the front line against infectious diseases, which are always with us [11, 12].

OVERVIEW OF EMERGING AND PANDEMIC INFECTIOUS DISEASES

This part of the study gives a detailed analysis of recent outbreaks and their impacts on emerging infectious diseases. It, therefore, points out how these threats have changed. It begins by spotlighting notable examples of recent outbreaks, including Ebola, Zika, and COVID-19 (Fig. **1**), each representing distinct challenges and global health concerns.

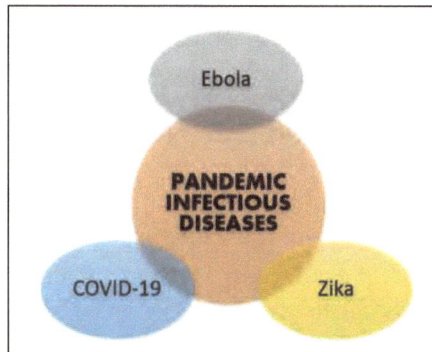

Fig. (1). Pandemic infectious disease.

Ebola

The serious problem that happened in Africa in 2014, which the rest of the world knew as the Ebola outbreak, is an example of how very harmful germs can be. The speed at which it spread, plus the lack of enough health facilities and few ways to cure it, led to many people falling sick and dying. That event showed that there was a great necessity for effective methods in responding to epidemics because many lives were lost [13].

Characteristics and Challenges of Ebola

Ebola virus disease (EVD) has a number of unique features and challenges that make it one of the most difficult infectious diseases to control. The high case fatality rate is particularly noteworthy; this can be anything between 25% and 90% depending on factors such as strain virulence and healthcare system capacity in affected areas. The importance of this death rate is that it shows how serious the sickness is and how much we need to do something about it as soon as possible. Besides, EVD symptoms are severe and incapacitating, which may include fever, tiredness, muscle ache, headache, vomiting, diarrhea, as well as later on in its course internal and external bleeding. They can advance quickly, resulting in the failure of multiple organs followed by fatal outcomes in a substantial number of instances [14].

Ebola has always been among the top challenges because of its way of spreading. It is mainly transmitted from one person to another through direct contact with body fluids like blood, saliva, vomit, feces, or objects contaminated by them. This means that healthcare providers and those who take care of patients in hospitals are at risk. Also, caregivers looking after their sick relatives at home face a high chance of getting infected as well. Additionally, Ebola frequently happens in distant and poor parts of sub-Saharan Africa, lacking the resources for proper healthcare. Suppose it is taken into account that in these regions, the medical infrastructure may not be enough to counteract the virus. In that case, it becomes clear why limited access to hospitals, labs, and trained personnel makes it even harder to confront this problem and offer prompt treatment [15].

The fact that Ebola has zoonotic origins makes it even more complicated in terms of its nature and the problems posed by this disease. The virus is thought to be present among different types of animals, with bats being the primary hosts where it can be detected naturally. Human beings get infected with Ebola after coming into contact with sickened or contaminated animals, such as monkeys found within forests inhabited by these creatures. In order to stop further outbreaks from happening and prevent infections from spreading between people, we need to know what causes them to appear first, which also helps us lower the chances of transmitting zoonoses to humans again [16].

Identifying Ebola is quite hard, especially in places where resources are scarce and laboratory tests, as well as professional medical personnel, are not easily accessible. Fever and fatigue, which are among the first symptoms of EVD, can also be observed in many other common diseases that usually occur in that area, thus making differential diagnosis more difficult. Additionally, at present, there are no authorized antiviral medicines for Ebola virus disease in particular, and supportive care continues to be an essential treatment. The development of effective therapeutics and vaccines against this disease is complicated by factors such as more demanding clinical trial requirements, regulatory clearance stages, or even industrial production expansion [17].

The urgent demand for continuous investment in public health infrastructure, research, and international cooperation to alleviate the effect of this ruinous communicable disease is indicated by the characteristics and challenges of Ebola, such as high mortality rate, severe symptoms, zoonotic origin, diagnostic intricacies as well as limited treatment modalities [18].

Zika Virus

The start of the Zika virus outbreak in the Americas during 2015-2016 drew attention to how infectious diseases, vector biology, and global travel are interconnected in complex ways. As neurological disorders such as microcephaly in babies were being linked with this infection, which spreads mainly through Aedes mosquito bites, its potential threat was realized worldwide, leading to massive interventions for public safety coupled with extensive studies [19].

Characteristics and Challenges of the Zika Virus

In the realm of global public health, the Zika virus (ZIKV) has attracted much interest due to its specific qualities and problems. One way that the Zika virus can be recognized is through its mode of transmission. This is mainly achieved by being bitten by an infected Aedes mosquito, especially the Aedes aegypti or Aedes albopictus species. The manner in which this virus is transmitted by vectors that move from one place to another over long distances affects its distribution around the world and makes it difficult to contain or control. Apart from this, Zika can be spread through sex between a person with the virus and their partner who does not have it, making prevention harder and increasing the risk of local infections in regions without these mosquitoes [20].

People who have been infected by the Zika virus usually suffer mild symptoms, which eventually disappear on their own. Most of them do not show any symptoms at all or have only a slight fever, rash, joint pain, and redness of the eyes. However, if a pregnant woman contracts this disease, it may lead to serious congenital disabilities in her baby, such as microcephaly (an abnormal smallness of the head) and brain malformation, among others. This peculiarity of the virus calls for more vigorous monitoring systems as well as preventive measures targeting expectant mothers or women planning to get pregnant soon [21].

The potential for asymptomatic transmission of Zika virus is one of the major challenges it poses. In this case, infected persons may not exhibit any signs but can still pass on the virus to others through mosquitoes or sex. Such silent spreading makes it difficult to detect and isolate cases and also to break chains of transmission through successful vector control strategies [22].

The global Zika virus is also a concern for the travel and tourism industry around the world. This is particularly worrying for areas that have been affected as visitors may be discouraged from visiting due to the possibility of getting infected and thus disrupting economies. Besides, when the Zika virus broke out in new countries, they realized that there were lapses in monitoring systems, laboratory tests, and healthcare services, which had never been addressed before since such regions did not recognize mosquito-borne diseases as key public health problems [23].

Creating effective vaccines and treatments for the Zika virus is also difficult, requiring rigorous clinical trials that demonstrate safety and efficacy, manufacturing scale-up, and regulatory approval processes. Despite these challenges, there have been more vaccine and therapeutic developments in recent times due to the global threat of the Zika virus [24].

Zika virus has exceptional qualities and complexities: the way it is transmitted, its potential for asymptomatic transferring, its impact on the results of pregnancy, and implications for journeys and the tourist industry. Responding to these difficulties needs surveillance systems; preventive measures need to be taken at various levels, such as research should be done internationally so as to prevent significant damage caused by this virus on worldwide public health [25].

COVID-19

Systems of health worldwide, economies, and societies have encountered unparalleled difficulties as a result of the COVID-19 pandemic. The rapid transmission of the new coronavirus, SARS-CoV-2, has revealed how closely connected we are in this modern world and also exposed weaknesses in our preparedness and response systems. The pandemic has stimulated remarkable activities toward vaccine production, diagnosis, and public health measures, thereby changing the manner in which we address infectious disease control during the 21st century [26].

Characteristics and Challenges of COVID-19

COVID-19 resulted from SARS-CoV-2, which is a new coronavirus and it has its distinctive features that pose unprecedented global health and social challenges.

The most notable feature of COVID-19 is how contagious it is, transmitted mainly through respiratory droplets released when people breathe out, talk, cough, or sneeze. This ease of transmission has led to quick worldwide distribution, resulting in community-wide infections and large outbreaks across different areas [27].

Symptoms of COVID-19 can be as mild as respiratory diseases or severe, like pneumonia, ARDS (acute respiratory distress syndrome), multiorgan failure, and death. Some people may have only a few symptoms or none at all; however, older adults and those with preexisting health problems are more likely to suffer from severe illness or mortality. This heterogeneity in clinical presentation poses challenges for diagnosis, triage, and clinical management, as well as for estimating disease burden and mortality rates [28].

The asymptomatic and pre-symptomatic transmission of SARS-CoV-2 further complicates containment efforts, as individuals infected with the virus may unknowingly spread it to others before developing symptoms or in the absence of symptoms altogether. This silent transmission poses challenges for identifying and isolating cases, contact tracing, and implementing effective infection control measures to break transmission chains [29].

The social and economic impacts of the pandemic have been one of the most significant things about COVID-19. Lockdowns, travel bans, and physical distancing measures have all interrupted normal life, overburdened healthcare systems, and caused global economic downturns. The pandemic has hit vulnerable populations harder than any other groups, such as low-income communities, essential workers, or marginalized individuals, thereby making worse existing health and social inequalities [30].

The COVID-19 pandemic is complicated by the sudden appearance of fresh strains of SARS-CoV-2 that may affect infectivity, severity, immunization efficiency, and diagnosis. As such, it becomes more difficult to respond to public health interventions and vaccine plans without continuous monitoring and comprehension of how these variants emerge or change in relation to different vaccine strategies [31].

Dealing with COVID-19 demands an approach that is unified and covers many areas; this includes the measures of public health, campaigns for vaccination, testing as well as surveillance, building healthcare capacity, and research and development, among others. Also, international cooperation should be taken into consideration. The creation and use of vaccines that are safe and work well against COVID-19 have given us some hope in our battle with this pandemic. However, efforts still need to be made to make sure all people get fair chances worldwide through vaccination access while grappling with new problems like logistic distribution or vaccine reluctance [32].

Public health, society, and the international community should not underestimate COVID-19. It is a very contagious disease that has many peculiarities, such as heterogeneous clinical presentation, asymptomatic transmission, social and economic consequences, emergence of new variants, unprecedented global scale, *etc.* Overcoming these difficulties will need continuous dedication, creativity, and unity in order to solve what could be considered one of the most significant global health emergencies in history [33, 34].

Global Impact of Pandemics

Pandemics' worldwide effect touches all human life, changing everything from economies to social systems in ways never seen before. Global health is profoundly influenced by pandemics like the recent COVID-19 pandemic, which often stretches healthcare systems beyond their capacity. Hospitals get crowded with patients; medical equipment runs out while doctors work until they cannot take it anymore. The death toll is overwhelming; millions fall sick and die, leaving behind mournful families and communities [35].

Apart from the present health emergency, pandemics lead to economic disorder, which interferes with trade, supply chains, and the lives of people across the world. Economic activity is halted by confinement measures, travel bans, and social distancing rules, leading to many people losing jobs, businesses closing down, and financial insecurity. Sectors depending on tourism and traveling record huge losses, whereas weak communities suffer most from poverty hence increasing disparities among countries as well as within nations themselves [36].

Socially, pandemics tend to cause fear, mistrust, and division among people by fostering stigma and discrimination towards victims or groups. Communities are broken apart by uncertainty and isolation, which strains their social support systems to the maximum. Schools close down, thereby denying millions of kids educational opportunities, thus worsening inequality in academic performance between advantaged and disadvantaged students [37].

Pandemics have an effect on the world, which can be seen worldwide across political borders and geopolitical divides. They show how interconnected our modern world is. The whole international community closes down its travel, shuts its borders, and causes supply chains to collapse, leading to a breakdown in the movement of goods, services as well as information. Nations need to work jointly to share resources, skills and best practices in fighting against a mutual foe for global cooperation and solidarity to become more important than ever [38].

Also, pandemics expose how weak global governance systems are and the failures of our preparedness actions. Requests for change are reverberating all over international bodies as they try to deal with the faults brought on by this calamity. The requirement for stronger health systems, sustainable supply chains, and synchronized responses to pandemics becomes clearly visible, thereby pushing the world into an epoch of worldwide health safety [39].

The global impact of pandemics is deep and wide, leaving an indelible imprint on mankind long after the immediate disaster has passed. In facing the issues of emerging and pandemic transmissible diseases, we should take notice of what past calamities have taught us and engage in creating a more capable, equitable, and sustainable tomorrow for posterity [40, 41].

IMMUNE RESPONSES AT MUCOSAL SURFACES

Mucosal Immunity

The body's defense system relies heavily on mucosal immunity, which protects against pathogens in the respiratory, digestive, and urogenital tracts. In contrast to systemic immunity, which primarily operates in the bloodstream and tissues, mucosal immunity is designed to address challenges encountered at various mucosal barriers, which are typically used by most infectious agents to enter the body [42].

The immune system of the mucous membrane is composed of a complex network of specialized cells, secretory factors, and tissues whose purpose is to recognize, neutralize, and remove harmful microorganisms that invade the body while still being able to tolerate harmless antigens like commensal bacteria or food proteins. Epithelial cells are among the most important components in this system since they serve as physical barriers against pathogens by producing mucus and antimicrobial peptides; innate immune cells such as macrophages, neutrophils, and dendritic cells detect pathogens through pattern recognition receptors (PRRs); adaptive immunity is responsible for mounting specific antibody-based immune responses mediated by T-cells, B-cells, and plasma cells [43].

The theory of mucosal immunity revolves around the idea of immune exclusion. The mucosal barrier stops infectious agents from destroying epithelial cells and moving into underlying tissues. It does this by using tight junctions between epithelial cells as well as a variety of resident immune cells, which orchestrate dynamic immune responses. During the pathogen invasion, the cells of the mucosal immune system respond quickly and locally to the specific pathogens they encounter; these include generating secretory IgA antibodies that can neutralize pathogens and prevent them from attaching to mucosal surfaces as well as attracting inflammatory cells to infected areas in order for there to be easy elimination of pathogens [44, 45].

There must be a balance between immunity and tolerance of harmless antigens. Otherwise, the immune system will be triggered inappropriately, leading to tissue damage. Moreover, a malfunctioning mucosal immune response can cause chronic inflammatory diseases, autoimmunity, and vulnerability to repetitive infections [46].

Mucosal immunity is the first defense against pathogens that are met at mucosal surfaces. It does this by using diverse cellular and molecular mechanisms to identify, disarm, and remove threats while still recognizing harmless antigens. Knowing the complexities of mucosal immunity is critical in creating vaccines and treatments for new or widespread infectious diseases that affect these areas [47].

Importance of Mucosal Immunity in Protection Against Pathogens

Mucosal immunity is vital in safeguarding the body from a variety of threats; it is, therefore, a key element in the body's defense system. What makes it so important is its capacity to offer first-line defense at mucosal surfaces, which are the major points of entry for several microorganisms such as viruses, bacteria, fungi, and parasites. (Fig. **2**) highlights the importance of mucosal immunity in protection against pathogens.

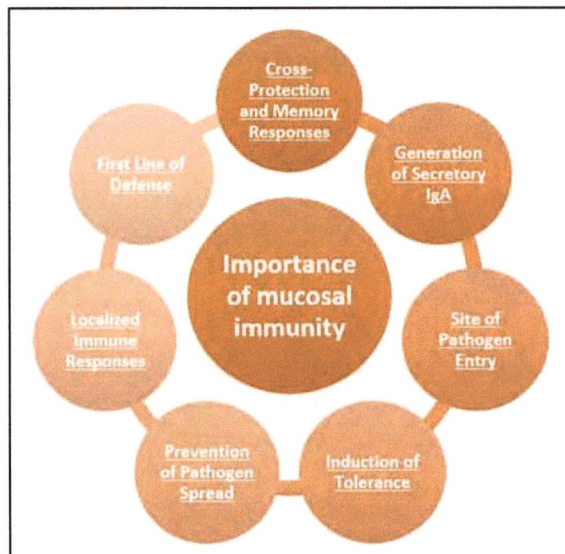

Fig. (2). Importance of mucosal immunity.

First Line of Defense

The first defense against pathogens is known as mucosal immunity, which is also responsible for safeguarding the organism from infections in the respiratory, digestive, and urinary tracts. This system is crucial because it can detect various kinds of pathogens that may invade through these points and provide quick protection locally [48].

The mucous membrane immune system is comprised of unique cells, glands, and substances that identify, disintegrate, and remove pathogenic microorganisms while responding to harmless antigens. Some of the most important elements are the epithelial cells that prevent pathogens from entering body tissues, mucus that traps and eliminates them, antimicrobial peptides that kill them instantly, and sIgA antibodies that stop their attachment to or colonization within host tissues [49].

The reason why this immune response is so important is that mucosal surfaces are the main places in which pathogens enter the body. By stopping them and making them harmless right at these points, immunity of the mucous membranes prevents their spreading to inner organs or around the whole organism through blood, so it also decreases the chances of getting infected systemically or infecting other people. Moreover, overall protective reactions, as well as the balance between defense and tolerance, greatly depend on such local defense mechanisms [50, 51].

The first line of defense against infection is mucosal immunity. This shows how important it is to protect yourself from different types of pathogens that can be found on the surface of your body. Knowing about and using this knowledge will help us find ways in which we can fight back against new diseases or ones that spread all over the world quickly [52, 53].

Site of Pathogen Entry

Mucosal immunity is vital to protecting the body from pathogens that enter through its surfaces: it is the first and main line of self-defense. Respiratory, alimentary, and urogenital tracts are mucosal surfaces that come into contact with countless numbers and types of microbes. Knowing why it safeguards against such infections in these areas is key to understanding its role as our lives' front guard [54].

This is because pathogens can easily invade these tissues since they are exposed directly to the outside environment. In the case of these entry sites, microorganisms like bacteria, viruses, fungi, and protozoa find their way into and establish themselves in the body. Therefore, an efficient mucosal defense system can prevent microbial colonization and invasion to stop a disease from beginning [55].

This is accomplished by the latter through a complicated set of actions that are designed to tackle the specific difficulties encountered in each mucosal point. The penetration of germs into underlying tissues cannot be allowed, therefore, but they can be made ineffective *via* epithelial cells, which constitute the lining of mucosal surfaces. These fortify tight junctions and, therefore, manufacture antimicrobial peptides and proteins to prevent microbial propagation [56].

Another reason is that mucosal surfaces have many special immune cells and tissues, for example, MALT, placed on them to promptly react to invading pathogens. Such immune cells, including B cells, dendritic cells, and T-cells, together with macrophages, play a significant role in coordinating adaptive and innate immunological responses aimed at preventing the establishment of pathogenic organisms within the host [57].

Mucosal immunity also creates sIgA antibodies that are useful in fighting pathogens at mucosal surfaces. These antibodies are secreted to the mucosal lumen in response to mucosal antigens, and they attach themselves to pathogenic organisms, preventing their attachment and colonization [58].

Mucosal immunity is the first line of defense against pathogens at the mucosal surfaces. It acts as a critical barrier against infections and thus plays a key role in preventing microbial colonization. Appreciating the significance of mucosal immunity at sites of pathogen entry is important for effective strategies to improve defenses against infectious diseases [59].

Generation of Secretory IgA

Mucosal immunity is reliant on sIgA antibodies that defend against specific pathogens in the respiratory and gastrointestinal tracts. They are produced locally in response to antigens of the mucosa, hence attaching to the invading organisms, inhibiting their attachment or colonization, and enhancing their removal from the body. Immune exclusion is the process that helps maintain mucosal integrity and prevents infections from establishing. sIgA antibodies are considered to be broad-spectrum with regard to pathogen activity, and thus, they provide long-lasting protection against recurrent infections. It is essential to understand the significance of sIgA in mucosal immunity in order to develop strategies for boosting mucosal defenses as well as fighting infectious diseases effectively [60, 61].

Localized Immune Responses

The significance of localized immune responses at mucosal surfaces in the defense against pathogens cannot be overemphasized. They are responsible for prompt detection and reaction towards intruders by specialized immune cells, which triggers a series of events aimed at nullifying and eradicating threats. This involves, among others, bringing on board more defenders like dendritic cells or macrophages from the innate immunity and mounting an antigen-specific response through adaptive immune cells such as B or T lymphocytes. The reaction should not only limit inflammation but also offer durable protection from recurrent infections. Realizing how important it is for mucosal immunity to coordinate these reactions can help us come up with methods that will work best against infectious diseases [62, 63].

Cross-Protection and Memory Responses

Mucosal immunity is the key to cross-protection as well as memory responses against pathogens, which are experienced in mucosal surfaces that line the respiratory, gastrointestinal, and urogenital tracts. This part of the immune system allows for identification and protection from many types of infectious organisms, including those with antigenic variability or close relationships with each other. Common antigens and the long-term presence of memory B cells and T cells enable rapid, strong reactions by the immune system when it encounters a known enemy again, thereby lessening the severity of infection and curtailing the dissemination of pathogens [64, 65].

The ability of mucosal immunity to confer cross-protection and memory responses is particularly important when considering vaccination strategies. Mucosal vaccines are formulated to induce immune responses at these surfaces that will help stimulate local immunity against specific pathogens when delivered nasally or orally. These vaccines have the potential to fight infectious diseases and decrease their worldwide burden by using the natural power of mucosa-based immunity to trigger broad and long-lasting immune responses [66, 67].

Prevention of Pathogen Spread

Mucosal immunity needs to act as a crucial obstacle against the spread of pathogens from the surfaces of the mucosa into systemic blood circulation. It has been established that the immune system functioning at such points of entry, including the respiratory, gastrointestinal, and urogenital tracts, helps in blocking and deactivating pathogens from being transferred to different body parts, thereby decreasing the threat to the entire body by systemic infections and transmission to other people. This localized defense mechanism involves an integrated attack by specialized immune cells and molecules located in positions where they can recognize invading pathogens before these can establish infection [68, 69].

Also, the key role in the clearance of pathogens from mucosal surfaces and the limitation of their colonization and replication is played by mucosal immunity. For example, the elimination of pathogens from the human body can be done through mechanisms like peristalsis of the gastrointestinal tract or mucociliary clearance in the respiratory. By effectively confining pathogens at the mucosal surface to facilitate their removal, the general contributions of host defense are made by this kind of immunity for public healthcare providers involved in infectious disease control [70, 71].

Induction of Tolerance

The significance of mucosal immunity is that it creates a peaceful coexistence with harmless antigens and fights off dangerous organisms that invade the mucosal surfaces. The immune system must ensure the right balance between these two functions so that it does not overreact to harmless things or attack itself but also reacts appropriately when faced with infection [72]. Respiratory, gastrointestinal, and urogenital tracts are all examples of mucosal tissues that are always being exposed to a range of foreign antigens; this includes friendly microorganisms and proteins that come from the diet. These protective immune responses against pathogens can be triggered by the same tolerant mechanisms towards harmless antigens orchestrated by mucosal immune cells like dendritic cells or regulatory T cells when necessary [73].

The process, therefore, is characterized by this ability to suppress inflammatory reactions and enhance the development of regulatory pathways that attenuate immune activation and preserve the equilibrium of tissues. In addition, mucosal immunity prevents abnormal immune responses like allergies and autoimmune diseases while still allowing for efficient defense against infectious agents by promoting tolerance to harmless antigens [74]. It is necessary to comprehend the significance of mucosal immunity in terms of tolerance and immunity equilibrium for the sake of mucosal health and the general immune system. A tabular representation of the types of mucosal immune responses is shown in Table **1**.

Table 1. Types of Mucosal Immune Responses

Type of Response	Description
Innate Immune Response	Immediate innate immunity is characterized by quick, non-specific defense mechanisms that protect against pathogens. It comprises physical barriers, antimicrobial peptides, and cells of the innate immune system [75, 76].

Type of Response	Description
Adaptive Immune Response	Specific immune responses tailored to the antigens encountered at mucosal surfaces. Involves activation of B cells and T cells, antibody production, and generation of immunological memory [77].
Secretory IgA Production	The plasma cells in mucosa-associated lymphoid tissue (MALT) generate sIgA antibodies. The purpose of these sIgA antibodies is to provide local immune defense against pathogens [78].
Inflammatory Response	Inflammation pathways become activated in response to infection, leading to immune cell recruitment and production of cytokine and chemokine [79, 80].
Tolerance Induction	The goal is to prevent incorrect immune responses by inducing tolerance towards harmless antigens like commensal microorganisms and dietary proteins [81].

RATIONALE FOR MUCOSAL VACCINATION

The rationale for mucosal vaccination is strong because it uses the natural defense of the body in mucosal areas. Mucosal vaccines target the respiratory, gastrointestinal, and urogenital tracts and, therefore, induce strong immune responses that are specific to the major sites of pathogen entry [82]. These vaccines also promote the production of secretory IgA antibodies, which are essential for pathogen neutralization and blocking infection establishment. Besides, mucosal vaccines elicit both local and systemic immunity, giving wide coverage against the mucosal and systemic pathogens. Their needle-free administration also facilitates their use in large-scale immunization campaigns [83]. In addition, these vaccines can provide cross-protective immunity against other related pathogens as well as confer long-lasting immunity that is associated with memory cells, which contributes to herd immunity. The above attributes highlight the importance of mucosal vaccination in global health efforts targeted at infectious diseases [84].

Advantages of Mucosal Vaccination Compared to Systemic Vaccination

The mucosal vaccine is preferred to systemic vaccination because of its several benefits, thus making it an appealing option for evoking immune responses at the mucosal surfaces like respiratory, gastrointestinal, and urogenital tracts. The benefits of mucosal vaccination compared to systemic vaccination are discussed below.

Site-Specific Immune Responses

The immune responses that mucosal vaccines can generate at the site of entry of a pathogen help to improve protection against infections by pathogens in the mucosa. This method enables the production of secretory IgA antibodies and mucosal T cells, thus preventing the colonization of pathogens on the mucosal surface and subsequent infection [85].

Needle-Free Administration

Mucosal vaccines are administered non-invasively using methods like oral, nasal, or intranasal delivery; hence, there is no need to inject with needles and syringes. This needle-free administration is also less painful and more convenient, making it ideal for mass immunization campaigns and conquering the fear of injections [86].

Enhanced Mucosal Immune Responses

Mucosal vaccination can induce robust mucosal immune responses, including the production of secretory IgA antibodies and activation of Mucosal T Cells, which offer immediate and localized protection against pathogens. These responses better serve mucosal pathogens than systemic immune responses elicited by conventional parenteral vaccines [87].

Cross-Protection at Mucosal Surfaces

Mucosal vaccines can achieve cross-protection against related pathogens found at mucosal surfaces. They can provide a wider range of defense by immunizing against shared conserved epitopes among related pathogens, which also leads to greater protection against various strains and variants [88].

Stimulation of Systemic Immunity

Mucosal vaccination can also cause immune responses throughout the body through the production of antibodies that travel through the blood vessels and the activation of T cells all over the body. This double-pronged immune response guarantees protection against both mucosal and systemic pathogens [89].

Need for Targeting Mucosal Surfaces in Preventing Infectious Diseases

Various essential elements make it imperative to focus on protecting mucosal surfaces from infectious diseases. These are the most common entry points for the majority of pathogens, such as the respiratory, urogenital, and gut tracts [90]. Therefore, controlling infection at these sites is critical to lessening disease prevalence and managing outbreaks. Moreover, mucosal immunity seems to be an effective way of defending against the pathogens that are encountered on these surfaces, thus emphasizing the need for immune response stimulation in these areas [91].

There are other advantages to mucosal vaccination over systemic vaccination, such as the generation of IgA antibodies and the possibility of cross-protection against related pathogens. Robust, long-lasting immune responses can be mounted by vaccines specifically delivered at mucosal surfaces that would afford protection from both mucosal and systemic infections. For global health security to be enhanced and for impacts of emerging or pandemic pathogens to be mitigated, infectious diseases must be stopped by targeting mucosal surfaces [92].

Examples of Successful Mucosal Vaccines

Several successful mucosal vaccines have been developed, demonstrating the efficacy of targeting mucosal surfaces in preventing infectious diseases.

Oral Polio Vaccine (OPV)

OPV is one of the most efficacious mucosal vaccines and has been effective in protecting against poliovirus infections. When administered by mouth, OPV causes both systemic and mucosal immune responses, resulting in a high level of immunity in the gut. OPV contributed significantly to global eradication campaigns against poliovirus, which greatly reduced the occurrence of polio worldwide [93, 94].

Rotavirus Vaccine

Rotarix and RotaTeq are examples of rotavirus vaccines given orally to protect against the disease, which is the main cause of severe diarrhea among newborns and infants. They stimulate immune responses in the gut mucosa, preventing infection by rotavirus and lowering the intensity of diarrhea illness. Consequently, there has been a large global decrease in morbidity and mortality relating to rotavirus on account of vaccination [93, 95].

Intranasal Influenza Vaccine (FluMist)

FluMist is a live attenuated influenza vaccine given through the nose to cause the immune system in the respiratory tract to react. It also triggers a response from the mucous membrane and other parts of the body to protect against strains of flu. Children and adults have been proven to avoid Influenza, which is considered an alternative to injectable influenza vaccines when taking FluMist [96, 97].

Oral Cholera Vaccine (OCV)

Dukoral and Shanchol are some examples of oral cholera vaccines that are taken through the mouth to prevent cholera infection. The vaccines result in mucosal responses taking place within the gastrointestinal tract, including the production of secretory IgA antibodies against Vibrio cholerae. Oral cholera vaccines have been used for interventions during outbreaks of cholera, thereby contributing to the reduction in its prevalence in endemic areas [98, 99].

Intranasal COVID-19 Vaccines

Numerous COVID-19 vaccines, which can be administered through the nose, are in development or under investigation in clinical studies. Such vaccines are aimed at inducing mucosal immunity that shields against SARS-CoV-2 infection and transmission *via* the respiratory tract. The intranasal COVID-19 vaccines could work alongside current injections and strengthen the protective effect of the mucosal immune system against the virus [100, 101].

MUCOSAL VACCINE DELIVERY SYSTEMS

Mucosal vaccine delivery systems are fabricated to deliver antigens to mucosal surfaces, such as respiratory, gastrointestinal, and urogenital tracts, and induce immune responses to protect against infectious diseases. (Fig. **3**) represents common mucosal vaccine delivery systems.

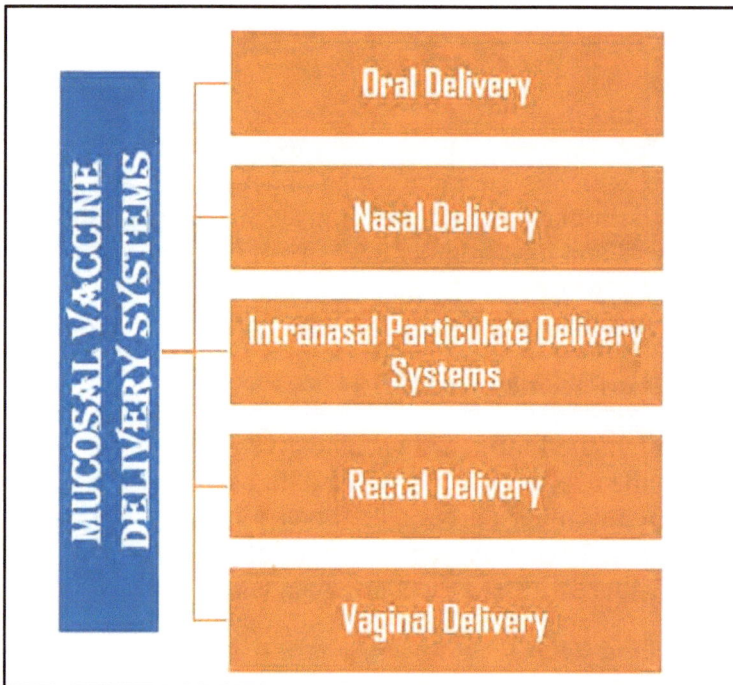

Fig. (3). Mucosal vaccine delivery systems.

Oral Delivery

Oral vaccines are administered by mouth and target the mucosal surfaces of the gastrointestinal tract. They can be in liquid form, as tablets or capsules containing antigenic proteins or live attenuated pathogens. Oral delivery has many benefits, such as ease of administration, patient compliance, and the potential for mass vaccination campaigns. Examples are oral polio vaccine (OPV), oral cholera vaccine (OCV), and oral rotavirus vaccine [102].

Nasal Delivery

These nasal vaccines are given intranasally to target the respiratory tract's mucosal surfaces. Such vaccines can be supplied as aqueous sprays, droplets, or powders that hold antigenic proteins or live attenuated pathogens. Nasal administration is advantageous due to its swift absorption through the nasal mucosa, which also induces both mucosal and systemic immune responses apart from being needle-free. Some instances include intranasal influenza vaccine (FluMist) and intranasal COVID-19 vaccines [103].

Intranasal Particulate Delivery Systems

Intranasal particulate delivery systems are based on a variety of particulate carriers, such as liposomes, nanoparticles, and microparticles, that serve as delivery vehicles for encapsulating proteins or DNA vaccines that can be delivered *via* the nasal route. These agents safeguard antigens from being destroyed, improve their movement across mucus membranes, and stimulate their intake by mucosal immune cells. They offer advantages such as controlled antigen release, better immunogenicity, and potential for use as mucosal adjuvants [104, 105].

Vaginal Delivery

The mucosa of the female reproductive tract is targeted by intravaginal administration of vaginal vaccines. These vaccines can take the form of gels, creams, or suppositories containing antigenic proteins or DNA vaccines. Due to the induction of local immune responses in genital mucosa and the likelihood of safeguarding against sexually transmitted infections, vaginal delivery is beneficial. For instance, there are experimental vaccines for human papillomavirus (HPV) and herpes simplex virus (HSV) [106, 107].

Rectal Delivery

Rectal vaccines are given through the rectum to target the mucous membrane surfaces of the lower parts of the gastrointestinal tract. These vaccines can be suppositories or enemas containing antigenic proteins or live attenuated pathogens. Some of the benefits associated with rectal administration include inducing mucosal and systemic immune responses, the potential for no needles, and improved patient adherence. Some examples include HIV experimental vaccines and those that combat enteric viral infections [108].

Challenges in Mucosal Vaccine Delivery

Mucosal vaccine delivery faces many barriers that must be traversed to ensure the development of efficacious vaccines. A major obstacle is overcoming the protective barriers at mucosal surfaces, such as mucus layers and epithelial cell linings, that may obstruct the penetration of vaccine antigens [109]. Another crucial challenge is the maintenance of antigen stability and activity during storage and administration due to their vulnerability to conditions like pH variations and enzymatic degradation typical for mucosal vaccines. Furthermore, achieving sufficient immunogenicity is also a challenge, mainly due to antigens that can confer weak mucosal immune responses. This is because of the mucosal surface area variability and its non-uniform tolerance to various delivery approaches, thereby rendering it difficult to establish appropriate dosages and routes of administration for mucosal vaccines. Besides, there are additional hurdles like regulatory concerns and modes of suppression of mucosal immunity that should be carefully thought out during vaccine development. Finally, the translation of preclinical discoveries to clinical practice calls for a rigorous examination in human trials that entails logistic and ethical intricacies. Meeting these difficulties requires pioneering ways, strong research drives, and collaborations with stakeholders to unleash the potential of mucosal vaccines against infections and global health progress [110, 111].

Strategies to Enhance Mucosal Vaccine Efficacy

To improve the effectiveness of mucosal vaccines, it is necessary to take into account all aspects of mucosal immune response. The best way to do this is to increase antigen delivery efficiency as it counteracts strong opposition of mucus layers or epithelial cell linings found in the mucosae. Among them are different types of particulate carriers, such as liposomes and nanoparticles, which are able not only to stabilize antigens but also better their penetration through these barriers, making vaccines more accessible for presentation by cells responsible for immunity in mucosal tissues [112].

Furthermore, the use of additives may also enhance mucosal vaccine immunogenicity. Adjuvants chosen with care can trigger regional immunity, help capture antigens, and produce cytokines essential for effective immune response stimulation. Important are those adjuvants that can change mucosal defenses against infection without causing too much inflammation at the same time [113].

To enhance the efficacy of mucosal vaccines, these could be directed towards specific sites. This involves making vaccine formulations and delivery routes correspond with the anatomical location of the pathogens being targeted so as to optimize their uptake and effectiveness in preventing infections. Another strategy may be to investigate live attenuated vaccines, which mimic natural infections, thereby provoking wide-ranging immunization that lasts for a long time on mucous membranes [114].

Strategies for improving the effectiveness of mucosal vaccines also encompass provoking the secretion of IgA that neutralizes pathogens at mucosal surfaces. Robust secretory IgA responses can be triggered by vaccines that are designed in a way that directs them toward lymphoid tissues associated with mucosa and induces class switching to IgA [115].

In addition, combination vaccines targeting multiple pathogens or antigens at once stimulate the immune system to provide protection against a number of different diseases. The challenge now is to integrate these approaches into the development and clinical testing of mucosal vaccines so that they can induce stronger immunity in mucosal surfaces, which will help prevent many types of infections [116].

Development of Mucosal Vaccines

Vaccine Development Process for Mucosal Vaccines

The production of mucosal vaccines undergoes a progression similar to that of conventional vaccine development but with particular features designed to target the mucosal aspects. Below is an overview of the vaccine development process for mucosal vaccines.

Antigen Selection

It is necessary to determine the right antigens for a particular pathogen in the same way traditional vaccines do. In order to stimulate protective immune responses on mucosal surfaces, antigens should be conserved and immunogenic [117].

Formulation Design

Vaccine delivery to mucosal surfaces requires an optimized formulation to increase antigen immunogenicity and delivery to mucosal surfaces. This entails selecting suitable adjuvants, carriers, and delivery systems that will improve antigen stability, immune activation, and penetration through the mucosa [118].

Preclinical Evaluation

Preclinical studies involve testing candidate vaccines on animals to determine their safety, efficacy, and immunogenicity. Through these studies, researchers can determine which vaccines have the potential for further development, refine formulation strategies, and better understand the immune mechanisms that underlie mucosal protection [119].

Clinical Trials

Potential vaccines are tested on animals before being administered to humans to ascertain their safety, immunogenicity, and efficacy. Human clinical trials usually have three phases: phase I, II, and III, each focusing on distinct aspects of vaccine development. These include dose escalation, immunogenicity assessment, and large-scale efficacy trials [120].

Regulatory Approval

This enables the successful completion of clinical trials, which lead to government agencies' regulatory review and approval, such as the FDA or EMA. Regulatory approval ensures that mucosal vaccines meet stringent safety, efficacy, and manufacturing standards prior to licensing for public use [121].

Manufacturing Scale-up

Upon regulators' approval, manufacturing procedures are upscaled to enable mass production of mucosal vaccines. To meet global demands, this includes optimizing production methods, ensuring uniformity in immunization qualities, and establishing tough quality control measures [122].

Post-marketing Surveillance

Post-licensure mucosal vaccines undergo post-marketing surveillance to monitor their long-term safety, effectiveness, and adverse event reporting in the real world. Surveillance systems help identify rare or unexpected adverse events and guide continuous vaccine safety monitoring efforts [123].

Global Distribution and Access

Mucosal vaccines are distributed worldwide through vaccination campaigns, public health initiatives, and international partnerships to ensure global reach. To increase vaccine access, they aim to work with governments, NGOs, and international agencies to promote equity in distribution and coverage [124, 125].

Preclinical and Clinical Studies of Mucosal Vaccines

In the development of these vaccines, preclinical and clinical assessment is an extremely important stage aimed at determining their safety, immunogenicity as well as efficacy prior to experimental formulations that could be moved into possible public health interventions. Animal models are employed in evaluating candidate mucosal vaccines through preclinical studies to determine their profile in terms of immunogenicity, safety, and potential protective efficacy. These studies are very useful when it comes to vaccine dosing, optimizing formulation, and understanding immune mechanisms associated with mucosal protection. Moreover, preclinical assessment helps to identify prospective vaccine candidates for human clinical trials [126].

Mucosal vaccines in human clinical trials are categorized into phases I, II, and III, which serve specific roles in the evaluation of vaccine immunogenicity, safety, and efficacy. Phase I studies mainly focus on evaluating the vaccine's tolerability and safety using a few healthy volunteers, as well as immune responses and dosage regimens that would be optimal. Phase II trials increase population sizes to expand safety and test for immunogenicity in larger groups, as well as to begin dose-ranging studies and alternative administration routes. Phase three trials consist of large-scale efficacy studies performed in populations at risk from diseases aimed at showing that these vaccines provide defense against infection or lower disease severity compared with the control group. These investigations yield crucial information regarding vaccination's efficiency, actual-world effectiveness, and safety record, hence helping regulatory bodies make decisions concerning licensing and implementation requirements [127].

There is a significant focus on issues of safety, adverse event reporting, and ethical concerns in the course of preclinical and clinical trials aimed at protecting the welfare of study subjects. Moreover, characterizing vaccine-induced immune responses by biomarker analysis and immune correlates of protection are valuable tools for assessing their efficacy. Suppose a successful completion of the preclinical and clinical stages is achieved. In that case, it not only shows that mucosal vaccines are safe but also allows them to be approved by regulatory authorities and manufactured for global distribution, especially in combating infectious diseases, thereby improving public health globally [128].

Regulatory Considerations and Challenges

Mucosal vaccine development must navigate a complex regulatory environment, taking into account specific issues and problems unique to directing the vaccine at mucosal surfaces. Below, we elaborate on the regulatory considerations and challenges.

Regulatory Considerations

Safety Assessment

In vaccine development, regulatory bodies prioritize safety. In the case of mucosal vaccines, safety evaluation has to consider possible mucosal administration-associated hazards that include local inflammation, disruption of the integrity of the mucosal barrier, and systemic adverse events. Extensive preclinical studies and clinical trials are mandatory for a thorough assessment of vaccine safety profiles.

Immunogenicity Evaluation

For regulatory approval, it is necessary to show that mucosal vaccines can elicit strong and long-lasting immune responses in the surfaces of these tissues. Immunogenicity evaluations should also incorporate estimations of antibodies both within the mucosal plane as well as at systemic levels. Uniform tests for appraising the state of immunity in mucosa may be considered to ensure uniformity and comparability across various experimental systems [129].

Efficacy Determination

Regulatory agencies demand evidence of vaccine efficacy before licenses are granted. Clinical trials are conducted on these vaccines to show that they can prevent infection, reduce the severity of disease, or stop transmission at mucosal sites. To ensure reliable safety assessments, it is advisable to carefully consider endpoint selection, study design, and statistical analysis plans.

Quality and Manufacturing Standards

To make mucosal vaccines that are safe, effective, and consistent, there is a need to comply with good manufacturing practices (GMP) and have stringent quality control measures in place. Vaccine manufacturers have to design strong manufacturing processes, conduct thorough quality assessments, and keep comprehensive records for regulatory standards to be met.

Clinical Trial Design and Ethics

The protocol may need a thorough review before any regulatory body gives its approval to clinical trials. Thus, there is a strong need for the design of clinical trials that must take into account some dosing regimens, participant selection criteria, and endpoints relevant to mucosal vaccine safety and efficacy. Concerns on ethical issues include informed consent procedures, risk-benefit assessments, and protection of vulnerable populations [130].

Regulatory Challenges

Complexity of Mucosal Immunity

Designing appropriate endpoints and evaluating vaccine efficacy is difficult because of the complexities of understanding mucosal immune responses. The interdisciplinary nature of standardizing assays for measuring mucosal immune responses and establishing correlates of protection can necessitate joint research by many scientists and consensus building with regulatory agencies.

Sampling and Assay Standardization

Variability in sampling methods, sample processing techniques, and assay protocols can complicate the determination of mucosal immune responses. Standardizing sampling procedures, assay protocols, and validation standards is crucial to ensure the homogeneity and reliability of immunogenicity data collected from different labs [131].

Lack of Regulatory Guidelines

The absence of particular regulations for mucosal vaccines may raise doubts and delay regulatory consent. Safety, immunogenicity, efficacy, and manufacturing issues pertaining to mucosal vaccines should be addressed by regulatory agencies through clear and comprehensive guidelines.

Risk-Benefit Assessment

Deliberate balancing of the risks and gains of mucosal vaccines, especially in vulnerable populations, demands critical thought about factors like age, health status, and possible vaccine-attributable adverse events. For them to make regulatory decisions that will enable the safe and effective use of these mucosal vaccines, regulatory agencies must conduct robust risk-benefit assessments [132].

CHALLENGES AND FUTURE DIRECTIONS

In the field of mucosal vaccination, there are several challenges, including antigen selection and formulation complexities, that need to be addressed. It is indeed a daunting task to strategically identify antigens that can induce strong immune responses at the mucosal surface while providing multiple defenses against diverse pathogens. Additionally, there is an ongoing challenge of optimizing vaccine formulations for improved antigen stability, mucosal penetration, and immunogenicity [133].

However, with difficulties come chances for innovation and betterment. Advanced delivery systems like nanoparticles-based carriers and adjuvants for the mucosal hold good promise for enhancing vaccine efficacy and (for) modulation of immune responses. Additionally, new vaccine platforms such as viral vectors and mRNA can potentially advance the development and deployment of mucosal vaccines faster.

In the future, mucosal vaccines will be an encouraging therapy for handling new and widespread types of diseases. By using different strategies that are pioneering and global cooperation, all these vaccine types can avail the chance to protect many people, decrease response period, and thus improve public health in light of changing infectious disease threats. Ongoing research activities should help to deal with remaining gaps, take advantage of emerging prospects, or any other opportunity to realize mucosal immunization potentials as a way of maintaining global health.

CONCLUSION

This chapter has extensively analyzed mucosal vaccination as an intervention for emerging and pandemic infectious diseases. Additionally, it has highlighted the complex issues surrounding antigen selection and formulation while at the same time emphasizing new avenues for vaccine development. The key importance of mucosal vaccination in public health strategies is to help block pathogens at their points of entry, thereby providing better protection than traditional vaccines do. Incorporating mucosal vaccination into immunization programs will improve vaccine coverage, lessen disease burden, and strengthen global health security. In order to further mucosal vaccination, more research work is needed. This encompasses antigen identification improvement, formulation optimization, and delivery system innovation. Mucosal immune response comprehension and the development of pathogen-specific vaccines are crucial areas for exploration. By any measure, mucosal vaccination represents a major advance in the fight against infectious diseases, with better public health outcomes promised through scientific innovation and cooperation efforts.

ACKNOWLEDGEMENTS

Authors are highly thankful to their Universities/Colleges for providing library facilities for the literature survey.

REFERENCES

[1]   Russell M. Mucosal Immunology (Fourth Edition) [Internet]. 2015.

[2]   Pavot V. New insights in mucosal vaccine development - ScienceDirect. 2012.

[3]   Song Y, Mehl F, Zeichner SL. Vaccine Strategies to Elicit Mucosal Immunity. Vaccines. Multidisciplinary Digital Publishing Institute (MDPI), 2024; 12.
[http://dx.doi.org/10.3390/vaccines12020191]

[4]   Anggraeni R, Ana ID, Wihadmadyatami H. Development of mucosal vaccine delivery: an overview on the mucosal vaccines and their adjuvants. Clinical and Experimental Vaccine Research. Korean Vaccine Society; 2022; 11, 235–48.

[5]   Holmgren J, Czerkinsky C. Mucosal immunity and vaccines. Nat Med 2005; 11(S4) (Suppl.): S45-53.
[http://dx.doi.org/10.1038/nm1213] [PMID: 15812489]

[6]   Ogra PL, Faden H, Welliver RC. Vaccination strategies for mucosal immune responses. Clin Microbiol Rev 2001; 14(2): 430-45.
[http://dx.doi.org/10.1128/CMR.14.2.430-445.2001] [PMID: 11292646]

[7]   Morens DM, Fauci AS. Emerging Pandemic Diseases: How We Got to COVID-19. Cell. Cell Press; 2020; 182, 1077–92.

[8]   Bloom DE, Cadarette D. Infectious disease threats in the twenty-first century: Strengthening the global response. Frontiers in Immunology. Frontiers Media S.A.; 2019; 10.

[9]   Nii-Trebi NI. Emerging and Neglected Infectious Diseases: Insights, Advances, and Challenges. BioMed Research International. Hindawi Limited; 2017.

[10]   McArthur DB. Emerging Infectious Diseases. Nursing Clinics of North America. W.B. Saunders; 2019; 54, 297–311.

[11]   Fauci A. S. 04-1167. 2005.

[12]   Morse SS. Factors in the Emergence of Infectious Diseases. 1995.
[http://dx.doi.org/10.3201/eid0101.950102]

[13]   Zimmermann C. SARS-CoV and MERS-CoV [Internet]. Vol. 39, The Pediatric Infectious Disease Journal. 2020. Available from: www.pidj.com

[14]   Callegari B, Feder C. Entrepreneurship and the systemic consequences of epidemics: A literature review and emerging model. Int Entrep Manage J 2022; 18(4): 1653-84.
[http://dx.doi.org/10.1007/s11365-021-00790-2]

[15]   Willem L, Verelst F, Bilcke J, Hens N, Beutels P. Lessons from a decade of individual-based models for infectious disease transmission: a systematic review (2006-2015). BMC Infect Dis 2017; 17(1): 612.
[http://dx.doi.org/10.1186/s12879-017-2699-8] [PMID: 28893198]

[16]   Barrett R, Kuzawa CW, McDade T, Armelagos GJ. Emerging and re-emerging infectious diseases: the third epidemiologic transition. Annu Rev Anthropol 1998; 27(1): 247-71.
[http://dx.doi.org/10.1146/annurev.anthro.27.1.247]

[17]   Morens DM, Folkers GK, Fauci AS. Emerging infections: a perpetual challenge. Lancet Infect Dis 2008; 8(11): 710-9.
[http://dx.doi.org/10.1016/S1473-3099(08)70256-1] [PMID: 18992407]

[18]   Janes CR, Corbett KK, Jones JH, Trostle J. Emerging infectious diseases: The role of social sciences. The Lancet. Elsevier B.V. 2012; 380: pp. 1884-6.

[19]   Jones KE, Patel NG, Levy MA, *et al.* Global trends in emerging infectious diseases. Nature 2008; 451(7181): 990-3.
[http://dx.doi.org/10.1038/nature06536] [PMID: 18288193]

[20]   Mahajan R, Bakshi S, Chatterjee D, De D, Saikia UN, Handa S. Clinico-Epidemiologic Profile of Non-Syndromic Congenital Ichthyosis – A Retrospective Chart Review of 107 Patients. Indian J Dermatol 2024; 69(2): 113-8. https://journals.lww.com/ijd/Pages/default.aspx
[http://dx.doi.org/10.4103/ijd.ijd_412_23] [PMID: 38841231]

[21]   Reza S, Jangi H, Jangi RH. A Brief Overview of Clinical and Epidemiological Features, Mechanism of Action, and Diagnosis of Novel Global Pandemic Infectious Disease, COVID-19, And its Comparison with Sars, Mers, And H1n1 [Internet]. Vol. 2, World J Clin Med Img. 2023. Available from: https://www.researchgate.net/publication/373757017

[22]   Cunningham AA, Daszak P, Wood JLN. One health, emerging infectious diseases, and wildlife: Two decades of progress?, Philosophical Transactions of the Royal Society B: Biological Sciences. Royal Society; 2017; 372.

[23]   Galán-Huerta KA, Rivas-Estilla AM, Martinez-Landeros EA, Arellanos-Soto D, Ramos-Jiménez J. The Zika virus disease: An overview. Med Univ 2016; 18(71): 115-24.
         [http://dx.doi.org/10.1016/j.rmu.2016.05.003]

[24]   Atif M, Azeem M, Sarwar MR, Bashir A. Zika virus disease: a current review of the literature. Infection. Urban und Vogel GmbH 2016; 44: pp. 695-705.

[25]   Dasti JI. Zika virus infections: An overview of the current scenario. Asian Pacific Journal of Tropical Medicine. Elsevier (Singapore) Pte Ltd; 2016; 9, 621–5.

[26]   Ibrahim NK. Epidemiologic surveillance for controlling Covid-19 pandemic: types, challenges and implications. Journal of Infection and Public Health. Elsevier Ltd; 2020; 13, 1630–8.
         [http://dx.doi.org/10.1016/j.jiph.2020.07.019]

[27]   Malik YS, Kumar N, Sircar S, Kaushik R, Bhat S, Dhama K, *et al*. Coronavirus disease pandemic (Covid-19): Challenges and a global perspective. Pathogens. MDPI AG 2020; 9: pp. 1-31.

[28]   Ghosh S, Bornman C, Zafer MM. Antimicrobial Resistance Threats in the emerging COVID-19 pandemic: Where do we stand? Journal of Infection and Public Health. Elsevier Ltd; 2021; 14, 555–60.

[29]   Abbas J. Crisis management, transnational healthcare challenges and opportunities: The intersection of COVID-19 pandemic and global mental health. Research in Globalization. 2021; 3.

[30]   Marshall JC, Murthy S, Diaz J, Adhikari N, Angus DC, Arabi YM, *et al*. A minimal common outcome measure set for COVID-19 clinical research. The Lancet Infectious Diseases. Lancet Publishing Group 2020; 20: pp. e192-7.

[31]   Haider N, Rothman-Ostrow P, Osman AY, *et al*. COVID-19—Zoonosis or Emerging Infectious Disease? Front Public Health 2020; 8596944
         [http://dx.doi.org/10.3389/fpubh.2020.596944] [PMID: 33324602]

[32]   Chew QH, Wei KC, Vasoo S, Chua HC, Sim K. Narrative synthesis of psychological and coping responses towards emerging infectious disease outbreaks in the general population: Practical considerations for the COVID-19 pandemic. Singapore Medical Journal. Singapore Medical Association; 2020; 61, 350–6.

[33]   Agarwal P, Nieto JJ, Ruzhansky M, Torres DFM, editors. Analysis of Infectious Disease Problems (Covid-19) and Their Global Impact [Internet]. Singapore: Springer Singapore; 2021. (Infosys Science Foundation Series).
         [http://dx.doi.org/10.1007/978-981-16-2450-6]

[34]   Amin Tabish S. COVID-19 pandemic: Emerging perspectives and future trends. Vol. 9. J Public Health Res 2020.

[35]   Madhav N, Oppenheim B, Gallivan M, Mulembakani P, Rubin E, Wolfe N. Pandemics: Risks, Impacts, and Mitigation. In: Disease Control Priorities, Third Edition (Volume 9): Improving Health and Reducing Poverty. The World Bank; 2017. p. 315–45.

[36]   Gupta R, Sheng X, Balcilar M, Ji Q. Time-varying impact of pandemics on global output growth. Finance Res Lett 2021; 41101823
         [http://dx.doi.org/10.1016/j.frl.2020.101823] [PMID: 36568733]

[37]   Patterson GE, McIntyre KM, Clough HE, Rushton J. Societal Impacts of Pandemics: Comparing

COVID-19 With History to Focus Our Response. Front Public Health 2021; 9630449
[http://dx.doi.org/10.3389/fpubh.2021.630449] [PMID: 33912529]

[38]   Sharma SS, Rath BN, Devpura N. Pandemics and their impact on global economic and financial systems. MethodsX. Elsevier B.V. 2021; 8.

[39]   Jamal T, Budke C. Tourism in a world with pandemics: local-global responsibility and action. Journal of Tourism Futures 2020; 6(2): 181-8.
[http://dx.doi.org/10.1108/JTF-02-2020-0014]

[40]   Mascie TN, Pandemics MK. Journal for Peace and Nuclear Disarmament. Routledge 2021; 4: pp. 47-59.

[41]   Gray K, Gills BK, editors. Post-covid transformations. Routledge, Taylor & Francis Group; 2023.
[http://dx.doi.org/10.4324/9781003330752]

[42]   Rombout JHWM, Yang G, Kiron V. Adaptive immune responses at mucosal surfaces of teleost fish. Fish and Shellfish Immunology. Academic Press; 2014; 40, 634–43.
[http://dx.doi.org/10.1016/j.fsi.2014.08.020]

[43]   Duerkop BA, Vaishnava S, Hooper LV. Immune responses to the microbiota at the intestinal mucosal surface. Immunity 2009; 31(3): 368-76.
[http://dx.doi.org/10.1016/j.immuni.2009.08.009] [PMID: 19766080]

[44]   Tomasi TB Jr. Mechanisms of immune regulation at mucosal surfaces. Vol. 5 Suppl 4. Clin Infect Dis 1983; 5 (Suppl. 4): S784-92.
[http://dx.doi.org/10.1093/clinids/5.Supplement_4.S784]

[45]   Russell MW, Ogra PL. Mucosal decisions: tolerance and responsiveness at mucosal surfaces. Immunol Invest 2010; 39(4-5): 297-302.
[http://dx.doi.org/10.3109/08820131003729927] [PMID: 20450281]

[46]   Tlaskalová-Hogenová Ludm ila Tučková Rája Lodinová-Z ˇ H, Renata ˇ těpánková Bozena Cukrow ska David P Funda Ilja Střiž Hana Kozáková Ilja TrebichavskyáTrebichavská Dan Sokol Zuzana R ˇ eháková JiříŠ inkora Petra Fundová Dana Horáková Lenka Jelínková Daniel Sánchez dniková S, Tlaskalová -Hogenová H. M ucosal Im m unit y: It s Role in D ef ense and A llergy [Internet]. Vol. 128, Int Arch Allergy Im m unol. 2002. Available from: www.karger.com/journals/iaa

[47]   Kaetzel CS. The polymeric immunoglobulin receptor: bridging innate and adaptive immune responses at mucosal surfaces. Immunol Rev 2005; 206(1): 83-99.
[http://dx.doi.org/10.1111/j.0105-2896.2005.00278.x] [PMID: 16048543]

[48]   Mayer L. Mucosal Immunity [Internet]. 2003. Available from: https://publications.aap.org/pediatrics/article-abstract/111/Supplement_3/1595/28630/Mucosal-Immunity

[49]   Revaz V. Current Opinion in Immunology [Internet]. 2005. Available from: https://doi.org/./j.coi

[50]   Yuan Q, Walker WA. Innate Immunity of the Gut: Mucosal Defense in Health and Disease [Internet]. 2004. Available from: http://journals.lww.com/jpgn

[51]   Pitman RS, Blumberg RS. First line of defense: the role of the intestinal epithelium as an active component of the mucosal immune system. J Gastroenterol 2000; 35(11): 805-14.
[http://dx.doi.org/10.1007/s005350070017] [PMID: 11085489]

[52]   Perez-Lopez A, Behnsen J, Nuccio SP, Raffatellu M. Mucosal immunity to pathogenic intestinal bacteria Key Points [Internet]. Vol. 16, Nature Reviews Immunology. 2016. Available from: https://www.nature.com/articles/nri.2015.17

[53]   Forchielli ML, Walker WA. The role of gut-associated lymphoid tissues and mucosal defence. Br J Nutr 2005; 93(S1) (Suppl. 1): S41-8.
[http://dx.doi.org/10.1079/BJN20041356] [PMID: 15877894]

[54]   Griffin AJ, McSorley SJ. Development of protective immunity to Salmonella, a mucosal pathogen with a systemic agenda. Mucosal Immunology. Nature Publishing Group 2011; 4: pp. 371-82.

[55] Belyakov IM, Ahlers JD. What role does the route of immunization play in the generation of protective immunity against mucosal pathogens? J Immunol 2009; 183(11): 6883-92.
[http://dx.doi.org/10.4049/jimmunol.0901466] [PMID: 19923474]

[56] Kaiserlian D, Cerf-Bensussan N, Hosmalin A. The mucosal immune system: from control of inflammation to protection against infections. J Leukoc Biol 2005; 78(2): 311-8.
[http://dx.doi.org/10.1189/jlb.0105053] [PMID: 15894590]

[57] Soloff AC, Barratt-Boyes SM. Enemy at the gates: dendritic cells and immunity to mucosal pathogens. Cell Res 2010; 20(8): 872-85.
[http://dx.doi.org/10.1038/cr.2010.94] [PMID: 20603644]

[58] Dharmani P, Srivastava V, Kissoon-Singh V, Chadee K. Role of intestinal mucins in innate host defense mechanisms against pathogens 2009.
[http://dx.doi.org/10.1159/000163037]

[59] Aich P, Dwivedy . Importance of innate mucosal immunity and the promises it holds. Int J Gen Med 2011; (Apr): 299.
[http://dx.doi.org/10.2147/IJGM.S17525]

[60] Brandtzaeg P. Mucosal immunity: induction, dissemination, and effector functions. Scand J Immunol 2009; 70(6): 505-15.
[http://dx.doi.org/10.1111/j.1365-3083.2009.02319.x] [PMID: 19906191]

[61] Turula H, Wobus CE. The role of the polymeric immunoglobulin receptor and secretory immunoglobulins during mucosal infection and immunity. Viruses. MDPI AG 2018; 10.

[62] Belyakov IM, Ahlers JD. What role does the route of immunization play in the generation of protective immunity against mucosal pathogens? J Immunol 2009; 183(11): 6883-92.
[http://dx.doi.org/10.4049/jimmunol.0901466] [PMID: 19923474]

[63] Li Y, Jin L, Chen T, Pirozzi CJ. The Effects of Secretory IgA in the Mucosal Immune System. BioMed Research International. Hindawi Limited 2020; 2020.

[64] Zuercher AW, Jiang HQ, Thurnheer MC, Cuff CF, Cebra JJ. Distinct mechanisms for cross-protection of the upper versus lower respiratory tract through intestinal priming. J Immunol 2002; 169(7): 3920-5.
[http://dx.doi.org/10.4049/jimmunol.169.7.3920] [PMID: 12244191]

[65] Hasegawa H, van Reit E, Kida H. Mucosal immunization and adjuvants. Curr Top Microbiol Immunol 2014; 386: 371-80.
[http://dx.doi.org/10.1007/82_2014_402] [PMID: 25015787]

[66] Zuercher AW, Jiang HQ, Thurnheer MC, Cuff CF, Cebra JJ. Distinct mechanisms for cross-protection of the upper versus lower respiratory tract through intestinal priming. J Immunol 2002; 169(7): 3920-5.
[http://dx.doi.org/10.4049/jimmunol.169.7.3920] [PMID: 12244191]

[67] Wang Y, Jiang B, Guo Y, *et al.* Cross-protective mucosal immunity mediated by memory Th17 cells against Streptococcus pneumoniae lung infection. Mucosal Immunol 2017; 10(1): 250-9.
[http://dx.doi.org/10.1038/mi.2016.41] [PMID: 27118490]

[68] Jiang J, Zhang H, He W, *et al.* Adhesion of Microdroplets on Water-Repellent Surfaces toward the Prevention of Surface Fouling and Pathogen Spreading by Respiratory Droplets. ACS Appl Mater Interfaces 2017; 9(7): 6599-608.
[http://dx.doi.org/10.1021/acsami.6b15213] [PMID: 28121417]

[69] Frankel SJ, Conforti C, Hillman J, *et al.* Phytophthora introductions in restoration areas: Responding to protect California native flora from human-assisted pathogen spread. Forests 2020; 11(12): 1291.
[http://dx.doi.org/10.3390/f11121291]

[70] Ahmad MDF, Wahab S, Ali Ahmad F, Intakhab Alam M, Ather H, Siddiqua A, *et al.* A novel

perspective approach to explore pros and cons of face mask in prevention the spread of SARS-CoV-2 and other pathogens. Saudi Pharmaceutical Journal. Elsevier B.V. 2021; 29: pp. 121-33.

[71]   Landelle C, Pagani L, Harbarth S. Is patient isolation the single most important measure to prevent the spread of multidrug-resistant pathogens?. 2013.
[http://dx.doi.org/10.4161/viru.22641]

[72]   Steinbrink K, Wölfl M, Jonuleit H, Knop J, Enk AH. Induction of tolerance by IL-10-treated dendritic cells. J Immunol 1997; 159(10): 4772-80.
[http://dx.doi.org/10.4049/jimmunol.159.10.4772] [PMID: 9366401]

[73]   Nowak-Węgrzyn A, Chatchatee P. Mechanisms of Tolerance Induction. Ann Nutr Metab 2017; 70(2) (Suppl. 2): 7-24.
[http://dx.doi.org/10.1159/000457915] [PMID: 28521317]

[74]   Linda SC, *et al.* 123Library_ Aeroallergen and Food Immunotherapy, An Issue of Immunology and Allergy Clinics of North America. E-Book 2016.

[75]   Elias PM. The skin barrier as an innate immune element. Semin Immunopathol 2007; 29(1): 3-14.
[http://dx.doi.org/10.1007/s00281-007-0060-9] [PMID: 17621950]

[76]   Andrew Kiboneka . Principals of innate and adaptive immunity. Immunity to microbes & fundamental concepts in immunology. World Journal of Advanced Research and Reviews 2021; 10(3): 188-97.
[http://dx.doi.org/10.30574/wjarr.2021.10.3.0271]

[77]   Andrew Kiboneka . Principals of innate and adaptive immunity. Immunity to microbes & fundamental concepts in immunology. World Journal of Advanced Research and Reviews 2021; 10(3): 188-97.
[http://dx.doi.org/10.30574/wjarr.2021.10.3.0271]

[78]   Kim DH, Ewbank JJ. Signaling in the innate immune response. WormBook 2018; 2018: 1-35.
[http://dx.doi.org/10.1895/wormbook.1.83.2] [PMID: 26694508]

[79]   Giacomo Z. Fish defenses. Science Publishers 2009.

[80]   Martin N. Protective mechanisms of the body - ScienceDirect. 2006.

[81]   Diamond G, Beckloff N, Weinberg A, Kisich KO. The Roles of Antimicrobial Peptides in Innate Host Defense [Internet]. 2009. Available from: http://www.bbcm.univ.

[82]   Dedieu-Engelmann L. Contagious bovine pleuropneumonia: A rationale for the development of a mucosal sub-unit vaccine. Comp Immunol Microbiol Infect Dis 2008; 31(2-3): 227-38.
[http://dx.doi.org/10.1016/j.cimid.2007.07.009] [PMID: 17706775]

[83]   Aldovini A. Mucosal Vaccination for Prevention of HIV Infection and AIDS_ Ingenta Connect. 2016.

[84]   Kozlowski PA, Mantis NJ, Frey A. Editorial: Mucosal Vaccination: Strategies to Induce and Evaluate Mucosal Immunity. Frontiers in Immunology. Frontiers Media S.A. 2022; 13.

[85]   Highton AJ, Girardin A, Bell GM, Hook SM, Kemp RA. Chitosan gel vaccine protects against tumour growth in an intracaecal mouse model of cancer by modulating systemic immune responses. BMC Immunol 2016; 17(1): 39.
[http://dx.doi.org/10.1186/s12865-016-0178-4] [PMID: 27756214]

[86]   Shahiwala A, Vyas T, Amiji M. Nanocarriers for systemic and mucosal vaccine delivery. Recent Pat Drug Deliv Formul 2007; 1(1): 1-9.
[http://dx.doi.org/10.2174/187221107779814140] [PMID: 19075870]

[87]   Kour P, Rath G, Sharma G, Goyal AK. Recent advancement in nanocarriers for oral vaccination. 2018.
[http://dx.doi.org/10.1080/21691401.2018.1533842]

[88]   Crothers JW, Ross Colgate E, Cowan KJ, *et al.* Intradermal fractional-dose inactivated polio vaccine (fIPV) adjuvanted with double mutant Enterotoxigenic Escherichia coli heat labile toxin (dmLT) is well-tolerated and augments a systemic immune response to all three poliovirus serotypes in a randomized placebo-controlled trial. Vaccine 2022; 40(19): 2705-13.

[http://dx.doi.org/10.1016/j.vaccine.2022.03.056] [PMID: 35367069]

[89]   Huang Y, Lu L, Zhao J, Kim SN, Yu WL, Park JY, *et al.* Changes of local microenvironment and systemic immunity after acupuncture stimulation during inflammation: A literature review of animal studies 2023.

[90]   Lavelle EC, Ward RW. Mucosal vaccines — fortifying the frontiers. Nature Reviews Immunology. Nature Research 2022; 22: pp. 236-50.

[91]   Baker JR Jr, Farazuddin M, Wong PT, O'Konek JJ. The unfulfilled potential of mucosal immunization. J Allergy Clin Immunol 2022; 150(1): 1-11.
[http://dx.doi.org/10.1016/j.jaci.2022.05.002] [PMID: 35569567]

[92]   Kelly CG, Medaglini D, Younson JS, Pozzi G. Biotechnological approaches to fight pathogens at mucosal sites. Biotechnol Genet Eng Rev 2001; 18(1): 329-47.
[http://dx.doi.org/10.1080/02648725.2001.10648018] [PMID: 11530695]

[93]   Wright PF, Connor RI, Wieland-Alter WF, *et al.* Vaccine-induced mucosal immunity to poliovirus: analysis of cohorts from an open-label, randomised controlled trial in Latin American infants. Lancet Infect Dis 2016; 16(12): 1377-84.
[http://dx.doi.org/10.1016/S1473-3099(16)30169-4] [PMID: 27638357]

[94]   Hird TR, Grassly NC. Systematic review of mucosal immunity induced by oral and inactivated poliovirus vaccines against virus shedding following oral poliovirus challenge. PLoS Pathog 2012; 8(4)e1002599
[http://dx.doi.org/10.1371/journal.ppat.1002599] [PMID: 22532797]

[95]   Michael W. Russell. 4th ed., Mucosal Immunology 2015.https://doi.org/./B

[96]   Barría MI, Garrido JL, Stein C, *et al.* Localized mucosal response to intranasal live attenuated influenza vaccine in adults. J Infect Dis 2013; 207(1): 115-24.
[http://dx.doi.org/10.1093/infdis/jis641] [PMID: 23087433]

[97]   Prosper N. Boyaka main (1). 2020..

[98]   Raymond A. Strikas et al. 5th ed., Principles and Practice of Pediatric Infectious Diseases 2018.https://doi.org/./B

[99]   Thwaites RS, Uruchurtu ASS, Negri VA, *et al.* Early mucosal events promote distinct mucosal and systemic antibody responses to live attenuated influenza vaccine. Nat Commun 2023; 14(1): 8053.
[http://dx.doi.org/10.1038/s41467-023-43842-7] [PMID: 38052824]

[100]   Pilapitiya D, Wheatley AK, Tan HX. Mucosal vaccines for SARS-CoV-2: triumph of hope over experience. Vol. 92, eBioMedicine. Elsevier B.V.; 2023.

[101]   Song KR, Lim JK, Park SE, Saluja T, Cho S. Il, Wartel TA Oral cholera vaccine efficacy and effectiveness. Vaccines. MDPI 2021; 9.

[102]   Nagler C, *et al.* Cancer Immunotherapy. 2nd ed., 2013.https://doi.org/./B

[103]   Feng F, Wen Z, Chen J, Yuan Y, Wang C, Sun C. Strategies to Develop a Mucosa-Targeting Vaccine against Emerging Infectious Diseases. Viruses 2022; 14(3): 520.
[http://dx.doi.org/10.3390/v14030520] [PMID: 35336927]

[104]   Zhang Y. Advanced oral vaccine delivery strategies for improving the immunity - ScienceDirect. 2021.

[105]   Corthésy B, Bioley G. Lipid-based particles: Versatile delivery systems for mucosal vaccination against infection. Frontiers in Immunology. Frontiers Media S.A. 2018; 9.

[106]   Hannah M. VanBenschoten Vaginal delivery of vaccines - ScienceDirect. 2021.

[107]   Anggraeni R, Ana ID, Wihadmadyatami H. Development of mucosal vaccine delivery: an overview on the mucosal vaccines and their adjuvants. 2022.

[108] Kammona O. Recent advances in nanocarrier-based mucosal delivery of biomolecules - ScienceDirect. 2012.

[109] Newsted D. Advances and challenges in mucosal adjuvant technology - ScienceDirect. 2015.

[110] Sharma R. Polymer nanotechnology-based approaches in mucosal vaccine delivery_ Challenges and opportunities - ScienceDirect. 2015.

[111] Rosen RS, Yarmush ML. Current Trends in Anti-Aging Strategies. Annual Review of Biomedical Engineering. Annual Reviews Inc. 2023; 25: pp. 363-85.

[112] Fukuyama Y, Tokuhara D, Kataoka K, *et al.* Novel vaccine development strategies for inducing mucosal immunity. Expert Rev Vaccines 2012; 11(3): 367-79.
[http://dx.doi.org/10.1586/erv.11.196]

[113] Li M, Wang Y, Sun Y, Cui H, Zhu SJ, Qiu HJ. Mucosal vaccines: Strategies and challenges. Immunology Letters. Elsevier B.V. 2020; 217: pp. 116-25.

[114] Lycke N. Recent progress in mucosal vaccine development: potential and limitations. Nat Rev Immunol 2012; 12(8): 592-605.
[http://dx.doi.org/10.1038/nri3251] [PMID: 22828912]

[115] Longet S, Lundahl MLE, Lavelle EC. Targeted Strategies for Mucosal Vaccination. 2018.
[http://dx.doi.org/10.1021/acs.bioconjchem.7b00738]

[116] Chadwick S, Kriegel C, Amiji M. Delivery strategies to enhance mucosal vaccination. Expert Opin Biol Ther 2009; 9(4): 427-40.
[http://dx.doi.org/10.1517/14712590902849224] [PMID: 19344280]

[117] Mcghee JR, George-Chandy A, Holmgren J, Kieny MP, Fujiyashi K, Mestecky JF, Cecil Czerkinsky Fabienne Anjuere. 1999.

[118] Azegami T, Kiyono H. The Mucosal Immune System for Vaccine Development Aayam Lamichhane [Internet]. 2014. Available from: https://www.elsevier.com/open-access/userlicense/1.0/

[119] Wilkhu J, McNeil SE, Kirby DJ, Perrie Y. Formulation design considerations for oral vaccines. 2011.
[http://dx.doi.org/10.4155/tde.11.82]

[120] Pavot V. New insights in mucosal vaccine development - ScienceDirect. 2012.

[121] Li. M. Mucosal vaccines_ Strategies and challenges - ScienceDirect. 2020.

[122] Chen H. Recent advances in mucosal vaccine development - ScienceDirect. 2000.

[123] Kiyono H, Azegami T. The mucosal immune system: From dentistry to vaccine development. Vol. 91, Proceedings of the Japan Academy Series B: Physical and Biological Sciences. Japan Academy; 2015. p. 423–39.

[124] Ogra PL, Faden H, Welliver RC. Vaccination strategies for mucosal immune responses. Clin Microbiol Rev 2001; 14(2): 430-45.
[http://dx.doi.org/10.1128/CMR.14.2.430-445.2001] [PMID: 11292646]

[125] Hellfritzsch M, Scherließ R. Mucosal vaccination *via* the respiratory tract. Pharmaceutics MDPI AG. 2019; 11.

[126] Lavelle EC, Ward RW. Mucosal vaccines — fortifying the frontiers. Nature Reviews Immunology. Nature Research 2022; 22: pp. 236-50.

[127] Li M, Wang Y, Sun Y, Cui H, Zhu SJ, Qiu HJ. Mucosal vaccines: Strategies and challenges. Immunology Letters. Elsevier B.V. 2020; 217: pp. 116-25.

[128] Moore AC, Dora EG, Peinovich N, Tucker KP, Lin K, Cortese M, *et al.* Pre-clinical studies of a recombinant adenoviral mucosal vaccine to prevent SARS-CoV-2 infection. 2020.
[http://dx.doi.org/10.1101/2020.09.04.283853]

[129] Narag A. Pharmaceutical Development and Regulatory Considerations for Nanoparticles and Nanoparticulate Drug Delivery Systems - ScienceDirect. 2013.

[130] Shankar G, Shores E, Wagner C, Mire-Sluis A. Scientific and regulatory considerations on the immunogenicity of biologics. Trends Biotechnol 2006; 24(6): 274-80.
[http://dx.doi.org/10.1016/j.tibtech.2006.04.001] [PMID: 16631266]

[131] Taeihagh A, Ramesh M, Howlett M. Assessing the regulatory challenges of emerging disruptive technologies. Regul Gov 2021; 15(4): 1009-19.
[http://dx.doi.org/10.1111/rego.12392]

[132] Dwyer JT, Coates PM, Smith MJ. Dietary supplements: Regulatory challenges and research resources. Vol. 10, Nutrients. MDPI AG; 2018.

[133] Mettelman RC, Allen EK, Thomas PG. Mucosal immune responses to infection and vaccination in the respiratory tract. 2022.
[http://dx.doi.org/10.1016/j.immuni.2022.04.013]

CHAPTER 4

Mucosal Vaccination in Veterinary Medicine

Shekhar Singh[1], **Akanksha Sharma**[2], **Shaweta Sharma**[3] and **Akhil Sharma**[2,*]

[1] *Babu Banarasi Das Northern India Institute of Technology, Faculty of Pharmacy, Lucknow, Uttar Pradesh, 226028, India*

[2] *R. J. College of Pharmacy, 2HVJ+567, Raipur, Gharbara, Tappal, Khair, Uttar Pradesh 202165, India*

[3] *School of Medical and Allied Sciences, Galgotias University, Yamuna Expressway, Gautam Buddha Nagar, Uttar Pradesh-201310, India*

Abstract: Mucosal vaccination is emerging as a paradigm shift in veterinary medicine that gives a non-traumatic and efficient way to immunize animals against different infections. Unlike traditional injectable vaccines, mucosal vaccines focus on the mucosal surfaces, which are the preferred entry points for several pathogens. This chapter explains how mucosal immunity works and highlights some ways mucosal vaccination can be done, such as orally, nasally, and sublingually administered routes. All these routes have benefits, such as easy administration, a high chance of compliance, and strong immune responses without injection-related anxieties. The chapter also discusses the contemporary uses of mucosal vaccines in veterinary medicine, emphasizing their successful application in poultry, cattle, and pigs (livestock) and companion animals such as dogs and cats. Mucosal vaccines have several limitations, however, including the need to maintain formulation stability, develop effective delivery systems, and manage immune response variations across various animal species. Furthermore, utmost care is needed to ensure safety, and the possibility of side effects needs to be ensured. Such innovative technologies in vaccine production, such as nanotechnology-based delivery systems, genetic/recombinant vaccines, and new adjuvants, have improved mucosal vaccine efficacy and their range. To address emerging infectious diseases and improve animal health, researchers continue to generate new knowledge through ongoing studies and clinical trials. In conclusion, vaccination *via* the mucosal route represents an important breakthrough in veterinary medicine that could revolutionize animal healthcare with less invasive and highly effective immunization strategies. There is a chance for future advances in this area where integrated vaccination programs or individualized animal healthcare systems would lead to better global welfare of animals.

* **Corresponding author Akhil Sharma:** R. J. College of Pharmacy, 2HVJ+567, Raipur, Gharbara, Tappal, Khair, Uttar Pradesh 202165, India; E-mail: xs2akhil@gmail.com

Shaweta Sharma, Aftab Alam & Akhil Sharma (Eds.)

Keywords: Animal, Biotechnology, Clinical trial, Gut-associated lymphoid tissue, Genetic, Health, Immunity, Livestock, Personalized medicine, Mucosal vaccine, Nasopharynx-associated lymphoid tissue, Oral vaccine, Recombinant, Technology, Veterinary medicine.

INTRODUCTION

Mucosal immunization refers to delivering vaccines through mucosa such as the respiratory, gastrointestinal, and genitourinary tracts. These vaccines are designed to generate immunity at the site of pathogen entry, providing local protection against infections. The mucosal immune system has a key role in protecting the body from pathogens; it includes tissues like Gut Associated Lymphoid Tissues (GALT) and Nasopharynx Associated Lymphoid Tissue (NALT) [1]. They may be delivered by mouth, nose, rectum, or vagina and work by stimulating the mucosal immune response that is characterized by the production of secretory immunoglobulin A (sIgA) antibodies that neutralize pathogens before they can reach deeper tissues [2, 3].

Importance in Veterinary Medicine

Mucosal vaccination is significant in veterinary medicine due to several unique advantages and its critical role in animal health management [4], which is discussed below in detail and summarized in Fig. (**1**).

Enhanced Immune Response

The main advantage of mucosal vaccines is their ability to promote both mucosal and systemic immunity. In contrast, injectable vaccines are designed to promote only systemic immunity. Mucosal vaccines, on the other hand, elicit a strong immune response at the site of infection, unlike traditional injected vaccines, which induce systemic immunity only. This dual effect is especially useful in preventing infections that invade through the respiratory or gastrointestinal systems. For example, oral vaccination against rotavirus can control severe diarrheal outbreaks, reducing animal morbidity and mortality rates [5].

Ease of Administration

It is easier to administer mucosal vaccines than injectable ones, especially in big animals. Oral vaccines can be mixed with feed or water, allowing for a less labor-intensive and more feasible mass vaccination drive. The result is that, in this way, the ease of administration reduces stress for animals and handlers while at the same time increasing compliance and guaranteeing a more uniform vaccine coverage. For instance, nasal vaccines used against respiratory diseases found among cattle and swine have been administered without using needles, hence reducing handling time and related stress [6].

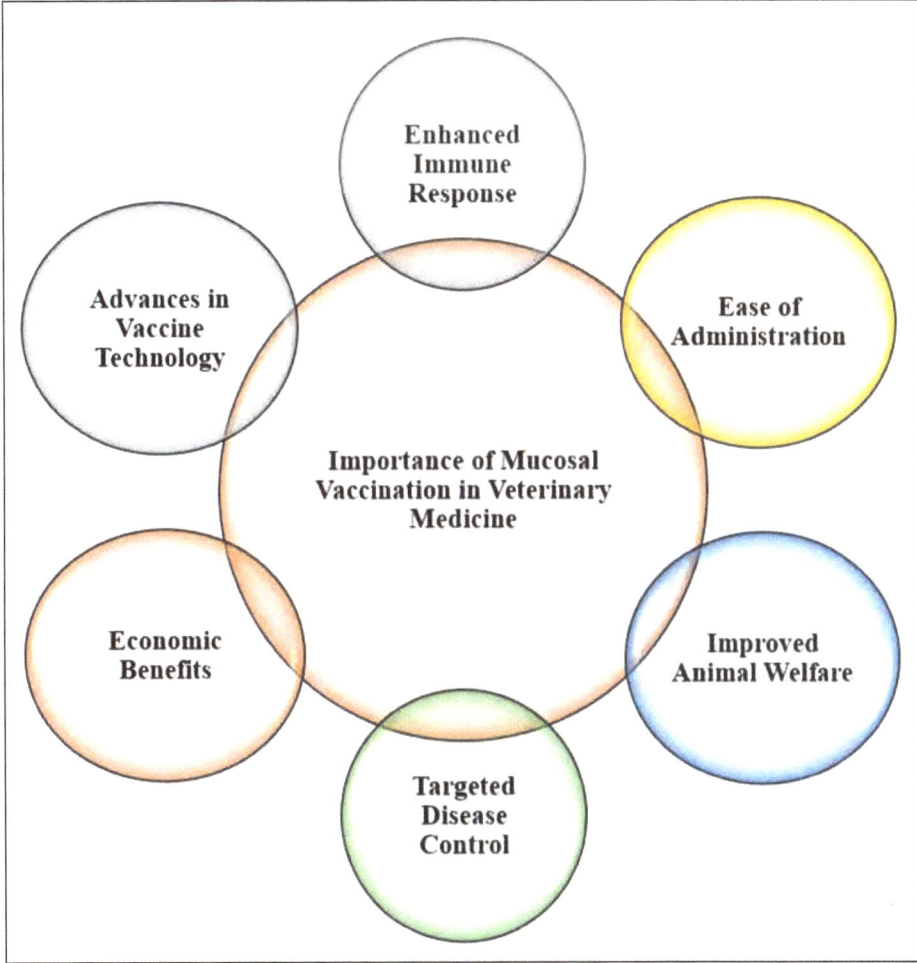

Fig. (1). Importance of mucosal vaccination in veterinary medicine.

Improved Animal Welfare

Mucosal vaccination avoids the use of needles and, therefore, improves animal welfare by eliminating the painful and stressful aspects of injection. This is especially crucial in pets and wild animals, where injecting them is tough and stressful. Unlike restraining the animal for injections, mucosal vaccines are given without it, thus reducing both discomfort and chances of injury to animals or human beings taking care of them. Besides, there are no dangers involved with needle-related diseases such as abscesses or infections [7].

Targeted Disease Control

Mucosal vaccines are specifically effective in diseases that target mucosal surfaces. For example, intranasal vaccines for infectious bovine rhinotracheitis (IBR) provide immunity targeted at the respiratory tract where virus replication occurs initially. This specificity-based method can help reduce the incidence of cases and transmission within herds, thus improving overall herd productivity and health [8].

Economic Benefits

Mucosal vaccination can bring great economic benefits to the livestock sector by enhancing the prevention and control of diseases. This implies that healthier animals will incur lower veterinary costs, have reduced death rates, and increase production. To illustrate, when it comes to poultry farming, higher survivability percentages may be achieved through the use of enteric vaccines administered orally, resulting in more profitable weight gains at the farm level. In terms of preventing outbreaks among livestock while minimizing the use of antibiotics or other drugs in treatment, mucosal vaccines are highly cost-effective [9].

Advances in Vaccine Technology

Lately, vaccine technology has increased the possibility of mucosal vaccination in veterinary medicine. These developments include, but are not limited to, new delivery methods like nanoparticles, recombinant vaccines, and adjuvants, which stimulate immune responses, thereby making them more effective against different diseases. This is also accompanied by an increase in stability and shelf life, thus broadening applicability across diverse veterinary environments [10, 11].

BACKGROUND AND SIGNIFICANCE

History of Vaccination in Veterinary Medicine

Veterinary medical vaccination history is a wealth of stories similar to those of human medicine, which portray scientific advancements and changing knowledge about infectious diseases. The history of vaccination-related to veterinary medicine is summarized in Table **1**.

Table 1. History of vaccination related to veterinary medicine.

Period	Key Developments
18th and 19th Centuries	In early inoculation practices, farmers realized that exposing their animals to less virulent disease could give them immunity. - Edward Jenner's smallpox work affected how veterinarians work [12].
Late 19th Century	**Louis Pasteur's Work:** - Chicken Cholera Vaccine (1879): Developed the first successful live attenuated vaccine for chicken cholera. - Anthrax Vaccine (1881): Sheep public vaccination was carried out effectively [13].
Early 20th Century	- Rabies Vaccine (1885): It was initially tried on dogs before it became crucial in the fight against rabies transmission. - Foot-and-Mouth Disease: First, attempts to prevent epidemics by vaccination [14].
Mid-20th Century	Expansion of mass vaccination campaigns for livestock diseases can improve food security and increase animal health. - Develop vaccines for poultry diseases such as Newcastle disease and Marek's disease [15].
Late 20th Century	**Biotechnology and Molecular Advances:** - Recombinant DNA Technology: Development of genetically modified vaccines for diseases such as rabies and feline leukemia. - Subunit and Conjugate Vaccines: Enhanced safety and efficacy [16].
Modern Era	**Novel Delivery Systems:** Enhance vaccine stability and efficacity through applying nanoparticles and biodegradable polymers [17]. -**One Health Approach**: Strategies for zoonotic disease control. -**Global Disease Eradication**: Success in eradicating diseases like rinderpest (declared eradicated in 2011) [18].

Mucosal Surfaces and their Role in Immunity

Mucosal surfaces are critical to the immune system because they allow pathogens to enter the body. The gastrointestinal, respiratory, and genitourinary tracts are among these surfaces. They are covered in specialized tissues that come into contact with many different types of germs all the time. Therefore, strong and flexible methods must be used by our bodies to stop infections in their tracks. This is where things get interesting. The mucous membrane, also known as GALT or NALT, can start or control immunity responses, which makes them very important [19].

Secretory IgA (sIgA) antibodies characterize mucosal immunity. These antibodies are essential for neutralizing pathogens on the mucosal surfaces before transgressing into deeper tissues and causing systemic infections. For instance, sIgA antibodies link up with and prevent the adherence of pathogens to epithelial cells, thereby preventing their invasion, which is a vital step in many infections. Secondly, there are different types of immune cells on the surfaces of mucus membranes, including dendritic cells, macrophages, and T-cells. These cells interact to detect, capture, and bring antigens to the immune system, which starts an adaptive immune response [20].

Located in the mucosal tissues, dendritic cells are crucial because they collect antigens directly from the mucosal surfaces and move to nearby lymphoid tissues to stimulate T-cells. This leads to the production of particular antibodies and immunological memory, which ensures long-term protection against other species of harmful pathogens. The mucosal surfaces also perform a key role in destroying pathogens after engulfing them, while T-cells regulate immune responses [21].

Mucosal immunization uses the body's natural defense mechanism in epithelial surfaces by directly delivering antigens to these areas. This approach results in local and systemic immune responses that protect against pathogens invading by mucosal routes. They effectively prevent infections at their entry point by stimulating the production of secretory IgA and activating immune cells. It is preferable to use this form of immunization in veterinary medicine because it makes administration easier and enhances compliance compared to traditional injection vaccination techniques [22].

The mucosal surfaces help the immune system protect against infections. They act as an initial barrier by producing sIgA antibodies and activating immune cells that can respond to invading pathogens promptly. This natural defense mechanism during mucosal vaccination boosts immunity against various diseases, emphasizing the significance of maintaining good health *via* mucosal immunity [23].

Comparison with Traditional Vaccination Methods

The aim of mucosal vaccination and traditional vaccination methods, mainly injectable vaccines, is protection against animal diseases. However, they do that through different mechanisms and with various pros and cons. Mucosal vaccines are given *via* mucosal surfaces such as oral, nasal, or intrarectal routes. They provoke local immunity towards mucosal surfaces where most pathogens invade the body when they trigger the production of sIgA antibodies [24].

It neutralizes pathogens at their entry points as a first line of defense and also helps in comprehensive protection by causing systemic immune responses. On the other hand, traditional vaccines are injected intramuscularly, subcutaneously, or intradermally, which primarily induce systemic immunity characterized by circulating IgG antibodies. Usually, traditional vaccines do not elicit strong mucosal immunity, leaving mucosal entry sites less protected [25].

The mucosal vaccine regime is not done by needle, which reduces the suffering of animals while improving animal welfare. This convenience may be especially useful for large groups where it can be supplied through feed, drinking water, or nasal sprays, reducing the chances of needle-related injuries and infections. Traditional vaccines require that an injection be made with a needle; thus stresses and hurts any large animal and requires more labor in vaccinating big numbers together. In addition, there is a possibility of abscesses, infections as well as physical damage caused by needles [26].

By overcoming the natural barriers of the mucosal immune system, Mucosal vaccines provide both local and systemic immunity, which effectively prevents diseases such as respiratory and gastrointestinal infections. Traditional vaccines efficiently control Bloodborne and systemic infections, which give strong system immunities for many diseases as they have been well established over time. Some traditional vaccines can require adjuvants to boost the immune response, causing side effects [27].

Manufacturers create oral vaccines for diseases like rotavirus in livestock and poultry, nasal vaccines for respiratory diseases such as infectious bovine rhinotracheitis (IBR) or Bordetella in dogs, and edible vaccines under development to address various pathogens found in livestock and poultry. Traditional vaccines include injectable ones against rabies, foot-and-mouth disease, and anthrax. These types of vaccines are commonly used on both pet and domesticated animals, such as the distemper vaccine on dogs and feline leukemia vaccination on cats [28].

Therefore, mucosal vaccine formulations must be developed to optimize stability in the mucosal environment, which is not easy and may necessitate special stabilizers or delivery systems. Traditional vaccines are quite stable and easily stored, often requiring refrigeration but nothing beyond standard cold chain practices with set protocols for storage and handling [29].

In terms of cost, mucosal vaccines are inexpensive to administer because they are easier to deliver and do not require as many needles and syringes, so they are a cost-effective way of immunizing livestock and poultry on a large scale. On the other hand, conventional vaccines have known costs, mainly due to needle/syringe costs, but these are affordable, especially when produced in large quantities [30].

Veterinary medicine is an arena where both mucosal and traditional vaccination methods are important, each having advantages and challenges. The administration's convenience, better animal health status, and boosted mucosal immunity make mucosal vaccines ideal for preventing diseases associated with mucosal surfaces. Traditional vaccines, on the other hand, confer effective systemic immunity against a broad spectrum of diseases. The selection between these two approaches primarily hinges on the disease in question, the targeted population, and its level of practicality regarding vaccine delivery and effectiveness [31, 32].

TYPES OF MUCOSAL VACCINES IN VETERINARY MEDICINE

Veterinary medicine uses mucosal vaccines to encourage immune responses on the mucus membranes, consequently providing localized protection against pathogens that gain access to the body through these ways. Hence, diverse types of mucosal vaccines have been developed to fight a range of diseases and species [33]. The common types of mucosal vaccines used in veterinary medicine are described below and summarized in Fig. (2).

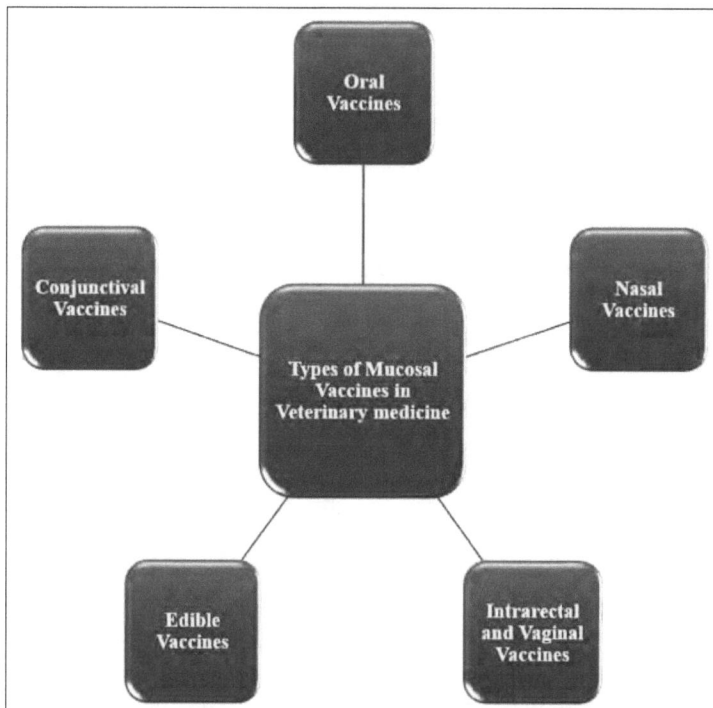

Fig. (2). Types of mucosal vaccines used in veterinary medicine.

Oral Vaccines

Veterinary medicine relies on oral vaccines as indispensable instruments that provide a reliable and suitable way of immunizing animals against different diseases. Oral vaccines can be given orally with food or water, thus providing a noninvasive method of vaccination, which is advantageous in vaccination campaigns targeted at large numbers of animals kept in livestock farms. For example, oral vaccines have effectively controlled poultry diseases like Newcastle, infectious bronchitis, and infectious bursal disease [34].

For example, by-mouth injections have reduced the mortality rate and financial risks for poultry industries globally regarding Newcastle disease. Likewise, oral vaccines have been employed in swine production to fight diseases such as transmissible gastroenteritis and porcine epidemic diarrhea, contributing to enhanced herd health and productivity. The simplicity of delivery and increased compliance rates linked to oral vaccines make them especially appropriate for extensive farming systems where handling animals individually may not be easy [35].

In addition, oral vaccines stimulate local and systemic immune responses that give extensive coverage against pathogens introduced through mucosal surfaces. However, formulation stability and vaccine efficacy can be issues, as current research shows improvements in developing and applying oral vaccines in veterinary medicine. Oral vaccines are a valuable means of preventing diseases and are used to protect animals' health and welfare across diverse agricultural systems [36].

Nasal Vaccines

Veterinary medicine cannot do without nasal vaccines since they enable the immunization of animals against respiratory diseases in a targeted and efficient manner. Thus, administered intranasally, these vaccines deliver antigens directly to the respiratory mucosa, where many pathogens initiate infections. These vaccines have revolutionized disease control strategies, particularly in cattle and swine. For example, the intranasal vaccination used to prevent infectious bovine rhinotracheitis (IBR) and bovine respiratory syncytial virus (BRSV) has effectively diminished the rate and seriousness of respiratory ailments experienced by cattle herds [37].

For instance, in swine farming, intranasal vaccines have been essential in controlling diseases like porcine reproductive and respiratory syndrome (PRRS) and swine influenza. Protection against respiratory pathogens through localized immune responses caused by nasal vaccines is key to preventing their establishment and spread among animal populations. Furthermore, noninvasive nasal vaccination eases the stress and suffering of these animals, thus enhancing their welfare and ensuring compliance [38].

As vaccine developers continue to focus on formulation stability and delivery efficiency, advances in vaccine technology are ongoing, resulting in improved efficacy and applicability of nasal vaccines for veterinary medicine. In general, nasal vaccines are a specific and efficient way to prevent respiratory diseases among animals, promoting healthier, sustainable livestock production methods [39].

Edible Vaccines

The promise of edible vaccines is slowly emerging in veterinary medicine as alternative ways to immunize animals from infectious diseases. These shots are grown in plants or other eatable materials that will allow for oral vaccination of animals. Research in this area has been going well, with the advantages of edible vaccines over injectable ones in terms of ease and, therefore, cost and practicability gaining momentum. Edible vaccines remain within the experimental confines for animal use, although they appear to hold great potential for diseases that affect livestock and poultry production industries [40].

Avian flu in birds and classical swine fever in pigs are crucial to animal health and global food safety. Such edible vaccines would change vaccination strategies for those diseases, offering a practical and sustainable approach to preventing disease occurrence in large populations of animals. Similarly, edible vaccines do not require injections, thus eliminating the need for these and the attendant injuries that occur when handling animals. Edible vaccines take advantage of the natural feeding behavior of animals, providing an easy, stress-free immunization option that can be particularly useful in extensive farming systems where individual animal management is sometimes difficult [41].

Nonetheless, antigens' stability, dosage uniformity, and regulatory requirements are major hurdles to accepting edible vaccines into mainstream veterinary medicine. Recent research and technological advancements have improved the development and practicability of edible vaccines, making them part of routine vaccination schemes for enhanced animal health and welfare [42, 43].

Intrarectal and Vaginal Vaccines

In veterinary medicine, intrarectal and vaginal vaccines are newly implemented methods of creating mucosal immunity in animals against gastrointestinal or reproductive pathogens. These vaccines are given through the anus or vulva to reach directly onto the lining of these anatomical parts. Intrarectal vaccines have been used in cattle farming to control diseases such as Bovine Viral Diarrhea (BVD) and Johne's Disease, which can cause huge financial losses for livestock producers [44].

Intrarectal vaccines deliver antigens to GALT, thus stimulating local immune responses that can protect the body from enteric pathogens. Similarly, vaginal vaccines have been used in pig production to prevent diseases like porcine reproductive and respiratory syndrome (PRRS), which is a highly contagious viral disease that causes pigs to have problems with reproduction and breathing. Vaginal vaccination focuses on the mucosal surfaces of the genitalia, where viruses such as PRRS enter and get established [45].

These vaccines develop mucosal immune responses, featuring the creation of sIgA antibodies that neutralize pathogens and prevent them from taking hold. Nonetheless, several aspects, such as formulation stability, dose accuracy, and route-specific immunity, must be considered to optimize their efficacies. Such intrarectal and vaginal vaccines have the potential to improve disease control strategies in veterinary medicine, thereby enhancing animal health and welfare in different agricultural settings [46].

Conjunctival Vaccines

Using conjunctival vaccines in veterinary medicine has resulted in many positive outcomes because they focus on the ocular mucosa's mucosal immunity and protect animals from eye diseases. The mucus of the ocular surfaces makes up the pathways through which these vaccines are administered by using conjunctiva directly targeting this structure. Additionally, conjunctival vaccines have been used to manage infectious bovine keratoconjunctivitis (IBK) among other animal species, such as horses suffering from equine influenza [47, 48].

IBK is a highly transmissible bacterial infection that leads to inflammation and ulceration of the cornea, causing impaired vision and economic losses in cattle herds. Conjunctival vaccination can reduce the incidence and severity of IBK, improving animal welfare and productivity. Similarly, for horses in the equine industry, this has been applied to prevent respiratory infections such as equine influenza, a viral disease that spreads quickly among horses, interfering with training and competition schedules [49].

Vaccination triggers the ocular mucosa immune response through the conjunctiva by particularly generating sIgA antibodies that are vital in pathogen deactivation and prevention of their entry into the eye. Conjunctival vaccines protect against particular ocular pathogens; however, they must overcome challenges regarding formulation stability, delivery efficiency, and potential adverse reactions for maximum results and safety. Nonetheless, the conjunctival vaccine constitutes a valuable component of disease preventive measures in veterinary medicine that leads to better health outcomes and increased animal welfare across different farming systems [50, 51].

Veterinary medicine has a variety of ways to protect animals from infectious diseases, including mucosal vaccines. Those vaccines that are meant for these areas elicit immune responses that are restricted to their area to offer effective protection where pathogen entry takes place. There are oral and nasal vaccination, intrarectal and vaginal including edible Formulations as well, all of which are considered mucosal vaccines that greatly contribute to maintaining the health and welfare of animals across different species and production systems [52, 53].

ADVANTAGES OF MUCOSAL VACCINATION IN VETERINARY MEDICINE

Mucosal vaccination offers several advantages in veterinary medicine, making it a valuable tool for preventing infectious diseases in animals. It is described below and summarized in Fig. (**3**).

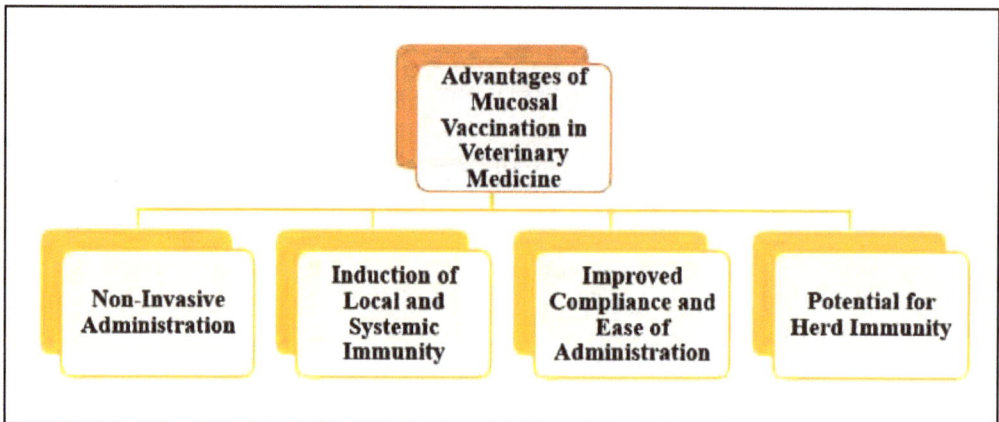

Fig. (3). Advantages of mucosal vaccination in veterinary medicine.

Non-Invasive Administration

Characterized by non-invasive administration routes like oral, nasal, or intrarectal delivery, mucosal vaccination changes the landscape of veterinary medicine by providing a less stressful and more comfortable alternative to traditional needle-based vaccinations. The use of this method eliminates the need for needles and injections that are usually associated with pain, fear, and stress in animals. For instance, restraining and injecting large animals such as cattle and pigs is problematic and laborious for farm animals, with risks of injury to both human beings working on them and themselves. By avoiding this invasive procedure, mucosal vaccines relieve strain and pain, improving animal welfare and reducing injuries caused during handling [54].

For example, oral vaccination incorporates the vaccine into feed or water so that animals can take it voluntarily without any restraint. Similarly, the nostrils administer the vaccine through nasal vaccination, and intrarectal vaccination is administered *via* the rectum. These are just a few examples of non-invasive methods that work well in extensive farming systems where handling each animal individually may be impossible or time-consuming. In addition to this advantage, the needle-less technique also eliminates dangers such as injury from needles themselves, abscesses caused by their use, and infections arising, thus protecting more animals' lives and minimizing veterinary involvement [55].

Additionally, mucosal vaccination is not invasive, so it helps with compliance among animal owners and producers. This convenience and simplicity of use linked to oral, intrarectal, and nasal delivery methods make vaccines given by these routes timely administered over larger areas, enhancing their efficiency in guarding against diseases. The non-invasive delivery method forms one of the basic principles behind veterinary medicine's mucosal vaccination as it provides care for animals without subjecting them to unnecessary suffering or risking their lives through conventional means of immunization [56, 57].

Induction of Local and Systemic Immunity

Mucosal vaccines are essential in veterinary medicine since they elicit strong immune responses at the entry points of pathogens into an animal's body through its respiratory, digestive, and reproductive systems. Such local immunization utilizes the body's natural defense mechanisms to make a protective barrier that blocks infectious agents from entering the body [58].

Mucosal vaccines, on the other hand, stimulate the production of sIgA antibodies at the mucosal surfaces. These antibodies act as a primary defense by neutralizing pathogens and preventing them from adhering to or penetrating through epithelial cells. This kind of local mucosal immunity is very important in preventing the initial stages of infection and blocking pathogen establishment in the body [59].

In addition to local immunity, mucosal vaccines also induce systemic immune responses, which encompass the activation of circulating immune cells and the synthesis of antibodies throughout the body. This systemic immunity provides a wider range of protection against pathogens that may traverse mucosal barriers and penetrate blood or other tissues. Affecting local and general immune system activities, mucous immunization ensures total defense against various infectious agents such as viruses, bacteria, and parasites [60].

It is important to note that mucosal immunization boosts the quality and sustains immune responses compared to injectable vaccines. Additionally, the mucosal immune system shows a high level of specialization and can produce memory responses that can be retained over time, thereby giving long-lasting protection against recurrent infections. Mucosal vaccines, which provoke local mucosal immunity and systemic immune responses, offer an all-out defense against infectious agents, thus making them highly valuable veterinary medicine tools for disease prevention and control [61].

Improved Compliance and Ease of Administration

The ease of access and convenience of using a mucosal vaccine is a major factor that makes animal keepers and producers comply with veterinary medicine. It's in the case of oral or nasal administrations, which are more convenient than traditional injections, especially in large-scale extensive farming where handling many animals can be problematic. Smoothing out the steps involved in vaccinations by removing the need for needles eases the process, even for untrained employees who have only received basic training. This modified system reduces needle-related injuries and increases safety levels among both animals and handlers [62].

Furthermore, the ease of managing mucosal vaccines contributes well to massive immunization programs in animal breeding and poultry industries. Vaccines can be disseminated to feed, water, or sprayed through an aerosol *via* oral or nasal routes, leading to a quick expansion of the vaccine coverage amongst animals. In this case, it may mean fast penetration of vaccination programs into remote locations or areas with densely populated populations, thus promoting infection control and reducing economic losses caused by breakouts [63].

Moreover, the simplicity of mucosal vaccine administration allows for timely vaccination schedules, given that it takes less time and effort than the injectable means. This timeliness is essential in maintaining herd or flock immunity and preventing disease outbreaks, especially in high-risk environments like intensive farming. Thus, by simplifying vaccinations and making them accessible, mucosal vaccines enable animal owners to proactively manage the risks of diseases and uphold the welfare standards set for animal health. Improved compliance and ease of administration related to mucosal vaccines are crucial in advancing disease control efforts and preserving animal populations' health in veterinary medicine [64, 65].

Potential for Herd Immunity

Through administering vaccines to large portions of a population, mucosal immunization offers hope for animal populations to gain herd immunity, which is pivotal in disease control in veterinary medicine. This means that if more animals on a farm are vaccinated using nasal or oral methods, then the transmissibility of pathogens will be disrupted and thus lower the overall burden of illness on the population. When many people are immune to certain infections, they cannot transmit them, and their chances of spreading are reduced significantly; both unvaccinated and immunized individuals are protected [66].

Mucosal vaccination's ability to trigger strong immune responses at the entry points of organisms such as respiratory, digestive, or reproductive tracts makes it a desirable way to attain herd immunity. By addressing these primary sites where most infectious agents launch infection and transmission, mucosal immunization can prevent the introduction and dissemination of pathogens through populations. It also breaks the chain of disease transmission, limiting the spread and reducing the total disease burden [67, 68].

The mucosal vaccination also has practical benefits for establishing herd immunity among animals in a veterinary context. The ease of application and scalability of mucosal vaccines make it possible to achieve quick, mass vaccination coverage in large animal populations. This implies that an appreciable percentage of the population can be vaccinated effectively, which increases the probability of reaching the status of herd immunity. The ability of mucosal immunization to promote herd immunity is useful in veterinary medicine against infectious diseases at the population level. Mucosal vaccines protect sick and healthy animals from infections, hence controlling disease and maintaining their well-being [69, 70].

CURRENT APPLICATIONS IN VETERINARY MEDICINE

Veterinarians use mucosal vaccines to treat a host of animal species, including poultry, cattle, and pigs, as well as pet animals such as dogs and cats.

Mucosal Vaccines for Livestock

Veterinary medicine relies on mucosal vaccines for livestock as indispensable tools to provide specific cover against several infectious diseases that often affect poultry, cattle, and pigs. The vaccines target the mucus membranes located at different sites, such as oral, nasal, or intrarectal regions [71]. In this way, immune reactions can be triggered at the points pathogens enter the body using the mucosal surfaces. Mucosal vaccines used in livestock are discussed below.

Poultry

Mucosal vaccines are important in the poultry industry for protecting birds against respiratory and gastrointestinal diseases that can ruin a flock's health and productivity. Two diseases significantly impacting the poultry sector are Newcastle disease and infectious bronchitis, which are effectively dealt with using mucosal vaccines [72].

Pouring disease is a great challenge to poultry globally as it is caused by virulent strains of avian paramyxovirus type 1 (APMV-1). Newcastle disease vaccines are given orally in drinking water or by spray methods soon after they have hatched. These vaccines contain live attenuated virus strains designed to specifically reproduce within the digestive tract, eliciting strong mucosal immune responses. Such vaccines, by giving local immunity in the respiratory and digestive tracts, can reduce the transmission and severity of Newcastle disease among chicken flocks. They control the dissemination of virulent strains of APMV-1, thereby checking death rates and production losses and safeguarding the general welfare of the flock [73].

The infectious bronchitis, caused by avian coronavirus in the same way, is another very contagious respiratory disease that results in many losses in poultry farming. Similar application techniques to the Newcastle disease vaccines are used when administering oral vaccines for infectious bronchitis in chicks. The vaccine comprises live attenuated strains of the virus that reproduce inside the respiratory system, causing mucosal immunity, thereby reducing the severity and longevity of respiratory infections. As a result, these vaccinations offer quick protection against infectious bronchitis through the target respiratory mucus, thus controlling the spread within flocks and guaranteeing sustainable well-being for poultry activities [74].

Cattle

Mucosal vaccines are very important in the livestock sector, especially in dealing with common diseases like bovine viral diarrhea (BVD) and bovine respiratory disease complex (BRDC). These have significant economic implications and affect animal welfare. Some of these mucosal vaccines target infectious bovine rhinotracheitis (IBR) and Johne's disease localized immunity, developed through strategic formulations in the respiratory or gastrointestinal tracts [75].

The bovine respiratory disease complex (BRDC) is a multifactorial respiratory disorder caused by several etiologies, including infectious agents such as bovine herpesvirus-1 (BoHV-1), bovine viral diarrhea virus (BVDV) and bacterial pathogens like Mannheimia hemolytic and Pasteurella multocida. Nasal vaccines for infectious bovine rhinotracheitis (IBR) form the basis of BRDC preventive measures. The intranasal route is used for the administration of these vaccines, which delivers attenuated or modified live IBR viruses directly to the respiratory mucosa, leading to a strong immune response in the mucosal system and production of sIgA antibodies, which are the first line of defense against respiratory pathogens. With such an approach, immunity is enhanced at the site of primary infection, thus lessening the severity and length of the respiratory infections with a subsequent reduction in outbreaks of BRDC and losses attributed to it in productivity [76].

There are many cases of Johne's disease in cows, brought about by Mycobacterium avium subspecies paratuberculosis (MAP), a chronic stomach sickness that causes diarrhea, weight loss, and reduced milk yield. Intrarectal vaccines for Johne's disease aim to provoke mucosal immunity within the gut region, where MAP first colonizes and remains in. These vaccines typically have attenuated or killed MAP antigens in them, and they should be introduced through the anus. In these cattle, intrarectal vaccination helps to decrease the shedding of MAP by eliciting mucosal immune responses similar to those seen when MALT is activated/produced, thereby limiting the progression of Johne's disease [77].

Pigs

Among the major infectious diseases that significantly impact the health and productivity of herds, mucosal vaccines are very important in the pig production business. They include porcine reproductive and respiratory syndrome (PRRS) as well as transmissible gastroenteritis (TGE), which can result in serious economic losses and poor animal welfare. To control these diseases, mucosal vaccines are used to induce immune responses in pigs' respiratory and gastrointestinal tracts.

PRRS is caused by a highly contagious virus called PRRS virus (PRRSV) that mainly affects pigs' respiratory and reproductive systems. Intranasal vaccines for swine influenza, commonly given intranasally to pigs, are integral to PRRS prevention programs. These vaccines contain live attenuated or inactivated strains of influenza virus, which replicate within the respiratory mucosa and cause induction of mucosal immune responses. Swine flu immunizations assist in priming the mucosal immune system, decreasing the severity and length of respiratory infections, thereby reducing the harmful effects of PRRS on herd health and productivity [78].

Another major pig gastrointestinal disease is transmissible gastroenteritis (TGE), which can cause severe diarrhea, vomiting, and dehydration, particularly in young piglets. Oral TGE vaccines are given to the little pigs *via* drinking water or feed, and they are administered live attenuated or inactivated TGE virus directly to their gastrointestinal tract. These vaccines induce mucosal immune responses within the intestinal mucosa, protecting against TGE virus infection and decreasing clinical signs' severity. By increasing mucosal immunity in the gut, these vaccines help reduce economic losses related to TGE outbreaks and stop swine herds from spreading the virus [79].

Vaccination Strategies for Companion Animals

Dogs

When it comes to dog health, mucosal vaccines are indispensable in fighting against diseases that affect the respiratory system, especially canine parainfluenza virus (CPIV) and Bordetella bronchiseptica, which contribute largely to kennel cough syndrome. Kennel cough is a highly infectious condition marked by chronic hacking coughs and mostly occurs in areas with high densities of dogs, like kennels, shelters, and dog parks [80].

Mucosal vaccines can be applied to kennel cough in a targeted way by stimulating local immunity in the respiratory tract, where CPIV and Bordetella bronchiseptica are mostly colonized. Nasal vaccines for CPIV and Bordetella bronchiseptica are given to puppies and adult dogs using a nasal spray or dripper. This means introducing live attenuated or inactivated virus particles directly into the nasal mucosa, which evokes an efficient response from the mucosal immune system [81].

When administered, mucosal vaccines initiate sIgA antibody production, which acts as the main defense against respiratory pathogens. These substances disable bacteria and viruses from attaching and invading respiratory epithelial cells. Additionally, MALT is activated by mucosal vaccines, thereby bolstering local immunity because it is found in the respiratory mucosa [82].

Mucosal vaccines help decrease the severity and duration of respiratory infections in dogs by quickly and selectively protecting against CPIV and Bordetella bronchiseptica. This diminishes clinical symptoms and reduces the rate at which canine populations are infected. Similarly, mucosal vaccines have the advantage of being easily administered and more convenient to use; hence, they can be employed in various contexts like veterinary clinics, boarding facilities, and shelters.

Mucosal vaccines for CPIV and Bordetella bronchiseptica guard canine respiratory health in dogs that live in different areas. These are priceless instruments for kennel cough prevention and control, as they can provide localized immunity in the respiratory tract. This can improve the quality of life for both dog owners and their pets [83].

Cats

Through mucosal vaccines, cats are protected from upper respiratory infections caused by feline calicivirus (FCV) and feline herpesvirus (FHV), which are important diseases in the complex syndrome called FVR. The disease is easily spread and causes sneezing, running nose, inflamed eyes, and, in severe cases, pneumonia [84].

Shelters, catteries, and multicat households are environments with many cats, and as such, intranasal vaccines for FCV and FHV have become a must-have preventive care. This route of administration is used to give kittens or adult cats attenuated or inactivated virus particles through a nasal dropper or spray; this method allows the vaccine to stimulate mucosal immunity in the nasal passages where infection by FCV and FHV begins and replication takes place [85].

Mucosal vaccines begin the immune response localized in the nasal mucosa, producing sIgA antibodies. These proteins are important for stopping FCV and FHV from invading nasal epithelial cells by neutralizing them. Mucosal vaccines can minimize replication and transmission of FCV and FHV by attacking their primary site of infection, thus reducing the severity and duration of upper respiratory infections in cats [86].

Moreover, the mucosal vaccines for FCV and FHV have an added advantage: They are quick to start immunization, thus protecting against respiratory pathogens within days after administration. This rapid immune response is a great advantage, especially in high-risk environments where cats may be exposed to infected individuals. Additionally, these mucosal vaccines are well accepted and easy to administer, making them appropriate for use on all age groups of cats, including seniors and kittens.

In cats, FCV and FHV vaccines for mucosa help them stay free of upper respiratory tract infections, contributing to their general health status. Vaccinating through the nasal passages stimulates the production of mucosal immunity, thus reducing the dangers of respiratory disease and improving a cat's quality of life in different environments [87].

RECENT ADVANCES AND RESEARCH

Innovations in Vaccine Technology

Innovations in vaccine technology are rapidly transforming the landscape of disease prevention and control, offering novel approaches to vaccine design, delivery, and efficacy, as discussed below.

Nanotechnology

Innovative platforms that help antigen presentation and immune stimulation have revolutionized vaccine delivery in nanotechnology. Nanoparticles and nanocarriers provide various benefits, such as antigen protection from degradation, targeted delivery to specific tissues or cells, and controlled release kinetics. Nanoscale carriers could be designed to replicate pathogens or hold multiple antigens, thus increasing their immunogenicity and efficiency. Furthermore, nanotechnology has also made using adjuvants or immunomodulatory agents in vaccine formulations feasible, enhancing the immune system. This holds promise for improving vaccine efficacy against a wide range of infectious diseases in human and animal medicine due to the optimization of antigen presentation and immune activation using vaccination systems based on nanotechnologies [88].

mRNA Vaccines

The development of mRNA vaccines has been transformed by using the body's inbuilt cellular machinery to produce antigenic proteins and elicit immune responses. These vaccinations contain synthetic mRNA molecules that encode particular viral or bacterial antigens enclosed within lipid nanoparticles for transport. After being administered, host cells take up the mRNA and translate it into antigenic proteins, which can prompt a defensive action against the marked pathogens. Rapid progression and scalability of the mRNA vaccine technique enabled an immediate response to any new infectious disease outbreak, such as COVID-19. In addition, the mRNA vaccines are adaptable; hence, they can be used in veterinary applications; this indicates that they have a possibility of generating vaccines against different animal infections. mRNA-based vaccines can potentially improve the prevention and control of human and veterinary diseases [84].

Vector-Based Vaccines

The vector-based vaccines utilize the natural infectiousness of viral or bacterial vectors to introduce antigenic proteins into the host cells that will induce strong defensive reactions. Often, these vectors are made replication-deficient or non-pathogenic and are used to carry foreign antigens into target cells. Within the host, the vector expresses this antigen, thereby inducing both humoral and cellular immune responses. There are two ways by which broad and complete protection from the targeted pathogen can be ensured. According to veterinary medicine, vector-based vaccines have been found to work efficiently against various infectious disorders such as rabies, influenza, and the West Nile virus. The main idea of these vaccines is to use viral or bacterial vectors as immune response inducers that prevent and control several animal infections, thereby improving animal health and welfare [89].

Adjuvant Development

New adjuvants have been discovered because the development of vaccine immune response stimulators has gone a step further. These adjuvants aim to cause lasting, strong, and safe immunological responses. This can be done in various ways, like mimicking natural immune stimulators or targeting specific immune pathways. They improve vaccine efficacy and enhance protection against infectious diseases by modulating the immune system's response to vaccine antigens. Developing adjuvants with improved safety profiles is essential for expanding vaccine use into vulnerable populations like children, elderly individuals, and immunocompromised patients. As a result, continued innovations in adjuvant design have great promise in advancing vaccine development efforts and effectively addressing global health challenges [90].

Computational Vaccine Design

The power of bioinformatics and structural biology is used in computational vaccine design to hasten the development of more effective and specific vaccines. Using computational approaches, scientists can identify antigenic epitopes within pathogens, create antigen constructs that mimic natural immune targets, and optimize vaccine formulations for improved immunogenicity. Such strategies enable vaccines to be designed rationally to elicit strong immune responses against particular pathogens or strains, improving their efficiency. Computational vaccine design also allows the identification of conserved epitopes that can provide broad protection against various strains of pathogens, thereby addressing antibody variance and newly evolving diseases. Computational approaches have been integrated into vaccine design for faster development, lessening costs for experimentation, and potential betterment in terms of global health challenges [91].

Plant-Based Vaccines

Plant-based vaccine technology is revolutionizing vaccine production through plant expression systems. Several advantages exist in using plants as platforms for vaccine production, such as cost, scale, and ease of administration. This is achieved through genetic manipulation that aims at exogenously producing viral or bacterial antigens, which can be proteins within plants at a high density. In addition, plant vaccines have the advantage of being inherently safe because they lack mammalian pathogens and do not require elaborate purification techniques [92].

In veterinary medicine, plant-based vaccines are effective in fighting against different infectious diseases in animals, such as foot-and-mouth disease and avian influenza. Rather than using traditional methods for making vaccines, this type of vaccine is available easily and can be used for scaling purposes in the prevention of diseases among animals. Moreover, this technology has the potential for managing new infections seen in poor countries due to low vaccination rates; this development could lead to better animal health and food security worldwide.

Innovations in vaccine technology offer great hope as they strive to improve the prevention and management of diseases in human beings and animals. Researchers are moving forward on product development through the use of the latest technologies and new approaches that will produce vaccines that are more secure, efficient, and available globally [93].

Genetic and Recombinant Vaccines

The development of vaccines using genetic and recombinant approaches that employ the skill of gene engineering to produce antigens has led to new strategies in vaccinology. In this case, genes encoding specific antigens are inserted into host cells or organisms to manufacture recombinant proteins capable of stimulating immune responses.

Recombinant Antigen Production

Genetic and recombinant vaccine development relies on the production of recombinant antigens, which involves genetically modifying host cells or organisms to make them express certain antigenic proteins. This starts with identifying and choosing target antigens sourced from pathogens, toxins, or other immunogenic molecules. Through recombinant DNA technology, these antigens' genes are inserted into either host cells or organisms [94].

Upon integration, the host cells or organisms are modified to generate the recombinant antigens that are later processed into vaccines. Creating recombinant antigens has many benefits compared to traditional vaccine development methods because it is scalable, flexible, and able to produce antigens, which may be difficult or hazardous for conventional production approaches [95].

Genetic engineering, with the help of recombinant antigen production, can develop vaccines with improved security, efficiency, and specificity, paving the way for preventing and managing infectious diseases [96].

Host Systems

In the production of genetic and recombinant vaccines, host systems are essential; these offer a variety of platforms with specific preferences. Bacteria like Escherichia coli are often used for their fast-growing rates, scalability, and ease of genetic manipulation. Saccharomyces cerevisiae is one of the best yeasts for efficient protein expression, proper protein folding, and glycosylation capabilities. Among the insect cells derived from the baculovirus expression system, the ones that have been developed have high protein yields similar to those obtained in mammalian cells, as well as post-translational modifications [97].

Chinese hamster ovary (CHO) cells, among other mammalian cells, are favored to produce complex proteins with correct folding and human-like glycosylation patterns. Tobacco and maize plants, on the other hand, are advantageous in regard to cheap manufacturing techniques that can be scaled up and the possible use of vaccines through the mouth. Although each model has its individual challenges and factors to consider, together, they offer flexible grounds for making recombinant epitopes meant for specific vaccine demands [98, 99].

Vector-Based Vaccines

Vector-based vaccines use the infectiousness of viral or bacterial vectors to introduce recombinant antigens and cause immunological reactions on particular pathogens. These transgenic vectors express the antigenic proteins originating from the pathogen in view. Adenovirus-based vaccines, for instance, employ replication-defective adenoviral vectors to inoculate antigens that activate immune responses. Adenoviral vectors have been reported to be efficient in infecting host cells and can induce strong immune responses, thus making them good candidates as vaccine delivery systems [100].

On the other hand, bacteria-based vectors such as Salmonella and Listeria have been genetically modified to produce and transfer recombinant antigens into host cells. This is because they can specifically interact with mucosal surfaces, leading to systemic immune responses that they elicit. Besides, bacterial vectors can be engineered to express antigens from diverse pathogens, thus offering hope for general protection against infectious diseases. In summary, vector-based vaccines stand out as one of the most exciting prospects in vaccine development because they offer specific pathogen-directed and potent immune responses [101].

DNA Vaccines

DNA vaccines, a hopeful group of genetic vaccines, use plasmid DNA encoding antigenic proteins to cause immune responses. The DNA vaccine is then taken up by muscle cells or dendritic cells in the host cell and expressed as plasmid DNA. Then, this host cell machinery transcribes and translates the DNA into these antigenic proteins, which will be presented on the surface of the cell, initiating immune responses [102].

DNA vaccines' foremost benefits are their ability to induce both humoral and cellular immune responses. It is necessary to combat intracellular pathogens and provide long-lasting immunity through this two-fold immune system stimulation. In addition, there are some other advantages associated with DNA vaccines, such as easy production, stable nature, safety, *etc.* Nevertheless, optimizing DNA vaccine delivery and improving their immunogenicity continues to be a topic of active research aimed at maximizing their effectiveness in preventing infectious diseases. They hold much potential as a flexible platform for making vaccines against a broad range of pathogens [103].

RNA Vaccines

Additionally, RNA vaccines constitute a new variety of viral vaccines that rely on mRNA, which encodes antigenic proteins to promote immune responses. After being given, these vaccines are taken up by cells within the body, where the ribosomes found in these host cells translate mRNA into antigenic proteins. Consequently, these antigens are revealed on the plasma membrane and consequently evoke immunity, including humoral and cellular immunity [104].

The quickness of development is the major benefit of RNA vaccines. Unlike traditional vaccine production methods, this can be quickened by the ease of mRNA synthesis and the absence of the need for viral propagation. Furthermore, they do not integrate into the host genome, eliminating the worries about genomic integration and potential long-term effects. Such an aspect makes them safer while allowing fast access to new infectious disease threats worldwide. RNA vaccines offer a positive approach to immunizing against many infectious diseases, thereby giving hope in terms of vaccine development [105].

Customization and Flexibility

Genetic and recombinant vaccines offer an exclusive opportunity for the customization of antigens and design flexibility compared to any other vaccine, which in turn allows for the production of pathogen or strain-specific vaccines. Researchers can develop immune responses against desired threats by optimizing vaccine efficacy and specificity using antigens relevant to the target pathogen [106].

It is flexible and thus can be employed to deal with the emergence of infectious diseases and antigenic variations. Traditional vaccines took long to develop, but the same cannot be said about genetic and recombinant ones; these can be made quickly for use in urgent cases. This quickness is helpful when dealing with pathogens that change over time or break out suddenly because it allows for timely vaccination required to control the transfer and stop the progress of ailments.

Additionally, the customizable nature of genetic and recombinant vaccines enables the incorporation of several antigens or epitopes within a single vaccine formulation to provide wider protection against various strains or variants caused by a pathogen. The customization and flexibility provided by genetic and recombinant vaccines are, therefore, great resources in the fight against infectious diseases [107].

FUTURE PROSPECTS

The future of veterinary medicine is intricately tied to the ever-changing field of emerging diseases and the demand for innovative vaccine solutions. New vaccines are essential as zoonotic infections continue to pose risks to animal health and human beings, too. In this respect, mucosal vaccines that can mount strong immune responses at sites of pathogen entry have high prospects. Existing vaccination programs can be built around mucosal vaccines to enhance disease prevention and control. By working with traditional parenteral vaccines, mucosal vaccination may help broaden protection against diseases primarily infecting mucosal surfaces. This integration also offers chances to design more all-encompassing immunization strategies that are specific to the disease ecologies and epidemiological problems [108].

Innovation in bovine vaccine development is driven by biotechnology, a field that makes it possible to have personalized medicine. Using genomic tools, bioinformatics, and proteomics provide discoveries on antigens and enable the production of vaccines that meet specific needs for each animal or even the animal population. Using personalized vaccines not only boosts immunity but also reduces side effects while enhancing vaccine performance. However, as the field moves forward, ethical and regulatory issues become more prominent. It is necessary to balance scientific advancement and ethical values to guarantee animal welfare, maintain professional integrity in the veterinary profession, and preserve public confidence in Veterinary Medicine [109].

Ethical considerations include animal rights, informed consent, and open research practices. Regulatory frameworks must adapt to new vaccine technologies while maintaining strict safety and efficacy regulations. Moreover, it is important to ensure that inventive vaccines are easily available to various animal species, such as those in economically deprived areas. To handle the intricate moral and regulatory web within which veterinary medicine functions regarding vaccines, there has to be collaboration among regulators, veterinary practitioners, investigators, and policymakers [110].

Emerging diseases, the development of technology, ethical considerations, and regulation frameworks determine the direction of veterinary medicine tomorrow. Disease prevention is a major front in mucosal vaccines, which offer selective protection against pathogens. Integrating mucosal vaccines into vaccination campaigns, biotech advances towards personalized medication, and various questions about ethics and regulations should be taken into account while creating animal health care priorities and promoting veterinary vaccine innovations in the future [111].

CHALLENGES AND LIMITATIONS

Many challenges and limitations to mucosal vaccines must be surmounted for their full potential to be realized in veterinary medicine. Vaccine formulation stability is a key drawback, notably within the mucosal environment characterized by enzymatic degradation and varying pH levels. Guaranteeing vaccine antigen's stability and potency under these conditions has been a major drawdown in vaccine development. Another problem is that developing suitable delivery systems and dosage-tracking mechanisms has logistical complexities. Thus, mucosal surfaces differ in anatomy and physiology, requiring customized delivery strategies for effective vaccination optimization. This means that the administration of a mucosal vaccine must also be complicated by the need to achieve exact dosing and uniform distribution of antigens [112].

Additionally, the variation of mucosal immunity between diverse animal species and individuals is quite a big problem. For example, age, health condition, genes, and the environment can influence the intensity and duration of mucosal immune response, thus complicating predictions about vaccine efficiency and the development of uniform vaccines. Additionally, care should be taken when considering the safety profiles of mucosal vaccines and possible side effects. Mucosal administration routes may cause unintentional local inflammation or immune responses, necessitating extensive evaluation for vaccine safety and immunogenicity in preclinical and clinical trials [113].

These obstacles require interdisciplinary collaboration and inventive vaccine research and development. New adjuvants, stabilizers, or delivery systems can stabilize the vaccines, increasing their effectiveness and storage life. This approach will also maximize the potential of mucosal antigen uptake in nasal, pulmonary, and vaginal routes through delivery technologies such as nanoparticles, microspheres, and mucosal adhesive. Additionally, predictive models that account for immune mechanisms occurring at the mucosa level can guide vaccine design and optimization by clearly showing how vaccines affect these regions [114].

In addition, very stringent preclinical and clinical examination methods must be used to evaluate the safety of vaccines, immunogenicity (the ability of vaccines to stimulate the immune system), efficacy, and performance in different animal populations. It is vital for a vaccine to be safe; organized monitoring of adverse effects and long-term immunity response which minimize possible dangers. In reality, mucosal vaccines' difficulties and restrictions can only be addressed by using several techniques that bring together scientific creativity, regulatory control mechanisms, and ethical issues advanced within the development of veterinary vaccines, leading to improved animal welfare standards [115].

CONCLUSION

In veterinary science, vaccines that target the mucosa are a potentially effective preventive measure and remedy for some diseases. When directed at mucous membranes, these vaccines generate effective immune responses where the infections start, which offers a total safeguard against different contagious illnesses. Integrating mucosal vaccines into present vaccination plans may improve efforts to manage diseases more effectively, especially against pathogens predominantly involving the mucosa. Challenges that must be tackled include vaccine formulation stability, delivery mechanisms, mucosal immune response variations, and safety concerns. Interdisciplinary liaisons must be established, notable research must be conducted, and stringent assessment criteria must be set to counter these challenges and ascertain the practicality, efficiency, and safety of mucosal vaccines on different animal groups. As we look forward to future developments in vaccine technology, biotechnology, and personalized medicine, the various possibilities for improving mucosal vaccines are quite apparent. Researchers can improve the stability and effectiveness of vaccines if they leverage innovative delivery systems, adjuvants, and antigen design strategies. The other way to customize vaccination strategies for different animal populations is by taking into account personalized medicine approaches and insights into mucosal immune mechanisms. To protect animal health, welfare, and productivity and mitigate the effects of new and existing pathogens, mucosal vaccination is a powerful tool that can be employed extensively in veterinary medicine. Mucosal vaccination can significantly safeguard animal populations and enhance global health through cooperation among veterinarians, policymakers, and regulators.

ACKNOWLEDGEMENTS

Authors are highly thankful to their Universities/Colleges for providing library facilities for the literature survey.

REFERENCES

[1]   Huang M, Zhang M, Zhu H, Du X, Wang J. Mucosal vaccine delivery: A focus on the breakthrough of specific barriers. Acta Pharmaceutica Sinica B. Chinese Academy of Medical Sciences; 2022; 12, 3456–74.

[2]   Lavelle EC, Ward RW. Mucosal vaccines — fortifying the frontiers. Nature Reviews Immunology. Nature Research 2022; 22: pp. 236-50.

[3]   Anggraeni R, Ana ID, Wihadmadyatami H. Development of mucosal vaccine delivery: an overview on the mucosal vaccines and their adjuvants. Clinical and Experimental Vaccine Research. Korean Vaccine Society; 2022; 11, 235–48.

[4]   Rhee JH. Current and new approaches for mucosal vaccine delivery. Mucosal Vaccines. Academic Press 2020; 1: pp. 325-56.

[5]   Abdulhaqq SA, Weiner DB. DNA vaccines: developing new strategies to enhance immune responses. Immunol Res 2008; 42(1-3): 219-32.
       [http://dx.doi.org/10.1007/s12026-008-8076-3] [PMID: 19066740]

[6]   Karam EG, Mneimneh ZN, Salamoun MM, Akiskal HS, Akiskal KK. Suitability of the TEMPS-A for population-based studies: Ease of administration and stability of affective temperaments in its Lebanese version. J Affect Disord 2007; 98(1-2): 45-53.
       [http://dx.doi.org/10.1016/j.jad.2006.06.029] [PMID: 16949160]

[7]   Kauppinen T, Vainio A, Valros A, Rita H, Vesala KM. Improving animal welfare: qualitative and quantitative methodology in the study of farmers' attitudes. Anim Welf 2010; 19(4): 523-36.
       [http://dx.doi.org/10.1017/S0962728600001998]

[8]   Tian L, Li J, Xu Y, Qiu Y, Zhang Y, Li X. A MAP kinase cascade broadly regulates the lifestyle of *Sclerotinia sclerotiorum* and can be targeted by HIGS for disease control. Plant J 2024; 118(2): 324-44.
       [http://dx.doi.org/10.1111/tpj.16606] [PMID: 38149487]

[9]   Borjas GJ. The Economic Benefits from Immigration. J Econ Perspect 1995; 9(2): 3-22.
       [http://dx.doi.org/10.1257/jep.9.2.3]

[10]   Josefsberg JO, Buckland B. Vaccine process technology. Biotechnol Bioeng 2012; 109(6): 1443-60.
       [http://dx.doi.org/10.1002/bit.24493] [PMID: 22407777]

[11]   Francis MJ. Recent Advances in Vaccine Technologies. Veterinary Clinics of North America - Small Animal Practice. W.B. Saunders, 2018; 48, 231–41.
       [http://dx.doi.org/10.1016/j.cvsm.2017.10.002]

[12]   Smith DF. Lessons of history in veterinary medicine. J Vet Med Educ 2013; 40(1): 2-11.
       [http://dx.doi.org/10.3138/jvme.1112.04] [PMID: 23470241]

[13]   Lombard M, Pastoret P-P, Moulin AM. A brief history of vaccines and vaccination. Rev Sci Tech
       2007; 26(1): 29-48.
       [http://dx.doi.org/10.20506/rst.26.1.1724] [PMID: 17633292]

[14]   Aida V, Pliasas VC, Neasham PJ, North JF, McWhorter KL, Glover SR, *et al.* Novel Vaccine
       Technologies in Veterinary Medicine: A Herald to Human Medicine Vaccines. Frontiers in Veterinary
       Science. Frontiers Media S.A. 2021; 8.

[15]   Gehrig AC, Hartmann K, Günther F, Klima A, Habacher G, Bergmann M. A survey of vaccine history
       in German cats and owners' attitudes to vaccination. J Feline Med Surg 2019; 21(2): 73-83.
       [http://dx.doi.org/10.1177/1098612X18759838] [PMID: 29529958]

[16]   Meeusen ENT, Walker J, Peters A, Pastoret PP, Jungersen G. Current status of veterinary vaccines.
       Clin Microbiol Rev 2007; 20(3): 489-510.
       [http://dx.doi.org/10.1128/CMR.00005-07] [PMID: 17630337]

[17]   Pal M. Perspective of Vaccination in Veterinary Medicine: A Review. 2022. Available from:
       www.microbiojournal.com

[18]   Cha SH. The history of vaccination and current vaccination policies in Korea. Clin Exp Vaccine Res
       2012; 1(1): 3-8.
       [http://dx.doi.org/10.7774/cevr.2012.1.1.3] [PMID: 23596573]

[19]   Pearson JP, Brownlee IA. Structure and Function of Mucosal Surfaces. Colonization of Mucosal
       Surfaces. ASM Press 2014; pp. 1-16.
       [http://dx.doi.org/10.1128/9781555817619.ch1]

[20]   Durbin RK, Kotenko SV, Durbin JE. Interferon induction and function at the mucosal surface.
       Immunol Rev 2013; 255(1): 25-39.
       [http://dx.doi.org/10.1111/imr.12101] [PMID: 23947345]

[21]   Cerutti A, Chen K, Chorny A. Immunoglobulin responses at the mucosal interface. Annu Rev
       Immunol 2011; 29(1): 273-93.
       [http://dx.doi.org/10.1146/annurev-immunol-031210-101317] [PMID: 21219173]

[22]   Knoop KA, Newberry RD. Goblet cells: multifaceted players in immunity at mucosal surfaces.
       Mucosal Immunology. Nature Publishing Group 2018; 11: pp. 1551-7.

[23]   Brown TA. Immunity at mucosal surfaces. Adv Dent Res 1996; 10(1): 62-5.
       [http://dx.doi.org/10.1177/08959374960100011201] [PMID: 8934927]

[24]   Mousel MR, Leeds TD, White SN, Herrmann-Hoesing LM. Technical Note: Comparison of traditional
       needle vaccination with pneumatic, needle-free vaccination for sheep1,2. J Anim Sci 2008; 86(6):
       1468-71.
       [http://dx.doi.org/10.2527/jas.2007-0839] [PMID: 18310489]

[25]   Jorge S, Dellagostin OA. The development of veterinary vaccines: a review of traditional methods and
       modern biotechnology approaches. Biotechnology Research and Innovation 2017; 1(1): 6-13.
       [http://dx.doi.org/10.1016/j.biori.2017.10.001]

[26]   Luman ET, Worku A, Berhane Y, Martin R, Cairns L. Comparison of two survey methodologies to
       assess vaccination coverage. Int J Epidemiol 2007; 36(3): 633-41.
       [http://dx.doi.org/10.1093/ije/dym025] [PMID: 17420165]

[27]   Legnardi M, Baranyay H, Simon C, *et al.* Infectious bronchitis hatchery vaccination: Comparison
       between traditional spray administration and a newly developed gel delivery system in field
       conditions. Vet Sci 2021; 8(8): 145.
       [http://dx.doi.org/10.3390/vetsci8080145] [PMID: 34437467]

[28]   Shi M, An Q, Ainslie KEC, Haber M, Orenstein WA. A comparison of the test-negative and the

traditional case-control study designs for estimation of influenza vaccine effectiveness under nonrandom vaccination. BMC Infect Dis 2017; 17(1): 757.
[http://dx.doi.org/10.1186/s12879-017-2838-2] [PMID: 29216845]

[29]   Gong W, Taighoon Shah M, Firdous S, *et al.* Comparison of three rapid household survey sampling methods for vaccination coverage assessment in a peri-urban setting in Pakistan. Int J Epidemiol 2019; 48(2): 583-95.
[http://dx.doi.org/10.1093/ije/dyy263] [PMID: 30508112]

[30]   Saha A, Sarker M, Hossen MT, Hassan Z, Adhikari JM, Latif MAHM. Digitalized to reach and track: a retrospective comparison between traditional and conditional estimate of vaccination coverage and dropout rates using e-Tracker data below one-year children in Bangladesh during-COVID and pre-COVID period. Lancet Reg Health Southeast Asia 2023; 16: 100252.
[http://dx.doi.org/10.1016/j.lansea.2023.100252] [PMID: 37529088]

[31]   Banks D, Woo EJ, Burwen DR, Perucci P, Braun MM, Ball R. Comparing data mining methods on the VAERS database. Pharmacoepidemiol Drug Saf 2005; 14(9): 601-9.
[http://dx.doi.org/10.1002/pds.1107] [PMID: 15954077]

[32]   Chiarella P, Fazio VM, Signori E. Application of electroporation in DNA vaccination protocols. Curr Gene Ther 2010; 10(4): 281-6.
[http://dx.doi.org/10.2174/156652310791823506] [PMID: 20504275]

[33]   Gerdts V, Mutwiri G, Tikoo S, Babiuk L, Mucosal LB, Mutwiri GK, *et al.* Mucosal delivery of vaccines in domestic animals 2006.
[http://dx.doi.org/10.1051/vetres:2006012]

[34]   Długońska H, Grzybowski M. Mucosal vaccination-an old but still vital strategy 1. Vol. 58. Ann Parasitol 2012.

[35]   Zainutdinov SS, Sivolobova GF, Loktev VB, Kochneva GV. Mucosal immunity and vaccines against viral infections. Problems of Virology. 2021; 66(6): 399-408.

[36]   Hodgins DC, Chattha K, Vlasova A, Parreño V, Corbeil LB, Renukaradhya GJ, Mucosal Veterinary Vaccines: Comparative Vaccinology. In: Mucosal Immunology: Fourth Edition. Elsevier Inc.; 2015. p. 1337–61.

[37]   Pabst R. Mucosal vaccination by the intranasal route. Nose-associated lymphoid tissue (NALT)—Structure, function and species differences - ScienceDirect. 2015.

[38]   Morein B. Advanced Drug Delivery Reviews. 2004. Available from: https://doi.org/./j.addr

[39]   Calderon-Nieva D, Goonewardene KB, Gomis S, Foldvari M. Veterinary vaccine nanotechnology: pulmonary and nasal delivery in livestock animals. Drug Delivery and Translational Research. Springer Verlag; 2017; 7, 558–70.

[40]   Borges O, Lebre F, Bento D, Borchard G, Junginger HE. Mucosal vaccines: recent progress in understanding the natural barriers. Pharm Res 2010; 27(2): 211-23.
[http://dx.doi.org/10.1007/s11095-009-0011-3] [PMID: 19953309]

[41]   Jogi Madhya Pradesh Pashu-Chikitsa Vigyan Vishwavidyalaya J, Chhabra Madhya Pradesh Pashu-Chikitsa Vigyan Vishwavidyalaya D, Sharda Madhya Pradesh Pashu-Chikitsa Vigyan Vishwavidyalaya R. Immunology of Edible Vaccines and its Veterinary Importance. 2023.
[http://dx.doi.org/10.5281/zenodo.10073185]

[42]   Jacob SS, Cherian S, Sumithra TG, Raina OK, Sankar M. Edible vaccines against veterinary parasitic diseases—Current status and future prospects. Vaccine 2013; 31(15): 1879-85.
[http://dx.doi.org/10.1016/j.vaccine.2013.02.022] [PMID: 23485715]

[43]   Kurup VM, Thomas J. Edible Vaccines: Promises and Challenges. Molecular Biotechnology. Humana Press Inc.; 2020; 62, 79–90.

[44]   Mesteckya J. Current options for vaccine delivery systems by mucosal routes - ScienceDirect. 1997.

[45]   Meeusen N. T. Advances in mucosal vaccination _ Animal Health Research Reviews _ Cambridge Core. 2007.

[46]   Mestecky J, Raska M, Novak J, Alexander RC, Moldoveanu Z. Antibody-mediated protection and the mucosal immune system of the genital tract: relevance to vaccine design. J Reprod Immunol 2010; 85(1): 81-5.
[http://dx.doi.org/10.1016/j.jri.2010.02.003] [PMID: 20236708]

[47]   Meeusen EN. Exploiting mucosal surfaces for the development of mucosal vaccines. Vaccine 2011; 29(47): 8506-11.
[http://dx.doi.org/10.1016/j.vaccine.2011.09.010] [PMID: 21945494]

[48]   Harandi M. Mucosal Adjuvants_ Ingenta Connect. 2010.

[49]   Seo KY, Han SJ, Cha HR, *et al.* Eye mucosa: an efficient vaccine delivery route for inducing protective immunity. J Immunol 2010; 185(6): 3610-9.
[http://dx.doi.org/10.4049/jimmunol.1000680] [PMID: 20709955]

[50]   Anthony B. Topical_Mucosal Delivery of Sub-Unit Vaccines That Stimulate the Ocular Mucosal Immune System - ScienceDirect. 2006.

[51]   van Ginkel FW, Gulley SL, Lammers A, Hoerr FJ, Gurjar R, Toro H. Conjunctiva-associated lymphoid tissue in avian mucosal immunity. Dev Comp Immunol 2012; 36(2): 289-97.
[http://dx.doi.org/10.1016/j.dci.2011.04.012] [PMID: 21641931]

[52]   Barisani-Asenbauer T, Inic-Kanada A, Belij S, *et al.* The ocular conjunctiva as a mucosal immunization route: a profile of the immune response to the model antigen tetanus toxoid. PLoS One 2013; 8(4): e60682.
[http://dx.doi.org/10.1371/journal.pone.0060682] [PMID: 23637758]

[53]   Kiyono H. Mucosal Vaccines - Hiroshi Kiyono - Google Books. 1996.

[54]   Khatri K. International Journal of Pharmaceutics. 2008. Available from: https://doi.org/./j.ijpharm

[55]   Partidos C. D. The bare skin and the nose as non-invasive routes for administering peptide vaccines - ScienceDirect. 2001.

[56]   Zhang YB, Xu D, Bai L, Zhou YM, Zhang H, Cui YL. A Review of Non-Invasive Drug Delivery through Respiratory Routes. Pharmaceutics. MDPI 2022; 14.

[57]   Harakuni T, Kohama H, Tadano M, *et al.* Mucosal vaccination approach against mosquito-borne Japanese encephalitis virus. Jpn J Infect Dis 2009; 62(1): 37-45.
[http://dx.doi.org/10.7883/yoken.JJID.2009.37] [PMID: 19168957]

[58]   Ádám AL, Nagy Z, Kátay G, Mergenthaler E, Viczián O. Signals of systemic immunity in plants: Progress and open questions. International Journal of Molecular Sciences. MDPI AG 2018; 19.

[59]   Maloy KJ, Donachie AM. Immune-stimulating complexes as adjuvants for inducing local and systemic immunity after oral immunization with protein antigens. Vol. 80. Immunology 1993.

[60]   Beverley PCL, Sridhar S, Lalvani A, Tchilian EZ. Harnessing local and systemic immunity for vaccines against tuberculosis. Mucosal Immunology. Nature Publishing Group 2014; 7: pp. 20-6.

[61]   Truman W, Bennett MH, Kubigsteltig I, Turnbull C, Grant M. *Arabidopsis* systemic immunity uses conserved defense signaling pathways and is mediated by jasmonates. Proc Natl Acad Sci USA 2007; 104(3): 1075-80.
[http://dx.doi.org/10.1073/pnas.0605423104] [PMID: 17215350]

[62]   Rapaport R, Saenger P, Schmidt H, *et al.* Validation and ease of use of a new pen device for self-administration of recombinant human growth hormone: results from a two-center usability study. Med Devices (Auckl) 2013; 6(1): 141-6.
[PMID: 24039458]

[63]   Indrajit A, Eresta Jaya V, Van Loenen B, Lemmen C, Van Oosterom P, Ploeger H, The role of the

revised land administration domain model and spatial data infrastructure in improving ease of doing business in indonesia. 2020. Available from: https://www.doingbusiness. org/en/about-us

[64]   Nordmann J. P. Impact of Xal-Ease ® on eyedrop administration. 2009.

[65]   Winblad B, Kawata AK, Beusterien KM, *et al.* Caregiver preference for rivastigmine patch relative to capsules for treatment of probable Alzheimer's disease. Int J Geriatr Psychiatry 2007; 22(5): 485-91.
[http://dx.doi.org/10.1002/gps.1806] [PMID: 17407176]

[66]   Frederiksen LSF, Zhang Y, Foged C, Thakur A. The Long Road Toward COVID-19 Herd Immunity: Vaccine Platform Technologies and Mass Immunization Strategies. Frontiers in Immunology. Frontiers Media S.A. 2020; 11.

[67]   Mallory ML, Lindesmith LC, Baric RS. Vaccination-induced herd immunity: Successes and challenges. Journal of Allergy and Clinical Immunology. Mosby Inc.; 2018; 142, 64–6.

[68]   Bhopal RS. COVID-19 zugzwang: Potential public health moves towards population (herd) immunity. Public Health Pract (Oxf) 2020; 1: 100031.
[http://dx.doi.org/10.1016/j.puhip.2020.100031] [PMID: 34173570]

[69]   Bhopal RS. COVID-19 zugzwang: Potential public health moves towards population (herd) immunity. Public Health in Practice. 2020; 1.

[70]   Flasche S, Van Hoek AJ, Goldblatt D, *et al.* The Potential for Reducing the Number of Pneumococcal Conjugate Vaccine Doses While Sustaining Herd Immunity in High-Income Countries. PLoS Med 2015; 12(6): e1001839.
[http://dx.doi.org/10.1371/journal.pmed.1001839] [PMID: 26057994]

[71]   Dunham S. P. The application of nucleic acid vaccines in veterinary medicine - ScienceDirect. 2002.

[72]   Heegaard PMH, Dedieu L, Johnson N, *et al.* Adjuvants and delivery systems in veterinary vaccinology: current state and future developments. Arch Virol 2011; 156(2): 183-202.
[http://dx.doi.org/10.1007/s00705-010-0863-1] [PMID: 21170730]

[73]   Dhama K, Mahendran M, Gupta PK, Rai A. DNA vaccines and their applications in veterinary practice: current perspectives. Vet Res Commun 2008; 32(5): 341-56.
[http://dx.doi.org/10.1007/s11259-008-9040-3] [PMID: 18425596]

[74]   Hodgins DC, Chattha K, Vlasova A, Parreño V, Corbeil LB, Renukaradhya GJ, Mucosal Veterinary Vaccines: Comparative Vaccinology. In: Mucosal Immunology: Fourth Edition. Elsevier Inc.; 2015. p. 1337–61.

[75]   El-Sayed A, Kamel M. Advanced applications of nanotechnology in veterinary medicine. Environ Sci Pollut Res Int 2020; 27(16): 19073-86.
[http://dx.doi.org/10.1007/s11356-018-3913-y] [PMID: 30547342]

[76]   Benjamin W. Potential applications for antiviral therapy and prophylaxis in bovine medicine _ Animal Health Research Reviews _ Cambridge Core. 2014.

[77]   Hocquette JF, Lehnert S, Barendse W, Cassar-Malek I, Picard B. Recent advances in cattle functional genomics and their application to beef quality. Animal 2007; pp. 159-73.

[78]   Douglas WR. O F P I G S A N D M E N A N D R E S E A R C H: A Review of Applications and Analogies of the Pig, sus scrofa, in Human Medical Research*. 1972.

[79]   Gruys E, Toussaint MJM, Upragarin N, van Ederen AM, Adewuyi AA, Candiani D, Acute phase reactants, challenge in the near future of animal production and veterinary medicine. J Zhejiang Univ Sci. 2005; 6 B(10):941–7.

[80]   Roth J. A. Duration of immunity induced by companion animal vaccines _ Animal Health Research Reviews _ Cambridge Core. 2010.

[81]   Dodds W. J. Guest editorial. 2001.

[82]   Day MJ, Horzinek MC, Schultz RD. Compiled by the Vaccination Guidlines Group (VGG) of the

World Small Animal Veterinary Association (WSAVA). J Small Anim Pract 2007; 48(9): 528-41.
[http://dx.doi.org/10.1111/j.1748-5827.2007.00462.x] [PMID: 17803726]

[83]   Dodds WJ. Early life vaccination of companion animal pets. Vaccines (Basel) 2021; 9(2): 92.
[http://dx.doi.org/10.3390/vaccines9020092] [PMID: 33513703]

[84]   Horzinek M. C. Vaccination Protocols for Companion Animals_ The Veterinarian's Perspective - ScienceDirect. 2010.

[85]   Hartmann K, Möstl K, Lloret A, Thiry E, Addie DD, Belák S, *et al.* Vaccination of Immunocompromised Cats. Viruses. MDPI 2022; 14.

[86]   Day MJ, Horzinek MC, Schultz RD. Guidelines for the vaccination of dogs and cats compiled by the vaccination guidelines group (vgg) of the world small animal veterinary association (WSAVA) Members of the VGG. Vol. 51, Journal of Small Animal Practice. 2010. Available from: www.bsava.com/

[87]   Day MJ, Horzinek MC, Schultz RD, Squires RA. WSAVA Guidelines for the vaccination of dogs and cats. J Small Anim Pract 2016; 57(1): E1-E45.
[http://dx.doi.org/10.1111/jsap.2_12431] [PMID: 26780857]

[88]   Malabadi RB, Meti NT, Chalannavar RK. Applications of nanotechnology in vaccine development for coronavirus (SARS-CoV-2) disease (Covid-19). Vol. VIII, International Journal of Research and Scientific Innovation (IJRSI). 2021. Available from: www.rsisinternational.org

[89]   Ghattas M, Dwivedi G, Lavertu M, Alameh MG. Vaccine technologies and platforms for infectious diseases: Current progress, challenges, and opportunities. Vaccines. MDPI 2021; 9.

[90]   Gebre MS, Brito LA, Tostanoski LH, Edwards DK, Carfi A, Barouch DH. Novel approaches for vaccine development. Cell. Elsevier B.V. 2021; 184: pp. 1589-603.

[91]   Rauch S, Jasny E, Schmidt KE, Petsch B. New vaccine technologies to combat outbreak situations. Frontiers in Immunology. Frontiers Media S.A. 2018; 9.

[92]   Takeyama N, Kiyono H, Yuki Y. Plant-based vaccines for animals and humans: recent advances in technology and clinical trials. Ther Adv Vaccines 2015; 3(5-6): 139-54.
[http://dx.doi.org/10.1177/2051013615613272] [PMID: 26668752]

[93]   Laere E, Ling APK, Wong YP, Koh RY, Mohd Lila MA, Hussein S. Plant-based vaccines: Production and challenges. Vol. 2016, Journal of Botany. Hindawi Publishing Corporation; 2016.

[94]   Stover CK, de Ia Cruz VF, Fuerst TR, Burlein JE, Benson L, Bennett LT, 47. Braithwaite, A. W. eta. Vol. 13, N. R. eta/. Proc. natn. Acad Sci. USA. 1989.

[95]   Roizman B, Palese P, Moss B. Co-chairs). Vol. 93. 1996. Available from: https://www.pnas.org

[96]   Yadav T, Srivastava N, Mishra G, *et al.* Recombinant vaccines for COVID-19. Hum Vaccin Immunother 2020; 16(12): 2905-12.
[http://dx.doi.org/10.1080/21645515.2020.1820808] [PMID: 33232211]

[97]   Barnard RT. Recombinant vaccines. In: Expert Review of Vaccines. 2010. p. 461–3.
[http://dx.doi.org/10.1586/erv.10.48]

[98]   Caron A, Cappelle J, Cumming GS, De Garine-Wichatitsky M, Gaidet N. Bridge hosts, a missing link for disease ecology in multi-host systems. Veterinary Research. BioMed Central Ltd. 2015; 46.

[99]   Twyman RM, Stoger E, Schillberg S, Christou P, Fischer R. Molecular farming in plants: Host systems and expression technology. Trends in Biotechnology. Elsevier Ltd; 2003; 21, 570–8.

[100] Chavda VP, Bezbaruah R, Athalye M, Parikh PK, Chhipa AS, Patel S, *et al.* Replicating Viral Vector-Based Vaccines for COVID-19: Potential Avenue in Vaccination Arena. Viruses. MDPI 2022; 14.

[101] Ura T, Okuda K, Shimada M. Developments in viral vector-based vaccines. Vaccines. MDPI AG 2014; 2: pp. 624-41.

[102] Liu MA. DNA vaccines: a review. J Intern Med 2003; 253(4): 402-10.
[http://dx.doi.org/10.1046/j.1365-2796.2003.01140.x] [PMID: 12653868]

[103] Donnelly JJ, Ulmer JB, Shiver JW, Liu MA. DNA vaccines. Annu Rev Immunol 1997; 15(1): 617-48.
[http://dx.doi.org/10.1146/annurev.immunol.15.1.617] [PMID: 9143702]

[104] Kramps T, Knut ·, Editors E. RNA Vaccines Methods and Protocols Methods in Molecular Biology 1499. 2017. Available from: http://www.springer.com/series/7651

[105] Sandbrink JB, Shattock RJ. RNA Vaccines: A Suitable Platform for Tackling Emerging Pandemics?. Frontiers in Immunology. Frontiers Media S.A. 2020; 11.

[106] Shi J, Huang F, Jia F, Yang Z, Rui M. Mass customization: the role of consumer preference measurement, manufacturing flexibility and customer participation. Asia Pac J Mark Log 2023; 35(6): 1366-82.
[http://dx.doi.org/10.1108/APJML-10-2021-0719]

[107] Fredriksson P. Flexibility and rigidity in customization and build-to-order production - ScienceDirect. 2005.

[108] Wenjun M. & Jurgen A. Swine influenza vaccines_ current status and future perspectives _ Animal Health Research Reviews _ Cambridge Core. 2010.

[109] Liu MA. DNA vaccines: an historical perspective and view to the future. Immunol Rev 2011; 239(1): 62-84.
[http://dx.doi.org/10.1111/j.1600-065X.2010.00980.x] [PMID: 21198665]

[110] Baron MD, Iqbal M, Nair V. Recent advances in viral vectors in veterinary vaccinology. Current Opinion in Virology. Elsevier B.V. 2018; 29: pp. 1-7.

[111] Hataminejad M, Anvari D, Khaleghi N, Nayeri T, Shirazinia R, Shariatzadeh SA, *et al.* Current status and future prospects of Echinococcus multilocularis vaccine candidates: A systematic review. Veterinary and Animal Science. Elsevier B.V. 2024; 24.

[112] Thomas S, Abraham A, Rodríguez-Mallon A, Unajak S, Bannantine JP. Challenges in Veterinary Vaccine Development. Methods in Molecular Biology. Humana Press Inc. 2022; pp. 3-34.

[113] Mucosal immunisation and adjuvants_ a brief overview of recent advances and challenges - ScienceDirect.

[114] Vaernewyck V, Arzi B, Sanders NN, Cox E, Devriendt B. Mucosal Vaccination Against Periodontal Disease: Current Status and Opportunities. Frontiers in Immunology. Frontiers Media S.A. 2021; 12.

[115] Munang'andu HM, Mutoloki S. Evensen Oø. An overview of challenges limiting the design of protective mucosal vaccines for finfish. Front Immunol 2015; 6(OCT)

CHAPTER 5

Innovation in Adjuvants for Mucosal Vaccine Enhancement

Akanksha Sharma[1], Sunita[2], Ashish[3], Shaweta Sharma[4] and Akhil Sharma[1,*]

[1] *R. J. College of Pharmacy, 2HVJ+567, Raipur, Gharbara, Tappal, Khair, Uttar Pradesh 202165, India*

[2] *Metro College of Health Sciences and Research, Greater Noida, India*

[3] *Mangalmay Pharmacy College, Plot No. 9, Knowledge Park II, Greater Noida, Uttar Pradesh, 201306, India*

[4] *School of Medical and Allied Sciences, Galgotias University, Yamuna Expressway, Gautam Buddha Nagar, Uttar Pradesh-201310, India*

Abstract: The growth of efficacious mucosal vaccines delivered through mucosal surfaces like oral and nasal routes is a major improvement in immunization strategies. These agents provide the possibility for non-invasive administration, ease of giving them out, and the capability to induce systemic and local immune responses. Nevertheless, the body's natural barriers and the necessity of potent adjuvants to trigger immune responses have historically hindered the mucosal vaccines' effectiveness. This abstract will discuss new developments in adjuvants that can transform mucosal vaccine adoption's effectiveness. Traditional adjuvants like aluminum salts and MF59 have proved ineffective in mucosal contexts because they cannot penetrate the mucosal barriers to elicit strong mucosal immunity. This led to the development of new adjuvants such as nanoparticles, liposomes, and Toll-like receptor (TLR) agonists that could address these challenges. An example of such adjuvants is nanoparticle-based ones, which aid in stabilizing antigens and enable targeted delivery, thus ensuring they reach correct immune cells. Adjuvants commonly used in adjuvant development, such as aluminum salts and MF59, have proved less effective in mucosal contexts due to their inability to penetrate the mucosal barriers and elicit strong mucosal immunity. For this reason, scientists have created new adjuvants, including nanoparticles, liposomes, and Toll-like receptor (TLR) agonists, which can potentially address these deficiencies. Nanoparticle-based adjuvants, for example, may improve antigen stability while promoting delivery to specific immune cells that require them. Additionally, the development of recombinant proteins and synthetic peptides with strong functions as mucosal adjuvants has been made possible through improvements in bioengineering. To study these new adjuvants that are under trial progressively in medical practice, it is essential to perform clinical trials and research continuously. The future of mucosal

---

* **Corresponding author Akhil Sharma:** R. J. College of Pharmacy, 2HVJ+567, Raipur, Gharbara, Tappal, Khair, Uttar Pradesh 202165, India; E-mail: xs2akhil@gmail.com

Shaweta Sharma, Aftab Alam & Akhil Sharma (Eds.)

vaccines is bright, and this could be achieved by employing novel materials and technologies to make more efficient vaccines that can be easily accessed by everyone, thereby enhancing global health outcomes.

Keywords: Adjuvant, Antigen, Health, Immunization, Immune cells, Liposomes, Mucosal-associated lymphoid tissue, Mucosal vaccine, Mucosal surfaces, Non-invasive delivery, Nanoparticles, Toll-like receptor agonists, Targeted delivery.

INTRODUCTION

In this case, mucosal vaccines are administered *via* the gastrointestinal (oral) and respiratory (nasal) tracts. These types of vaccines do not require a needle injection like most traditional injectable vaccines but aim to create immunity at the point of pathogen entry to generate both local mucosal and systemic immune responses. They guard against infections that breach the body *via* its mucosal surfaces, including influenza, rotavirus, and certain types of pneumonia [1].

Mucosal vaccines can be delivered in several forms, such as liquids, powders, or oral vaccines packaged as tablets and nasal vaccines as sprays or drops. This kind of delivery is less invasive and more user-friendly, not to mention better suited to the elderly and children; it also has the potential to elicit stronger and more specific immune responses at numerous infectious agent portals of entry [2].

Mucosal immunity describes the immune defenses on mucosal membranes like the gastrointestinal, respiratory, and urogenital tracts, eyes, and oral cavities. These interfaces are the primary window between our bodies and the external environment. It is crucial to understand that entry points are quite frequent for pathogens; hence, this type of immunity plays a very important role. The innermost linings of the mucosa have epithelial cells that serve as a barrier and are reinforced by mucus; this is a slimy fluid that entraps germs and also contains antimicrobial peptides and enzymes. In MALT, such as the tonsils, Peyer's patches in the intestines and lymphoid tissues in the respiratory tract are found. It comprises immune cells primed to detect and react against any infecting pathogen [3].

Secretory IgA, the primary antibody class in these areas, represents a fundamental aspect of mucosal immunity. The chief role played by IgA is neutralization of pathogens and preventing them from getting attached to or penetrating the epithelial cells. Additionally, various specialized immune cells are found in the mucosal immune system. Antigen-presenting cells, namely dendritic cells (DCs), are the ones that capture antigens from pathogens and then travel to the lymphoid tissues where they display these antigens to T and B cells to initiate adaptive immune responses. Th17 cells are among the mucosal T-cells that participate in maintaining mucosal barriers and responding to infections, whereas IgA-secreting B-cells transudate into the lumen of the epithelium at mucosa [4].

The mechanisms of the mucosal immune responses begin with sampling and presentation of antigens. M cells, specialized epithelial cells, sample antigens from the mucosal surface and transport them to underlying immune cells. Dendritic cells process these antigens and present them to T and B cells in the MALT. As a result of this interaction, secretory IgA is induced, and activated B cells turn into plasma cells that make IgA. The latter gets transferred *via* the epithelial layer to the mucosal surface, where it can attach to and deactivate pathogens. Furthermore, cell-mediated immunity is important, with MALT-activated T cells migrating to the mucosal surface for the direct killing of infected cells or coordinating other immune responses [5].

The significance of mucosal immunity in vaccination is that it can direct the immune response to the site of pathogen entry, thus providing local and systemic protection. Mucosal vaccines are modeled after natural infection routes, which trigger a powerful localized immune response leading to preventing pathogen entry and replication. In addition, their ability to cause systemic immunity offers all-inclusive security against pathogens. These vaccines can be taken through the mucosal route without any invasion; they can be given orally or nasally, and this is an alternative to needle administration that can help increase vaccine acceptance and compliance, especially among those who are afraid of needles. The immune system has a complicated aspect known as mucosal immunity that gives critical cover to the areas where our body easily gets infections. The potential to improve immunization strategies and public health outcomes through these vaccines depends on how best one utilizes their parts and functions from the immunological perspective [6].

Importance of Adjuvants

To improve the effectiveness and potency of vaccines, they are boosted with adjuvants that enhance their immuno-potency, leading to better immune responses. Adjuvants are designed to enhance immunity so as to make vaccines more effective in protecting against diseases with fewer antigens, which is important, especially in new or difficult-to-treat diseases [7].

Adjuvants are mainly used to boost the body's immune response to a vaccine antigen. Hence, adjuvants help stimulate innate immunity, which is usually the first line against infections. This includes the inducement of dendritic cells and macrophages necessary for antigen presentation before T and B cells. Antigen presentation carries out this purpose, and it is vital in starting adaptive immunity for long-term protection [8].

Additionally, adjuvants can change the kind of immunity that a vaccine stimulates. For example, certain adjuvants act to boost antibody production, while others are more effective in promoting T-cell-mediated immunity, which involves activating T-cells. Such modulation is especially crucial for vaccines against intracellular pathogens like viruses, for which a strong cellular immune response is important [9].

In addition, adjuvants further reduce the antigen needed per vaccine dose. Adjuvants enhance immune response, enabling dose sparing, which becomes critical during pandemics or outbreaks with an urgent need for faster vaccine production. This allows a population larger than that which could have been vaccinated using the available antigens to be immunized more broadly and quickly [10].

Moreover, adjuvants also help stabilize vaccines, which is important for their durability. They also play a big role in protecting antigens from degradation, hence maintaining the effectiveness of the vaccine over time. This feature becomes particularly crucial in cases where vaccines have to be kept for long durations or when they need to be transported in remote areas lacking advanced cold chain setups [11].

Adjuvants are important because they help improve the immune response of individuals with weak immune systems. This group includes the vulnerable elderly and those with weak immune systems. Adjuvants can help solve the difficulties that go with immunosenescence, which is the gradual decline of the body's defense system with age, thus keeping vaccines effective for all ages.

Modern vaccine development and delivery cannot be done without adjuvants, which make vaccines more effective, enable low doses, improve the stability of antigens, and ensure populations become highly immune to different diseases. Constant innovations in adjuvant technology are critical for addressing existing and emerging diseases, leading to better global health [12].

Role of Adjuvant in Vaccine Efficacy

Adjuvants play a crucial role in vaccine efficacy by enhancing and directing the immune response to the antigen. Their inclusion in vaccines is vital for several reasons:

Enhancing Immune Response

Adjuvants, which boost an immune response for a particular antigen, make possible higher levels of antibody production and activation of T cells. This is especially important for subunit vaccines that include only specific antigens rather than whole pathogens. Without adjuvants, these vaccines can evoke low immune responses. Adjuvants also help by creating more responses to make the pathogen visible to the immune system in case it is exposed again [13, 14].

Prolonging Immune Response

One of the main advantages of adjuvants is that they help prolong the immune response. They do this by causing a depot effect where antigens are released slowly to continue stimulating the immune system. This sustained release ensures that the immune system has a longer period to recognize and respond to the antigen, leading to the development of long-term immunity [15].

Dose Sparing

Adjuvants allow lower amounts of antigens to be used in vaccines without compromising the vaccine's efficiency. This is advantageous in circumstances like pandemic periods when there is high vaccine demand during manufacture. By lowering the quantity of antigen required, it is possible to make more doses of vaccines and thus increase accessibility and availability [16].

Modulating the Type of Immune Response

Effective protection against different pathogens requires varied kinds of immune responses. Some diseases can best be dealt with using a strong antibody response (humoral immunity), while there are others for which the most effective response will require stronger T-cell activity (cellular immunity). Vaccines may have adjuvants programmed in such a way as to tilt the immune reaction towards one specific type, thereby boosting their efficiency against particular pathogens. For example, some adjuvants encourage the development of Th1 cells, thus making them particularly useful in fighting off intracellular pathogens such as viruses, while others stimulate Th2 responses, which play an important role in eradicating extracellular bacteria [17].

Overcoming Immunosenescence

Vaccination might not produce enough immune response when the immune system is weak, such as in people who are either too old or whose immunity has been compromised. This problem can be overcome by using adjuvants that stimulate the immune systems of these individuals to receive adequate protection when vaccinated. This should be particularly noted for diseases that disproportionately affect this group [18].

Broadening Protection

Other substances added to vaccines can also improve their protection. By causing a more varied response in the immune system, they may raise the efficiency of a vaccine against different strains of particular pathogens. This is especially important when dealing with vaccines for viruses that undergo rapid mutation, such as influenza, where a wider immunity helps defend against multiple viral forms [19].

Historical Context and Traditional Adjuvants

The historical context and traditional adjuvants used in vaccines are summarized in Table 1.

Table 1. Historical context and traditional adjuvants used in vaccines.

Period	Historical Context	Traditional Adjuvants	Description
Early 20th Century	Enhanced vaccines need to be developed for promoting immune responses, including using adjuvants.	Aluminum Salts (Alum)	Alum was discovered in the 1920s and was the first widely used adjuvant. It enhances antibody production and is used in many vaccines [20].
1930s	Research into adjuvants continued, focusing on enhancing vaccine efficacy and safety.	Mineral Oil Emulsions	Freund's Complete Adjuvant (FCA) and Freund's Incomplete Adjuvant (FIA), containing mineral oil, were discovered. FCA contains killed forms of the mycobacteria that boost immune response [21].
1970s	Modern immunology has evolved to provide a greater knowledge of the immune systems and adjuvants' functions.	Aluminum Hydroxide and Phosphate	Enhanced alum forms with better profiles of safety and efficacy. Utilized in vaccines like DTP (Diphtheria, Tetanus, Pertussis) [22].
1980s	Attention has shifted towards searching for harmless and more efficient adjuvants for human vaccines.	MF59	An oil-in-water emulsion by Novartis used in influenza vaccines. It increases the immune response by recruiting immune cells to the injection site [23].
1990s	The development of recombinant vaccines has led to the emergence of new adjuvant types that can enhance their effectiveness.	AS04	The HPV vaccine combines aluminum hydroxide and monophosphoryl lipid A (MPL). MPL stimulates the immune system as a detoxified lipopolysaccharide (LPS) [24].

Period	Historical Context	Traditional Adjuvants	Description
2000s	Exploration of new adjuvants for a wider range of vaccines became possible with the onset of development in biotechnology.	AS03	The pandemic influenza vaccine has an oil-in-water emulsion that boosts the immune system by enhancing cytokine production and facilitating the mobilization of immune cells [25].
Present	The ongoing research puts all its effort into making adjuvants more effective, safer, and versatile for different types of vaccines, including those given through the mucosal route [26].	CpG Oligodeoxynucleotides	Synthetic DNA sequences can mimic bacterial DNA, stimulating a robust immune response. They are used in different experimental vaccines [27].

CHALLENGES IN MUCOSAL VACCINATION

Barriers to Effective Delivery

Mucosal Barriers

Various barriers protect mucosal surfaces, such as gastrointestinal and respiratory tracts, from pathogen invasion. Although these protections prevent infections, they make it difficult to deliver mucosal vaccines [28] effectively.

Mucus Layer

The mucus coating is a thick, jellylike matter of water, electrolytes, proteins, fats, and mucins. As a result, it shields the mucosal surfaces by blocking or eliminating pathogenic agents. Immunizations will not work if the mucus obstructs diffusion of their components to the epithelial cells beneath, which are ingested and processed by the immune system. The vaccines must pass through this dense fluid layer to work properly [29].

Enzymatic Degradation

Mucosal surfaces contain enzymes like proteases, lipases, and nucleases that digest proteins, fats, and nucleic acids. These enzymes can degrade vaccine antigens even before they reach their targeted sites, thereby reducing their efficacy. Therefore, formulations must protect antigens from enzymatic degradation to maintain their stability and potency [30].

Antigen Stability

For mucosal vaccines, antigens must be stabilized so that they work properly before any immune response happens. Several factors contribute to antigen instability at mucosal surfaces:

Physiological Conditions

The various mucosal surfaces have different pH levels. For instance, the stomach is highly acidic, while the small intestines exhibit a pH that is either neutral or slightly alkaline. Under such conditions, proteins can be denatured, and antigens can be degraded. Antigens that are sensitive to temperature can have their stability influenced by temperature fluctuations on the mucosal surfaces [31].

Physical and Chemical Degradation

Mucosal surfaces, for example, can lead to the degradation of antigens through oxidation or hydrolysis reactions. These processes are accelerated by contact with oxygen and water. As a result, antigenic substances may be insoluble or form large aggregates, making them less able to be taken up by immune cells [32].

Immune System Challenges

Immune system challenges in mucosal vaccination are discussed below and summarized in Fig. (1).

Low Immunogenicity at Mucosal Surfaces

Immunization cannot work effectively on mucosal surfaces found in the respiratory tract or gastrointestinal system since they have surpassed their goal of higher immunogenicity than those in systemic sites. Certain factors influence this low immunogenicity. It is vital to note that first, mucosal tissues are naturally oriented towards maintaining tolerance to harmless antigens so as not to react and cause inflammation [33]. Moreover, being also considered, there exist physical obstacles that hinder and obstruct the intake and exhibition of antigens. Additionally, enzymatic degradation in the mucosal environment can degrade vaccine protein antigens before they can even cause an immune response. Thus, vaccines may need to contain more antigens or adjuvants and delivery systems that will overcome these barriers for adequate immunity and vaccine efficacy [34, 35].

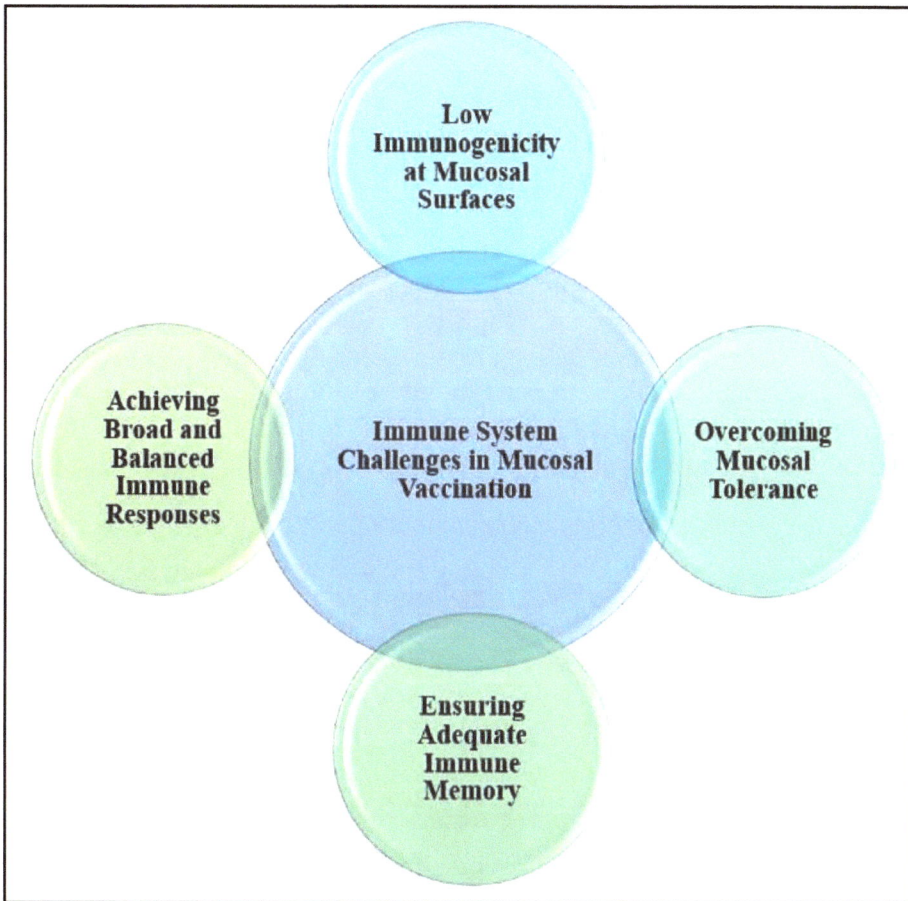

Fig. (1). Immune system challenges in mucosal vaccination.

Overcoming Mucosal Tolerance

In developing vaccines, overcoming mucosal tolerance is a crucial hurdle since harmless antigens can often induce immune tolerance through the mucosal immune system. Vaccines are not very effective as this tolerance mechanism tends to inhibit immune responses. In response to this problem, scientists are currently working on techniques that use only specific adjuvants and delivery systems for mucus. These strategies actively target mucosal sites where they facilitate antigen presentation and promote immunity activation in order to counteract its tendency toward tolerance induction [36].

Innate immune responses can be induced by mucosal-specific adjuvants, such as nanoparticles or Toll-like receptor agonists, which can also enhance antigen presentation to immune cells. In addition, liposomes or microparticles, as innovative delivery systems, may help deliver antigens specifically to the mucosal epithelium, thereby making them more visible to the immune system. As such, vaccine builders target these approaches to overcome the barriers of oral tolerance and reach maximal immunity against mucosal pathogens through vaccines [37].

Ensuring Adequate Immune Memory

Long-term protection from infection requires the development of a stable memory at mucosal sites. Mucosal immunity is transient since the tissues involved are continually changing, and there is a high turnover of immune cells. It, therefore, becomes necessary to set up and maintain memory T and B cells within the mucosa post-vaccination. This immune memory is developed through appropriate vaccine formulations. Principally, these include formulations that facilitate the formation of tissue-resident memory T-cells and long-lived plasma cells [38].

Mucosal tissue contains memory T cells that are permanent and can act rapidly by the body when a previously encountered pathogen is met again. However, long-lived plasma cells are responsible for making antibodies continuously to protect the system over a longer period. This ensures that vaccine developers who focus on producing these types of memory cells can increase the duration of mucosal immune memory, hence raising the effectiveness and longevity of various mucosal vaccines against pathogens [39].

Achieving Broad and Balanced Immune Responses

To gain complete infection protection, it is important to have a wide and balanced immune response. Both the arms of the immune system are involved in combating mucosal infections; thus, there is a need for strong induction of T cells as well as antibodies. Mucosal IgA antibodies form robust antibody responses that neutralize pathogens, preventing their binding and entry into mucosal epithelial cells. Again, infected cell clearance and coordination of immune responses involve T cell responses, including cytotoxic T cells and helper T cells [40].

Moreover, cross-protection towards a wide range of pathogens must be considered when dealing with the diversity of mucosal pathogens. Vaccine formulations offering broad-based immunity by targeting conserved antigens or incorporating multiple antigenic constituents from different strains or serotypes can boost vaccine efficacy against numerous pathogens. When they elicit responses that are protective and wide-ranging, mucosal vaccines offer complete protection against infections that occur inside the body lining and thus contribute to efforts aimed at controlling infectious diseases in the general population [41].

To deal with these challenges posed by the immune system, it is important to develop new strategies for making vaccines and delivering them to improve the efficacy of mucosal vaccination and make people more resistant to mucosal pathogens [42].

TYPES OF MUCOSAL ADJUVANTS

Mucosal adjuvants are substances that enhance immunity when they are presented through the mucus membranes of the nasal, oral, or genital mucous. These adjuvants can improve vaccine efficacy by promoting antigen uptake and presentation by mucosal-associated lymphoid tissues. Types of mucosal adjuvants are summarized in Fig. (**2**).

Types of Mucosal Adjuvants	Traditional Adjuvants	Cholera Toxin (CT) and Heat-Labile Enterotoxin (LT)
		Escherichia coli Heat-Labile Toxin (LT)
		Bacterial Lipopolysaccharides (LPS)
		Aluminum Salts (Alum)
		MF59
	Emerging Adjuvants	Toll-like Receptor (TLR) Agonists
		Nanoparticle-based Adjuvants
		Cytokine Adjuvants
		Virus-Vectored Adjuvants
		Pattern Recognition Receptor (PRR) Agonists
		RNA-based Adjuvants

Fig. (**2**). Types of mucosal adjuvants.

Traditional Adjuvants

Cholera Toxin (CT) and Heat-Labile Enterotoxin (LT)

CT and LT are powerful mucosal adjuvants that are derived from pathogenic bacteria, Vibrio cholerae and enterotoxigenic *Escherichia coli* (ETEC), respectively. These toxins have been widely studied for their ability to increase immune response, mainly in the mucosal surfaces that pathogens first attack following host infection [43].

They activate adenylate cyclase present in mucosal epithelial cells, leading to high levels of cyclic AMP (cAMP) that have a critical role in regulating immune responses by facilitating the production of pro-inflammatory cytokines, chemokines, and other immune mediators. Moreover, cAMP signaling can lead to the activation of antigen-presenting cells (APCs) and stimulate T and B lymphocytes' differentiation and proliferation, thus improving both humoral and cellular immune responses.

Their strong adjuvant activities notwithstanding, the adverse reactions of CT and LT, especially concerning their toxicity potential and side effects, restrict their use as human vaccines over the wider population. This results in safety concerns because such toxins can cause serious digestive system disorders, including dehydration and diarrhea, which are of particular concern for those who already have compromised health conditions, like aged people and children [44]. Therefore, safer alternatives of mucosal adjuvants, such as less toxic derivatives through detoxification or synthetic counterparts, are being sought after in place of CT and LT [45, 46].

Escherichia coli Heat-Labile Toxin (LT)

The powerful mucosal adjuvant derived from the pathogenic bacterium *Escherichia coli* Heat-Labile Toxin (LT) shares a lot of similarities with CT. LT, in the same way CT does, works by activating adenylate cyclase within mucosal epithelial cells, which enhances cyclic AMP (cAMP) production and subsequently activates the immune system. It also increases antigen expression, cytokine synthesis, and the migration of immune cells, thus leading to heightened immunity at mucosal surfaces [47].

However, LT may have certain benefits, such as being less toxic than CT. It is noted that it has been proposed by some scholars as a possible mucosal adjuvant in vaccines since it is considered to be less harmful than CT. The results of studies indicate that compared to the latter, LT might cause milder gut symptoms and have lesser effects on the host, thereby suggesting its potential use in vaccine formulations for children and older persons at risk [48].

However, despite its potential benefits, there are still concerns about the safety of LT, especially in terms of inducing side effects. Further research is required to elucidate its safety profile and optimize its use as a mucosal adjuvant in vaccine development [49].

Bacterial Lipopolysaccharides (LPS)

LPS is also called endotoxin and is a strong mucosal adjuvant found in the outer membrane of Gram-negative bacteria. Its ability to boost immune responses has made it popular in mucosal surfaces where most diseases initially attack the host. LPS acts as an adjuvant by activating Toll-like receptor 4 (TLR4) signaling that controls innate immunity. LPS, when bound to TLR4, triggers the transmission of a signal chain that eventually sets in motion the immune cells, for example, macrophages and dendritic cells. This being active inflames the production of pro-inflammatory cytokines such as interleukin-1 (IL-1), tumor necrosis factor-alpha (TNF-α), and interleukin-6 (IL-6), which play a role in inflammation and help to initiate and amplify adaptive immune responses [50].

In spite of its powerful adjuvant action, LPS has not been widely used in vaccines because of concerns about the potential to cause adverse reactions and pyrogenicity. LPS may cause fever, inflammation, and other systemic manifestations that are dependent on the dose, origin, and purity of the LPS preparation. To address these concerns, various safer alternative mucosal adjuvants to replace LPS have been identified, including detoxified derivatives and synthetic analogs with low toxicities [51].

Aluminum Salts (Alum)

Aluminum salts like aluminum hydroxide and aluminum phosphate are widely used in injectable vaccines as adjuvants to boost the immune system. These salts have also been scrutinized for their possible use in mucosal adjuvants, mostly for vaccines that target pathogens occurring on these surfaces. The way aluminum salts work is by causing inflammation at the site of injection, which attracts a number of antigen-presenting cells (APCs), such as dendritic cells and macrophages. This activation enhances the uptake, processing, and presentation of co-administered antigens to immune cells, which leads to stronger immunity responses [52].

Nevertheless, mucosal adjuvants made of aluminum salts may not be as effective as other substances. Even though they increase immune responses at the site of injection, their ability to activate the mucosal immune system, especially remotely from distant areas of the mucosa, is less definite. Moreover, injectable vaccines are mainly based on aluminum salts and may not work optimally when used in mucosal delivery systems. Because of these constraints, aluminum salts are still popularly used in vaccines because of their safety and efficacy in immune boosting. Nevertheless, further research is required to investigate other adjuvants that might have superiority in terms of mucosal adjuvant properties to those targeting mucosal pathogens [53].

MF59

MF59 is an oil-in-water emulsion adjuvant consisting of squalene oil, polysorbate 80, and sorbitan trioleate. By promoting the recruitment and activation of antigen-presenting cells (APCs) at the injection site, MF59 enhances immune responses. Additionally, it boosts the production of pro-inflammatory cytokines and chemokines that consequently activate and mature immune cells. Primarily used as an adjuvant in influenza vaccines to boost their immunogenicity specifically in populations with weak immune responses like elderly individuals, MF59 has been shown to improve vaccine efficacy and increase antibody response to influenza antigens [54].

Emerging Adjuvants

Toll-like Receptor (TLR) Agonists

As adjuvants, they mimic pathogen-associated molecular patterns (PAMPs) that boost immune responses. These PAMPS activate the receptors of innate immunity, such as Toll-like receptors, which are central for the recognition and initiation of immune responses towards microbial components. These TLR agonists, on binding to their respective TLRs, initiate signal transduction pathways leading to the production of pro-inflammatory cytokines, chemokines, and other immune mediators. This activation will enhance the recruitment and activation of antigen-presenting cells (APCs), which include dendritic cells and macrophages; subsequently, this promotes the activation required for adaptive immune response [55].

A good illustration of a TLR agonist is monophosphoryl lipid A(MPLA), an inactivated form of bacterial lipopolysaccharide (LPS). MPLA retains the immunostimulatory properties of LPS while significantly reducing its toxicity. For instance, MPLAs are in vaccines such as the AS04 HPV vaccine. Hence, through the AS04 adjuvant system, MPLA and aluminum salts have been combined to increase immune responses against human papillomavirus (HPV) infections, leading to stronger and more sustainable protection. Vaccination approaches offer hope with TLR agonists, for instance, MPLA which has the potential to stimulate the immune system strongly enough while keeping safety in check. There is a proven potential of these vaccines to increase vaccine efficacy especially in populations with poor immune responses [56, 57].

Nanoparticle-based Adjuvants

This is a highly modern way of producing vaccines whereby nanoparticles are used as adjuvants, which exploit the distinctive characteristics of these particles to empower immune responses. Both antigens and adjuvants can be delivered by such particles, thus guaranteeing targeted and slow release to immunity cells; in this way helping improve efficacy and safety in vaccination. One notable example is lipid nanoparticles (LNPs), which are particularly known for their use in mRNA vaccines such as those created for COVID-19. LNPs enfold mRNA, shielding it from rapid degradation and enhancing its translocation into host cells, where it undergoes translation into antigenic proteins that incite strong immune reactions [58].

In this case, polymeric nanoparticles could be taken into account, which are mainly formed of biodegradable polymers like PLGA (polylactic-co-glycolic acid. The encapsulation of antigens and adjuvants by these particles leads to sustained release as well as the promotion of their uptake by antigen-presenting cells (APCs). This feature is important for establishing potent and prolonged immune responses. They have the appearance of viruses but do not contain viral genetic material; hence are non-infectious and called virus-like particles (VLPs). VLPs have a repetitive surface that is highly immunogenic, activating the immune system effectively. They are known to be effective in promoting strong immune responses in vaccines for both hepatitis B and human papilloma virus (HPV) [59].

A versatile and powerful platform for enhancing vaccine efficacy is offered by nanoparticle-based adjuvants. This makes them a promising tool in the development of next-generation vaccines against a wide range of infectious diseases due to their ability to provide controlled release as well as targeted delivery [60].

Cytokine Adjuvants

Cytokine adjuvants are a hopeful variety of vaccine adjuvants that exploit the immune-modulating abilities of cytokines to enhance vaccine effectiveness. In a healthy body, there exist substances known as cytokines that play a role in regulating the intensity and kind of immune response, thus rendering them important in optimizing immunity triggered by vaccines. One potent cytokine adjuvant is Interleukin-12 (IL-12), which is renowned for its ability to stimulate Th1-type immune responses. These Th1 responses are associated with the secretion of interferon-gamma (IFN-γ), which prompts cytotoxic T cells and macrophages to become more active, leading to increased elimination of intracellular pathogens. Various formulations for vaccines have included IL-12 in an attempt to augment cell-mediated immunity and improve vaccine efficacy against diseases such as tuberculosis and HIV [61].

A number of other cytokines, like granulocyte-macrophage colony-stimulating factor (GM-CSF), can be used as adjuvant to increase the vaccine response. GM-

CSF actually promotes the differentiation and proliferation of dendritic cells and macrophages, which are key antigen-presenting cells (APCs) that initiate immune responses. GM-CSF then enhances the antigen presentation by increasing both the number and activity of APCs and, thereby, stimulating strong antigen-specific immune responses. This has been especially valuable with cancer vaccines, whereby GM-CSF is administered to strengthen the body's capacity to identify and invade tumor cells. Cytokine adjuvants, such as IL-12 and GM-CSF, have immense possibilities for vaccine enhancement by controlling the immune milieu, promoting specific immune pathways, and refining antigen-specific responses. The use of these is still an active area of study in the development of vaccines and has promising implications for bettering vaccine efficacy against infectious diseases and cancer [62].

Virus-Vectored Adjuvants

Novel antigen delivery systems using viruses have been developed to enhance vaccine immune responses. Examples of these viral vectors include adenoviruses and poxviruses, which can be genetically engineered to either express adjuvant molecules or deliver antigens directly into cells of the immune system. Thus, vaccination allows such genetic instructions to be expressed in host organisms [63].

Adenoviruses are typically employed as viral carriers due to their capacity to infect a wide array of cellular types and provoke strong immune reactions. Their use in vaccines for diseases like Ebola and COVID-19 has been successful. For example, the Ebola vaccine (rVSV-ZEBOV) involves using a recombinant vesicular stomatitis virus (VSV) vector expressing the Ebola virus glycoprotein to elicit vigorous immune responses, resulting in significant protection against disease. Similarly, COVID-19 vaccines such as AstraZeneca's (Vaxzevria) and Johnson & Johnson's (Janssen) utilize adenovirus vectors to carry the spike protein gene from SARS-CoV-2 virus, leading to potent immunogenicity and effective prevention [64].

Poxviruses, like modified vaccinia Ankara (MVA), are another subset of viral vectors that can be used as adjuvants. MVA vectors are altered to present antigens from pathogens, thereby increasing the immune system's ability to identify and fight these pathogens. They have found utility in experimental vaccines for diseases such as HIV and tuberculosis, displaying positive outcomes in preclinical and clinical work [65].

Pattern Recognition Receptor (PRR) Agonists

Novel adjuvants known as Pattern Recognition Receptor (PRR) agonists enhance the immune responses *via* stimulation of innate immune receptors like RIG-I-like receptors (RLRs) and NOD-like receptors (NLRs). These recognize pathogen-associated molecular patterns (PAMPs), starting an immune signaling pathway that boosts both innate and adaptive immunity [66].

Cytoplasmic sensors known as RLRs detect viral RNA, which can lead to the production of type I interferons and some other pro-inflammatory cytokines. The activation of RLRs, therefore, has the potential for improving immune response against viral infections and advancing vaccine efficacy. Vaccine adjuvants have been reported in literature where synthetic ligands have been used, such as Poly(I: C), a synthetic analog of double-stranded RNA that binds to RLRs. This implies that Poly (I: C) enhances the immune responses by copying the viral infection, stimulating RLR pathways, and improving vaccine efficacy [67].

NOD-like receptors (NLRs) detect danger signals and bacterial components, which are intracellular receptors. This leads to inflammasomes activation and production of interleukin-1β (IL-1β) and interleukin-18 (IL-18). Researchers have investigated the synthetic ligands for NLRs like muramyl dipeptide (MDP) regarding vaccine adjuvants. By activating NLR pathways, they increase immune responses that protect against bacterial and viral infections [68].

RNA-based Adjuvants

The class of RNA-based adjuvants is a novel sort of adjuvant that utilizes various RNA molecules, such as mRNA and RNA oligonucleotides, to boost immune responses. These kinds of RNA can provoke immunity by activating pattern recognition receptors (PRRs) such as Toll-like receptors (TLRs) and RIG-I-like receptors (RLRs) that respond to viral infection's signal in the form of the presence of RNA. When these trigger intracellular signaling pathways, they can produce type I interferons and other pro-inflammatory cytokines, boosting innate and adaptive immunity [69].

Adjuvants based on RNA are also observed in mRNA vaccines. The latter use artificial mRNA that codes viral antigens, which, once put into host cells, produce proteins that incite a strong immune response. Two best examples include Pfizer-BioNTech and Moderna COVID-19 vaccines that employ lipid nanoparticles for transporting SARS-CoV-2 spike protein-encoding mRNAs. These vaccines have proved to be highly effective and rapidly produced, thus contributing significantly to the global fight against the COVID-19 pandemic [70].

In addition to this, RNA oligonucleotides, which are smaller fragments of RNA, can also play the role of adjuvants by directly stimulating immune cells through PRR pathways. Additionally, these molecules can be engineered to resemble viral RNA, enhancing the immunogenicity of vaccines and encouraging a stronger and longer-lasting immune response.

Emerging adjuvants offer different mechanisms of action and are great hopes for improving vaccines' effectiveness, expanding immune responses, and dealing with vaccine development difficulties. For further development of new vaccines and solving global health issues, this domain needs to be developed and researched further [71].

MECHANISMS OF ACTION

Immune System Activation

It is through adjuvants that vaccine potency is increased since the immune system becomes active. This process begins when adjuvant molecules are identified by pattern recognition receptors (PRRs) on the immune cells. Pattern recognition receptors like Toll-like receptors (TLRs) and NOD-like receptors (NLRs) detect microorganisms containing pathogen-associated molecular patterns (PAMPs) and danger-associated molecular patterns (DAMPs), thereafter initiating immunity. As a result, this activation results in pro-inflammatory cytokines and chemokines being released, leading to the production of a strong response [72, 73].

Enhancing Antigen Presentation

Adjuvants enhance antigen presentation. They encourage the APCs, such as macrophages and dendritic cells, to pick up antigens. The antigens then undergo internalization, and later, they present on MHC molecules present on the surface of these APCs. These T cells, which are also important in cell-mediated immune response and humoral immunity, must first be activated to trigger this response [74].

Stimulating Dendritic Cells and Macrophages

Adjuvants directly stimulate dendritic cells and macrophages, primary effectors in evoking immune reactions. These cells are scouts that sense and trap antigens. On activation by adjuvants, dendritic cells and macrophages mature and leave for lymph nodes, where they present the antigens to T-cells. This connection is crucial to instigate and amplify adaptive immune responses that enable an effective immune system response against the pathogen [75].

Modulation of Immune Responses

Adjuvants change the way the immune system responds to infection, making it more efficient at fighting some germs. This modification also involves affecting the ratio of T helper cell types (Th1, Th2, and Th17) and prompting the production of certain heavy chain isotypes, such as IgA, for mucous membrane immunity [76].

Th1/Th2 Response Modulation

Generated by adjuvants, the nature of T helper (Th) cell response can be changed. The production of interferon-gamma (IFN-γ) is a characteristic feature of Th1 responses and is essential in combating intracellular pathogens like viruses and some bacteria. In this regard, Th2 responses are characterized by the synthesis and secretion of interleukins (IL-4, IL-5, and IL-13), which are important for immune defense against parasites that cause extracellular infections. By designing them properly, adjuvants may direct immune responses towards a Th1 or Th2 bias, depending on vaccine requirements [77].

Mucosal IgA Production

IgA production is the major objective in the cases of vaccines against pathogens that infect through mucosal surfaces. IgA is the leading type of antibody in these secretions and plays a significant role in pathogen clearance from mucosal areas. Some adjuvants are made purposely to boost the production of IgA; this eventually gives rise to efficient protection against immunity to infections that typically start at sites like the respiratory and gastrointestinal tracts [78].

RECENT INNOVATIONS AND RESEARCH

Nanotechnology-Based Adjuvants

Types

Nanotechnology-based adjuvants have various types, which are described below and summarized in Fig. (**3**).

Gold Nanoparticles (AuNPs)

Gold nanoparticles (AuNPs) are little gold particles of 1 to 100 nanometers. They have unique properties that make them easily synthesized and able to interact with different biological molecules like antigens and adjuvants. The ability to be functionalized in this way makes AuNPs highly adaptable for use in biomedicine. In vaccine development, AuNPs are employed as antigen carriers that can directly reach immune cells, leading to improved uptake and presentation of the antigens. AuNPs are very efficient and accurate in the immune response, so they can be used to develop better vaccines. They have been found useful in cancer vaccines, activating potent anti-tumor immunity and infectious disease vaccines, improving pathogen sensing and clearance by the body's defense system. AuNPs are an important step towards developing more potent and precise vaccines [79].

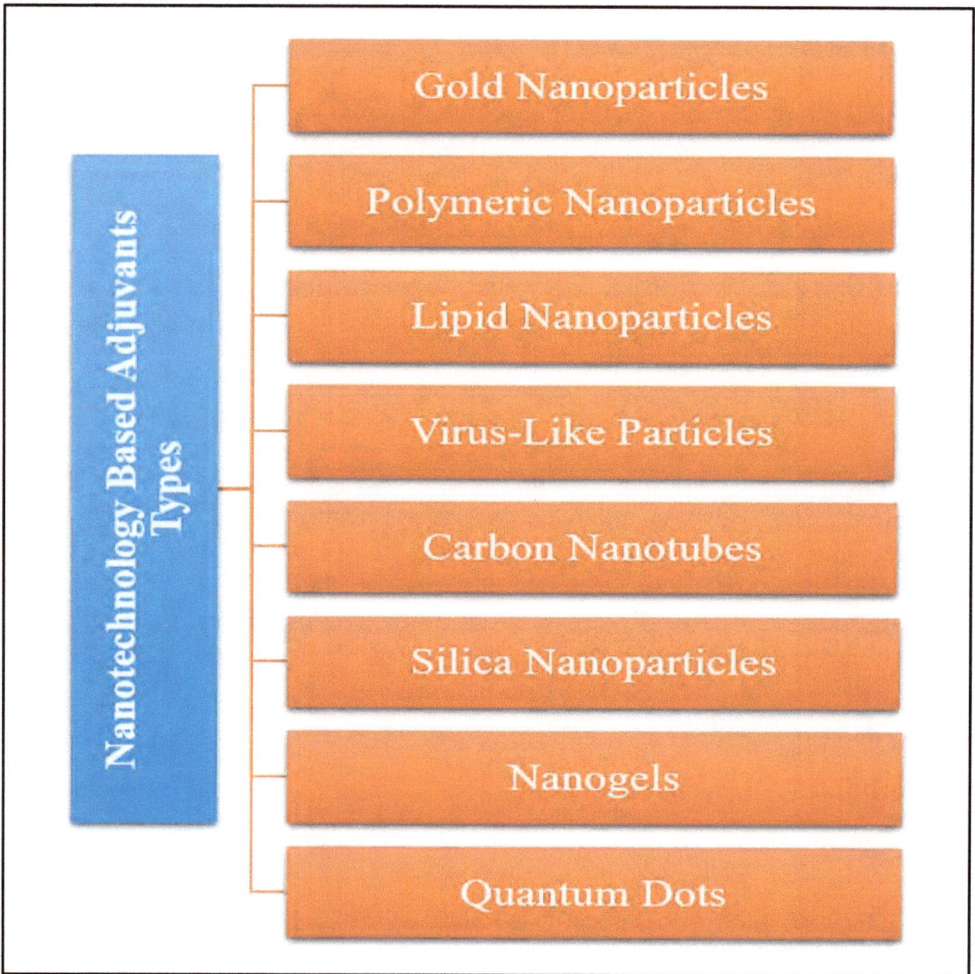

Fig. (3). Nanotechnology-based adjuvant types.

Polymeric Nanoparticles

Bio-degradable polymers such as PLGA, PLA, and chitosan are used to prepare polymeric nanoparticles. Because of this feature, these materials enable the particles to trap antigens and adjuvants inside them so that they do not decompose but remain stable. It also helps in the regulation of how much that vaccine component is released over time, thus giving an extended immune stimulation through release. It is a method of maintaining an optimum antigenic presence that boosts immunity and minimizes the number of booster doses. Nanoparticles made from polymers have been used in vaccine formulations for infectious diseases as well as cancer immunotherapy. Their versatility and strength in the delivery, protection, and controlled release of antigens make them useful tools for creating more efficient vaccines that elicit strong and sustained immunity [80].

Lipid Nanoparticles (LNPs)

However, LNPs are surrounded by lipids that create a bilayer that enables them to wrap nucleic acids like mRNA. This structure shields mRNA from degradation and allows it to enter host cells easily. This has made LNPs essential in producing RNA vaccines such as Pfizer-BioNTech and Moderna COVID-19 vaccine. These particles protect mRNA from enzymatic destruction or harsh conditions by adding stability to it so that it remains whole until reaching its destination. Furthermore, LNPs enhance delivery efficiency by promoting mRNA's uptake into cells and its subsequent release to the cytoplasm, where it can undergo translation for protein synthesis. Using these LNPs in mRNA vaccines has been a ground-breaking development that has greatly contributed to the rapid and effective response to the COVID-19 pandemic by ensuring consistent, powerful transportation of genetic materials needed for strong immune reaction [81].

Virus-Like Particles (VLPs)

Nanostructures resembling viruses are VLPs with viral organization and conformation but lack viral genetic material, thus rendering them non-infectious and safe for use in vaccines. Although VLPs do not have any genetic material, they keep the original virus's surface proteins and structural characteristics. Consequently, these particles closely resemble natural viruses and can effectively stimulate immune responses. VLPs have successfully been used for hepatitis B and human papillomaviruses and incite strong immune reactions against viral antigens. The repetitive shapes on the VLP's surface facilitate its engagement with immune cells, producing strong antibodies. The VLP is an efficient system of vaccination safe from various viral pathogens that leads to effective immune responses [82, 83].

Carbon Nanotubes (CNTs)

CNTs are cylindrical nanomaterials of carbon atoms with distinctive mechanical, electrical, and thermal properties. Because of their vast surface area and peculiar morphology, they can be used in various biomedical applications, including vaccine delivery. CNTs can be modified with antigens and adjuvants to direct them towards immune cells. Vaccines conjugated onto CNTs enable targeted delivery to antigen-presenting cells (APCs) like dendritic cells (DC), thereby improving immune responses. Moreover, the CNTs can also act as vehicles for adjuvants, augmenting vaccine immune-stimulatory qualities. Therefore, researchers are looking to improve the efficiency and safety of CNT-based vaccine delivery systems in this area. While encouraging, this approach must address biocompatibility and potential toxicity before it can be widely used in clinical settings. This signifies that CNTs present a novel approach for vaccine carriers that provide an avenue for improved immunity and treatment of infections caused by infectious organisms [84].

Silica Nanoparticles

The silica nanoparticles, consisting of silicon dioxide (SiO_2), can serve as a flexible base for vaccine delivery because they can adjust their size and surface. Silica nanoparticles are modified to encase or soak antigens and adjuvants to guard them from decay while assisting in the controlled release. This also results in stable administration of vaccines, hence maintaining their antigenicity and immunogenicity. Silica nanoparticles have been explored in several vaccine applications, such as cancer vaccines, where they can ably transport tumor antigens to immune cells, leading to vigorous cellular immunity against the tumor. Furthermore, silica nanoparticles also show potential in the transport of protein antigens. They may work as a stable and efficient vaccine platform to create vaccines against infectious diseases and other disorders. Further investigations on optimizing vaccine formulation through the controlled release of antigens formulated using silica nanoparticle-based vaccines may result in more stable, more potent, safer vaccine immunogenicity profiles [85].

Nanogels

Nanogels represent a very promising type of hydrogel nanoparticles with some unique vaccine delivery characteristics. Nanogels are cross-linked polymers that can swell and retain high amounts of water. This feature helps them effectively package antigens and adjuvants. They are used for the controlled release of vaccines to maintain immunity over time. Moreover, they are hydrophilic and biocompatible, making them suitable for preserving antigens' original structure and functionality. Nanogels have been notably used in mucosal vaccine delivery to effectively target mucosal surfaces like respiratory and gastrointestinal tracts. Encapsulating vaccine components within nanogels enables focused delivery to mucosal sites, facilitating vaccine uptake and immune activation at these critical entry points for pathogens. In conclusion, nanogels provide a promising approach to developing efficient mucosal vaccines with improved stability, controlled release kinetics, and enhanced immunogenicity [86].

Quantum Dots

Quantum dots are nanoscale semiconductors with unique optical and electronic properties, mainly used as imaging and tracking agents for vaccine studies. However, their exceptional characteristics also make them potential enhancers of immune responses by effective antigen delivery. Quantum dots can be linked to antigens to enhance the targeted transport of vaccines into immune cells. They are small and can modify their surface, making them suitable for accurately presenting antigens that may increase immunity. Although mainly looked into for their imaging functions, quantum dots have a great opportunity to improve vaccine performance by expeditiously bringing antigens to the immune system. More studies on their biocompatibility, safety, and immunostimulatory effects should be conducted to realize their complete application in vaccine development. Delivering vaccines through quantum dots is a ground-breaking approach that could offer new ways of developing more efficient and targeted immunization strategies [87].

Under the umbrella of nanotechnology-based adjuvants, a range of nanoparticle types are available, each with unique advantages for vaccine delivery and efficacy. These advanced materials, such as gold nanoparticles or polymeric nanoparticles, among others, enhance vaccines' targeting, stability, and immunogenicity, thereby facilitating more effective and efficient strategies for immunization [88].

Benefits

Targeted Delivery

Enhancing the delivery of antigens and adjuvants to specific immune cells can be done by targeting nanoparticles through ligand, antibody, or other molecule modifications on their surface that bind with target cell receptors. This eventually reduces off-target effects and produces an efficient and effective immune response, leading to a desired immune response [89].

Controlled Release

Nanoparticles can be modified to release their contents slowly over a given duration of time so that the antigens and adjuvants will still be present in the body. Controlled release maintains an ideal level of immune stimulation over time, cutting down on booster doses while promoting long-term immunity.

Furthermore, this strategy can also forestall early degradation and assure its delivery at the aimed site in active form [90, 91].

Bioengineered Molecules

Recombinant Proteins

Genetic engineering techniques are applied to produce recombinant proteins that enable the production of particular protein antigens in bulk. Thus, when these peptides are added to these nanoparticles, they have increased stability and delivery, resulting in more effective vaccines [92, 93].

Synthetic Peptides

Synthetic peptides are small chains of amino acids that may be made to resemble particular epitopes of pathogens. Peptides can be coated onto nanoparticles to enhance their immunogenicity. This method ensures accurate targeting of immune responses to particular regions within a pathogen [94, 95].

FUTURE PERSPECTIVES

The area of research into adjuvants for mucosal vaccines is ripe for breakthroughs due to advancements in new materials and technologies. Launching new nanoparticle formulations, including biodegradable polymer-based ones, lipid carriers using nanotechnology, and bioengineered molecules, may promote the delivery and efficacy of mucosal vaccines. These creative efforts should help circumvent obstacles such as the stability of antigens and efficient passage through the mucosa. For example, the evolution of smart nanoparticles that respond to environmental triggers or specific cells might transform vaccine design. Furthermore, bioinformatics and synthetic biology improvements are making it possible to create recombinant proteins and synthetic peptides that can cause stronger and more specific immune responses [96].

Another exciting domain is personalized mucosal vaccines. Through genetic and immunological profiling, it is possible to make customized vaccines that fit into each person's immune system, thus making them more effective and with lower side effects. This strategy could be useful for people from divergent immunological backgrounds or diseases with high genetic diversity. The technology provided by CRISPR and next-generation sequencing is advancing toward personalized vaccine components that are optimally matched to the recipient's immune system [97].

Substantial regulatory and safety issues have not yet been addressed besides these encouraging developments. Evaluating new adjuvants and vaccine formulations is a rigid process to guarantee safety and effectiveness. However, the intricacy of new materials and technologies can be problematic. Regulatory agencies should change how they assess such advanced products, which may demand modified guidelines and fresh testing protocols. Equally important is to ensure the long-term safety of new adjuvants. While preclinical and clinical trials can indicate short-term safety and efficacy, long-term monitoring is needed for possible delayed adverse effects. Such studies are essential, especially for new adjuvants that exhibit novel ways of interacting with the immune system [98].

Furthermore, the problem of making new adjuvants that can be scaled and manufactured must be faced. For mass adoption, new materials and technologies must be produced consistently at scale without quality compromises. How researchers, manufacturers, and regulatory agencies will work together to simplify shifting from laboratory research into clinical and commercial use is essential [99].

Mucosal vaccine adjuvants have a bright future, with many potential breakthroughs. Vaccine development is poised to be transformed by materials science, personalized medicine, and biotechnology advances. However, these innovations must be carefully navigated through regulatory landscapes and long-term safety evaluations to deliver on their promise of improving public health [100 - 102].

CONCLUSION

The progress in adjuvants for enhancing mucosal vaccines significantly advances immunology and vaccine fabrication science. In general, conventional vaccines have been aimed at systemic immunity, possibly overlooking the vital function of mucous membranes as prime ingress points for many pathogens. By creating adjuvants that specifically act on mucosal immunity, researchers hope to develop vaccines that stop systemic diseases and hinder pathogen access at their first site of contact. Nanotechnology, bioengineering, and synthetic biology have led to the development of new formulations of adjuvants that can increase immune responses in these sites. For example, nanoparticles promise to deliver antigens and control release for efficient stimulation of resilient and persistent immunity. In addition, such vaccines possess greater specificity and potency due to modified proteins like recombinant proteins or synthetic peptides produced through bioengineering techniques. Despite the promising developments, there are still significant challenges, with regulatory approval and long-term safety being the major ones. Therefore, a lot of testing through research and collaboration between scientists, regulatory bodies, and manufacturers is required to ensure that those novel adjuvants are safe enough to be used by humans. This means that it is important to have long-term studies that will enable us to know if these new adjuvants cause any negative effects to establish their overall safety profile. Consequently, ongoing innovation in mucosal vaccine adjuvants has great potential to change how we prevent and control infectious diseases. These developments can result in more efficient vaccines offering a wide range of pathogen protection if they focus on improving mucosal immunity. Long-term health benefits will depend on successfully incorporating these ideas into clinical practice as research evolves.

ACKNOWLEDGEMENTS

Authors are highly thankful to their Universities/Colleges for providing library facilities for the literature survey.

REFERENCES

[1]   Dotiwala F, Upadhyay AK. Next Generation Mucosal Vaccine Strategy for Respiratory Pathogens. Vaccines. Multidisciplinary Digital Publishing Institute (MDPI), 2023; 11.
[http://dx.doi.org/10.3390/vaccines11101585]

[2]   Lavelle EC, Ward RW. Mucosal vaccines — fortifying the frontiers. Nature Reviews Immunology. Nature Research 2022; 22: pp. 236-50.

[3]   Lin Y, Hu Z, Fu YX, Peng H. Mucosal vaccine development for respiratory viral infections. hLife. 2024; 2(2): 50–63.

[4]   Song Y, Mehl F, Zeichner SL. Vaccine Strategies to Elicit Mucosal Immunity. Vaccines. Multidisciplinary Digital Publishing Institute (MDPI), 2024; 12.
[http://dx.doi.org/10.3390/vaccines12020191]

[5]   Russell MW. Mucosal Immunology. 4th ed., 2015.https://doi.org/./B

[6]   Baker JR Jr, Farazuddin M, Wong PT, O'Konek JJ. The unfulfilled potential of mucosal immunization. J Allergy Clin Immunol 2022; 150(1): 1-11.
[http://dx.doi.org/10.1016/j.jaci.2022.05.002] [PMID: 35569567]

[7]   Holmgren J, Czerkinsky C. Mucosal immunity and vaccines. Nat Med 2005; 11(S4) (Suppl.): S45-53.
[http://dx.doi.org/10.1038/nm1213] [PMID: 15812489]

[8]   Kiyono H, Yuki Y, Nakahashi-Ouchida R, Fujihashi K. Mucosal vaccines: Wisdom from now and then. International Immunology. Oxford University Press; 2021; 33, 767–74.

[9]   Abu Khweek A, Kim E, Joldrichsen MR, Amer AO, Boyaka PN. Insights Into Mucosal Innate Immune Responses in House Dust Mite-Mediated Allergic Asthma. Front Immunol. 2020 Dec 7;11: 534501.
[http://dx.doi.org/10.3389/fimmu.2020.534501] [PMID: 33424827]

[10]   Holmgren J. Mucosal immunization and adjuvants_ a brief overview of recent advances and challenges - ScienceDirect. 2003.

[11]   Reed SG, Orr MT, Fox CB. Key roles of adjuvants in modern vaccines. Nat Med 2013; 19(12): 1597-608.
[http://dx.doi.org/10.1038/nm.3409] [PMID: 24309663]

[12]   Cuzzubbo S, Mangsbo S, Nagarajan D, Habra K, Pockley AG, McArdle SEB. Cancer Vaccines: Adjuvant Potency, Importance of Age, Lifestyle, and Treatments. Frontiers in Immunology. Frontiers Media S.A. 2021; 11.

[13]   Turley JL, Lavelle EC. Resolving adjuvant mode of action to enhance vaccine efficacy. Current Opinion in Immunology. Elsevier Ltd; 2022; 77.
[http://dx.doi.org/10.1016/j.coi.2022.102229]

[14]   Vogel FR. Improving Vaccine Performance with Adjuvants. 2000. Available from: https://academic.oup.com/cid/article/30/Supplement_3/S266/273084

[15]   de la Cruz-Merino L, Grande-Pulido E, Albero-Tamarit A, Codes-Manuel de Villena ME. Cancer and immune response: old and new evidence for future challenges. Oncologist 2008; 13(12): 1246-54.
[http://dx.doi.org/10.1634/theoncologist.2008-0166] [PMID: 19056856]

[16]   Smyth LM, Knight KA, Aarons YK, Wasiak J. The cardiac dose□sparing benefits of deep inspiration breath□hold in left breast irradiation: a systematic review. J Med Radiat Sci 2015; 62(1): 66-73.
[http://dx.doi.org/10.1002/jmrs.89] [PMID: 26229669]

[17]   Peñaflor-Téllez Y, Trujillo-Uscanga A, Escobar-Almazán JA, Gutiérrez-Escolano AL. Immune Response Modulation by Caliciviruses. Frontiers in Immunology. Frontiers Media S.A. 2019; 10.

[18]   Hieber C, Grabbe S, Bros M. Counteracting Immunosenescence—Which Therapeutic Strategies Are Promising? Biomolecules. Multidisciplinary Digital Publishing Institute (MDPI), 2023; 13.

[19]   Eichelberger MC, Monto AS. Neuraminidase, the Forgotten Surface Antigen, Emerges as an Influenza Vaccine Target for Broadened Protection. J Infect Dis 2019; 219 (Suppl. 1): S75-80.
[http://dx.doi.org/10.1093/infdis/jiz017] [PMID: 30715357]

[20]   Bragazzi NL, Watad A, Shoenfeld Y. Vaccine Adjuvants: History, Role, Mechanisms of Action, and Side Effects. In: Autoimmune Disorders. Wiley; 2024. p. 15–27. Available from: https://onlinelibrary.wiley.com/doi/10.1002/9781119858430.ch3

[21]   Bergmann-Leitner ES, Leitner WW. Adjuvants in the driver's seat: How magnitude, type, fine specificity, and longevity of immune responses are driven by distinct classes of immune potentiators. Vaccines. MDPI AG 2014; 2: pp. 252-96.

[22]   Pulendran BS, Arunachalam P, O'Hagan DT. Emerging concepts in the science of vaccine adjuvants. Nature Reviews Drug Discovery. Nature Research 2021; 20: pp. 454-75.

[23]   Kwissa M, Pai Kasturi S, Pulendran B. The science of adjuvants. Expert Rev Vaccines 2007; 6(5): 673-84.
[http://dx.doi.org/10.1586/14760584.6.5.673] [PMID: 17931149]

[24]   O'Hagan DT, Valiante NM. Recent advances in the discovery and delivery of vaccine adjuvants. Nature Reviews Drug Discovery. European Association for Cardio-Thoracic Surgery 2003; 2: pp. 727-35.

[25]   Garçon N, Di Pasquale A. From discovery to licensure, the Adjuvant System story. Human Vaccines and Immunotherapeutics. Taylor and Francis Inc.; 2017; 13, 19–33.

[26]   Yong WK. Books Animal Parasite Control Utilizing Biotechnology Selected pages Historical Context an. 1992. Available from: https://books.google.co.in/books?id=I3AqbnYq-UoC&dq=Historical+Context+and+Traditional+Adjuvants&lr=&source=gbs_navlinks_s

[27]   Kenney R. T. Adjuvants for the Future _ 29 _ v4 _ New Generation Vaccines_ Richard. 2010.

[28]   McCright JC, Maisel K. Engineering drug delivery systems to overcome mucosal barriers for immunotherapy and vaccination. Tissue Barriers. Taylor and Francis Inc.; 2020; McCright JC, Maisel K. Engineering drug delivery systems to overcome mucosal barriers for immunotherapy and vaccination. Vol. 8, Tissue Barriers. Taylor and Francis Inc., 2020. 8.
[http://dx.doi.org/10.1080/21688370.2019.1695476]

[29] Johansson MEV, Ambort D, Pelaseyed T, *et al.* Composition and functional role of the mucus layers in the intestine. Cell Mol Life Sci 2011; 68(22): 3635-41.
[http://dx.doi.org/10.1007/s00018-011-0822-3] [PMID: 21947475]

[30] Ernst S, Langer R, Cooney CL, Sasisekharan R. Enzymatic degradation of glycosaminoglycans. Crit Rev Biochem Mol Biol 1995; 30(5): 387-444.
[http://dx.doi.org/10.3109/10409239509083490] [PMID: 8575190]

[31] Le Basle Y, Chennell P, Tokhadze N, Astier A, Sautou V. Physicochemical Stability of Monoclonal Antibodies: A Review. Vol. 109, Journal of Pharmaceutical Sciences. Elsevier B.V.; 2020. p. 169–90.
[http://dx.doi.org/10.1016/j.xphs.2019.08.009]

[32] Gittleman CS, Coms FD, Lai YH. Membrane Durability: Physical and Chemical Degradation. Polymer Electrolyte Fuel Cell Degradation. Elsevier 2011; pp. 15-88.

[33] Yamamoto L, Amodio N, Gulla A, Anderson KC. Harnessing the Immune System Against Multiple Myeloma: Challenges and Opportunities. Frontiers in Oncology. Frontiers Media S.A. 2021; 10.

[34] Sinani G, Sessevmez M, Gök MK, Özgümüş S, Alpar HO, Cevher E. Modified chitosan-based nanoadjuvants enhance immunogenicity of protein antigens after mucosal vaccination. Int J Pharm 2019; 569: 118592.
[http://dx.doi.org/10.1016/j.ijpharm.2019.118592] [PMID: 31386881]

[35] Li M, Wang Y, Sun Y, Cui H, Zhu SJ, Qiu HJ. Mucosal vaccines: Strategies and challenges. Immunology Letters. Elsevier B.V. 2020; 217: pp. 116-25.

[36] Mann JFS, Acevedo R, Campo J, Pérez O, Ferro VA. Delivery systems: a vaccine strategy for overcoming mucosal tolerance? Expert Rev Vaccines 2009; 8(1): 103-12.
[http://dx.doi.org/10.1586/14760584.8.1.103] [PMID: 19093777]

[37] Mcghee JR, George-Chandy A, Holmgren J, Kieny MP, Fujiyashi K, Mestecky JF, *et al.* Cecil Czerkinsky Fabienne Anjuere. 1999.

[38] Palm AKE, Henry C. Remembrance of Things Past: Long-Term B Cell Memory After Infection and Vaccination. Frontiers in immunology. NLM (Medline), 2019; 10, 1787.

[39] AISB 2004 Convention Proceedings of the AISB 2004 Symposium on The Immune System and Cognition. 2004. Available from: http://www.aisb.org.uk

[40] Ekmekciu I, von Klitzing E, Fiebiger U, *et al.* Immune responses to broad-spectrum antibiotic treatment and fecal microbiota transplantation in mice. Front Immunol 2017; 8(APR): 397.
[http://dx.doi.org/10.3389/fimmu.2017.00397] [PMID: 28469619]

[41] McMichael AJ, Borrow P, Tomaras GD, Goonetilleke N, Haynes BF. The immune response during acute HIV-1 infection: clues for vaccine development. Nat Rev Immunol 2010; 10(1): 11-23.
[http://dx.doi.org/10.1038/nri2674] [PMID: 20010788]

[42] Viney ME, Riley EM, Buchanan KL. Optimal immune responses: immunocompetence revisited. Trends Ecol Evol 2005; 20(12): 665-9.
[http://dx.doi.org/10.1016/j.tree.2005.10.003] [PMID: 16701455]

[43] Clements JD, Norton EB. The Mucosal Vaccine Adjuvant LT(R192G/L211A) or dmLT. MSphere 2018; 3(4): e00215-18.
[http://dx.doi.org/10.1128/mSphere.00215-18] [PMID: 30045966]

[44] Holmgren J. Immunopotentiators in Modern Vaccines. 2006. Available from: https://doi.org/./B

[45] Pizza M. Mucosal vaccines_ nontoxic derivatives of LT and CT as mucosal adjuvants - ScienceDirect. 2001.

[46] Martin M, Metzger DJ, Michalek SM, Connell TD, Russell MW. Comparative Analysis of the Mucosal Adjuvanticity of the Type II Heat-Labile Enterotoxins LT-IIa and LT-IIb. Vol. 68, Infection and immunity. 2000. Available from: https://journals.asm.org/journal/iai

[47]   Dallas WS, Michael I), Ani G, Falkow' S. Cistrons Encoding Escherichia coli Heat-Labile Toxin. Journal of bacteriology. 1979. Available from: https://journals.asm.org/journal/jb

[48]   Norton EB, Lawson LB, Freytag LC, Clements JD. Characterization of a mutant Escherichia coli heat-labile toxin, LT(R192G/L211A), as a safe and effective oral adjuvant. Clin Vaccine Immunol 2011; 18(4): 546-51.
[http://dx.doi.org/10.1128/CVI.00538-10] [PMID: 21288994]

[49]   Yamamoto T, Yokota T. Sequence of Heat-Labile Enterotoxin of Escherichia coli Pathogenic for Humans. Vol. 155. 1983. Available from: https://journals.asm.org/journal/jb

[50]   Lasaro MA, Rodrigues JF, Mathias-Santos C, *et al.* Genetic diversity of heat-labile toxin expressed by enterotoxigenic Escherichia coli strains isolated from humans. J Bacteriol 2008; 190(7): 2400-10.
[http://dx.doi.org/10.1128/JB.00988-07] [PMID: 18223074]

[51]   Caroff M, Karibian D. Structure of bacterial lipopolysaccharides. Carbohydrate Research. Elsevier BV; 2003; 338, 2431–47.
[http://dx.doi.org/10.1016/j.carres.2003.07.010]

[52]   Lu Y, Liu G. Nano alum: A new solution to the new challenge. Human Vaccines and Immunotherapeutics. Taylor and Francis Ltd., 2022; 18.

[53]   Baylor NW, Egan W, Richman P. Aluminum salts in vaccines—US perspective. Vaccine 2002; 20: S18-23.
[http://dx.doi.org/10.1016/S0264-410X(02)00166-4]

[54]   O'Hagan DT, Ott GS, Nest GV, Rappuoli R, Giudice GD. The history of MF59 ® adjuvant: a phoenix that arose from the ashes. Expert Rev Vaccines 2013; 12(1): 13-30.
[http://dx.doi.org/10.1586/erv.12.140] [PMID: 23256736]

[55]   Bhagchandani S, Johnson JA, Irvine DJ. Evolution of Toll-like receptor 7/8 agonist therapeutics and their delivery approaches: From antiviral formulations to vaccine adjuvants. Advanced Drug Delivery Reviews. Elsevier B.V. 2021; 175.

[56]   Yang JX, Tseng JC, Yu GY, Luo Y, Huang CYF, Hong YR, *et al.* Recent Advances in Developing Toll-like Receptor Agonist-Based Vaccine Adjuvants for Infectious Diseases. Pharmaceutics. MDPI 2022; 14.

[57]   Kaur A, Baldwin J, Brar D, Salunke DB, Petrovsky N. Toll-like receptor (TLR) agonists as a driving force behind next-generation vaccine adjuvants and cancer therapeutics. Current Opinion in Chemical Biology. Elsevier Ltd, 2022; 70.

[58]   Bhagchandani S, Johnson JA, Irvine DJ. Evolution of Toll-like receptor 7/8 agonist therapeutics and their delivery approaches: From antiviral formulations to vaccine adjuvants. Advanced Drug Delivery Reviews. Elsevier B.V. 2021; 175.

[59]   Knuschke T, Epple M, Westendorf AM. The type of adjuvant strongly influences the T-cell response during nanoparticle-based immunization. Hum Vaccin Immunother 2014; 10(1): 164-9.
[http://dx.doi.org/10.4161/hv.26203] [PMID: 23982325]

[60]   Prashant CK, Kumar M, Dinda AK. Nanoparticle based tailoring of adjuvant function: The role in vaccine development. Journal of Biomedical Nanotechnology. American Scientific Publishers; 2014; 10, 2317–31.

[61]   Decker W. K. Cytokine adjuvants for vaccine therapy of neoplastic and infectious disease - ScienceDirect. 2011.

[62]   Barouch DH, Letvin NL, Seder RA. The role of cytokine DNAs as vaccine adjuvants for optimizing cellular immune responses. Immunol Rev 2004; 202(1): 266-74.
[http://dx.doi.org/10.1111/j.0105-2896.2004.00200.x] [PMID: 15546399]

[63]   Vnučák M, Graňák K, Beliančinová M, *et al.* Acute kidney rejection after anti-SARS-CoV-2 virus-vectored vaccine—case report. NPJ Vaccines 2022; 7(1): 30.

[http://dx.doi.org/10.1038/s41541-022-00445-5] [PMID: 35236844]

[64] Tripp RA, Mark Tompkins S. Virus-vectored influenza virus vaccines. Viruses. MDPI AG 2014; 6: pp. 3055-79.

[65] Choi Y, Chang J. Viral vectors for vaccine applications. Clin Exp Vaccine Res 2013; 2(2): 97-105.
[http://dx.doi.org/10.7774/cevr.2013.2.2.97] [PMID: 23858400]

[66] Vasou A, Sultanoglu N, Goodbourn S, Randall RE, Kostrikis LG. Targeting pattern recognition receptors (PRR) for vaccine adjuvantation: From synthetic PRR agonists to the potential of defective interfering particles of viruses. Viruses. MDPI AG 2017; 9.

[67] Ong GH, Lian BSX, Kawasaki T, Kawai T. Exploration of Pattern Recognition Receptor Agonists as Candidate Adjuvants. Frontiers in Cellular and Infection Microbiology. Frontiers Media S.A. 2021; 11.

[68] Shekarian T, Valsesia-Wittmann S, Brody J, Michallet MC, Depil S, Caux C, *et al*. Pattern recognition receptors: Immune targets to enhance cancer immunotherapy. Annals of Oncology. Oxford University Press; 2017; 28, 1756–66.

[69] Circelli L, Petrizzo A, Tagliamonte M, *et al*. Immunological effects of a novel RNA-based adjuvant in liver cancer patients. Cancer Immunol Immunother 2017; 66(1): 103-12.
[http://dx.doi.org/10.1007/s00262-016-1923-5] [PMID: 27832318]

[70] Alfagih IM, Aldosari B, Alquadeib B, Almurshedi A, Alfagih MM. Nanoparticles as adjuvants and nanodelivery systems for mRNA-based vaccines. Pharmaceutics. MDPI AG 2021; 13: pp. 1-27.

[71] Heidenreich R, Jasny E, Kowalczyk A, *et al*. A novel RNA□based adjuvant combines strong immunostimulatory capacities with a favorable safety profile. Int J Cancer 2015; 137(2): 372-84.
[http://dx.doi.org/10.1002/ijc.29402] [PMID: 25530186]

[72] Schiller M, Metze D, Luger TA, Grabbe S, Gunzer M. Immune response modifiers – mode of action. Exp Dermatol 2006; 15(5): 331-41.
[http://dx.doi.org/10.1111/j.0906-6705.2006.00414.x] [PMID: 16630072]

[73] Alonso-Torre S, Carrillo C, Cavia M del M. Papel del acido oleico en el sistema inmune; Mecanismo de acción; revisión científica. Vol. 27. Nutr Hosp 2012; 978-90.

[74] Ghimire TR, Benson RA, Garside P, Brewer JM. Alum increases antigen uptake, reduces antigen degradation and sustains antigen presentation by DCs *in vitro*. Immunol Lett 2012; 147(1-2): 55-62.
[http://dx.doi.org/10.1016/j.imlet.2012.06.002] [PMID: 22732235]

[75] Klinkert WEF, Labadie JH, Bowers{} WE. Accessory and stimulating properties dendritic cells and macrophages isolated from various rat tissues* of. 1982. Available from: http://rupress.org/jem/article-pdf/156/1/1/1663017/1.pdf

[76] Lynn DJ, Benson SC, Lynn MA, Pulendran B. Modulation of immune responses to vaccination by the microbiota: implications and potential mechanisms. Nature Reviews Immunology. Nature Research 2022; 22: pp. 33-46.

[77] Baranov MV, Kumar M, Sacanna S, Thutupalli S, van den Bogaart G. Modulation of Immune Responses by Particle Size and Shape. Frontiers in Immunology. Frontiers Media S.A. 2021; 11.

[78] Li Y, Jin L, Chen T, Pirozzi CJ. The Effects of Secretory IgA in the Mucosal Immune System. BioMed Research International. Hindawi Limited 2020; 2020.

[79] Johnson L, Duschl A, Himly M. Nanotechnology-based vaccines for allergen-specific immunotherapy: Potentials and challenges of conventional and novel adjuvants under research. Vaccines. MDPI AG 2020; 8.

[80] Kim MG, Park JY, Shon Y, Kim G, Shim G, Oh YK. Nanotechnology and vaccine development. Asian Journal of Pharmaceutical Sciences. Shenyang Pharmaceutical University, 2014; 9, 227–35.
[http://dx.doi.org/10.1016/j.ajps.2014.06.002]

[81]   Krishnan S, Thirunavukarasu A, Jha NK, Gahtori R, Roy AS, Dholpuria S, *et al.* Nanotechnology-based therapeutic formulations in the battle against animal coronaviruses: an update. Journal of Nanoparticle Research. Springer Science and Business Media B.V., 2021; 23.
[http://dx.doi.org/10.1007/s11051-021-05341-y]

[82]   Noad R, Roy P. Virus-like particles as immunogens. Trends in Microbiology. Elsevier Ltd; 2003; 11, 438–44.
[http://dx.doi.org/10.1016/S0966-842X(03)00208-7]

[83]   Zeltins A. Construction and characterization of virus-like particles: a review. Mol Biotechnol 2013; 53(1): 92-107.
[http://dx.doi.org/10.1007/s12033-012-9598-4] [PMID: 23001867]

[84]   Haddon RC. Carbon Nanotubes. Acc Chem Res 2002; 35(12): 997.
[http://dx.doi.org/10.1021/ar020259h] [PMID: 12484786]

[85]   Wu SH, Mou CY, Lin HP. Synthesis of mesoporous silica nanoparticles. Chem Soc Rev 2013; 42(9): 3862-75.
[http://dx.doi.org/10.1039/c3cs35405a] [PMID: 23403864]

[86]   Yallapu MM, Jaggi M, Chauhan SC. Design and engineering of nanogels for cancer treatment. Drug Discov Today 2011; 16(9-10): 457-63.
[http://dx.doi.org/10.1016/j.drudis.2011.03.004] [PMID: 21414419]

[87]   Reimann SM, Manninen M. Electronic structure of quantum dots. Rev Mod Phys 2002; 74(4): 1283-342.
[http://dx.doi.org/10.1103/RevModPhys.74.1283]

[88]   Jamieson T, Bakhshi R, Petrova D, Pocock R, Imani M, Seifalian AM. Biological applications of quantum dots. Biomaterials 2007; 28(31): 4717-32.
[http://dx.doi.org/10.1016/j.biomaterials.2007.07.014] [PMID: 17686516]

[89]   Nikam RR, Gore KR. Journey of siRNA: Clinical Developments and Targeted Delivery. Nucleic Acid Therapeutics. Mary Ann Liebert Inc., 2018; 28, 209–24.

[90]   Siegel RA, Rathbone MJ. Overview of controlled release mechanisms. Fundamentals and Applications of Controlled Release Drug Delivery. Springer US 2012; pp. 19-43.
[http://dx.doi.org/10.1007/978-1-4614-0881-9_2]

[91]   Shaviv A. Advances in controlled-release fertilizers. Advances in Agronomy. Academic Press Inc., 2001; 71, 1–49.
[http://dx.doi.org/10.1016/S0065-2113(01)71011-5]

[92]   Pillay P, Schlüter U, Van Wyk S, Kunert KJ, Vorster BJ. Proteolysis of recombinant proteins in bioengineered plant cells. Vol. 5. Bioengineered 2013.
[PMID: 23778319]

[93]   Jenkins N, Murphy L, Tyther R. Post-translational modifications of recombinant proteins: Significance for biopharmaceuticals. In: Molecular Biotechnology. 2008. p. 113–8.

[94]   Groß A, Hashimoto C, Sticht H, Eichler J. Synthetic peptides as protein mimics. Frontiers in Bioengineering and Biotechnology. Frontiers Media S.A. 2016; 3.

[95]   Noya O, Patarroyo M, Guzmán F, de Noya B. Immunodiagnosis of parasitic diseases with synthetic peptides. Curr Protein Pept Sci 2003; 4(4): 299-308.
[http://dx.doi.org/10.2174/1389203033487153] [PMID: 14529537]

[96]   Pippa N, Gazouli M, Pispas S. Recent advances and future perspectives in polymer based nanovaccines. Vaccines. MDPI 2021; 9.

[97]   Aribi M. New Topics in Vaccine Development [Working Title]. 2023. Available from: https://www.intechopen.com/online-first/88383

[98]   Ou B, Yang Y, Lv H, Lin X, Zhang M. Current Progress and Challenges in the Study of Adjuvants for Oral Vaccines. BioDrugs. Adis 2023; 37: pp. 143-80.

[99]   Sadeghi M, Keshavarz Shahbaz S, Dehnavi S, Koushki K, Sankian M. Current possibilities and future perspectives for improving efficacy of allergen-specific sublingual immunotherapy. International Immunopharmacology. Elsevier B.V. 2021; 101.

[100] Verma SK, Mahajan P, Singh NK, Gupta A, Aggarwal R, Rappuoli R, *et al.* New-age vaccine adjuvants, their development, and future perspective. Frontiers in Immunology. Frontiers Media S.A. 2023; 14.

[101] Wilson-Welder JH, Torres MP, Kipper MJ, Mallapragada SK, Wannemuehler MJ, Narasimhan B. Vaccine adjuvants: Current challenges and future approaches. Journal of Pharmaceutical Sciences. John Wiley and Sons Inc., 2009; 98, 1278–316.

[102] Facciolà A, Visalli G, Laganà A, Di Pietro A. An Overview of Vaccine Adjuvants: Current Evidence and Future Perspectives. Vaccines. MDPI 2022; 10.

CHAPTER 6

Bioprocessing and Scale-up Challenges in Mucosal Vaccine Production

Rupali Sharma[1,*], Koushal Dhamija[2], Sudhir Kumar[3], Shekhar Sharma[2] and **Alok Bhardwaj[2]**

[1] Amity University Haryana, Manesar, Gurugram, India

[2] Lloyd Institute of Management & Technology, Plot No.-11, Knowledge Park-II, Greater Noida, Uttar Pradesh-201306, India

[3] Faculty of Pharmaceutical Sciences, DAV University, Jalandhar, India

Abstract: Mucosal vaccination stimulates strong systemic and mucosal immune responses and presents a viable path for the fight against infectious diseases. To reach their full potential, mucosal vaccine production does, however, present major bioprocessing and scale-up hurdles. An outline of these difficulties and possible solutions is given in this abstract. The primary source of bioprocessing problems is the intricate structure of mucosal delivery channels. Specific needs relate to adjuvant selection, antigen stability, and formulation for the nasal, oral, and pulmonary routes. Moreover, maintaining sterility and controlling contamination present significant challenges for manufacturing mucosal vaccines. To overcome these obstacles, new strategies for adjuvant and antigen optimization are required, together with developments in formulation technologies. The difficulties associated with scaling up mucosal vaccination production add to its complexity. When moving from laboratory-scale to industrial-scale production, it is important to carefully handle equipment considerations, regulatory requirements, and process scalability issues. Economic issues are also significant, necessitating cost-effective measures that maintain the efficacy and quality of vaccines. Collaborative efforts between academia, industry, and regulatory bodies are frequently essential to successful scale-up plans. Emerging technologies, including advanced bioprocessing methods, computational modeling, and omics technologies, present viable ways to address these issues. Integrating nanotechnology and synthetic biology, along with the principles of Quality by Design (QbD), offers prospects for optimizing vaccine efficacy and production processes. Nonetheless, regulatory issues need to be properly taken into account to guarantee the security and effectiveness of innovative technologies. In conclusion, improving the production of mucosal vaccines requires tackling the issues of bioprocessing and scale-up. These challenges can be addressed, and the full potential of mucosal vaccination in

[*] **Corresponding author Rupali Sharma:** Amity University Haryana, Manesar, Gurugram, India; E-mail: rsharma9@ggn.amity.edu

the prevention of infectious diseases can be unlocked by utilizing cutting-edge technologies and collaborative methods.

Keywords: Adjuvant, Antigen, Bioprocessing, Immunity, Infectious diseases, Mucosal vaccine, Nasal delivery, Oral delivery, Pulmonary delivery, Quality by Design, Sterility.

INTRODUCTION

A class of vaccinations known as "mucosal vaccines" aims to produce protective immune responses at mucosal surfaces, including those lining the gastrointestinal, respiratory, and genitourinary tracts. Mucosal vaccines elicit both local mucosal and systemic immune responses, in contrast to traditional vaccines that are injected and mainly cause systemic immunity. This special characteristic is crucial to preventive medicine because mucosal surfaces are the main entry sites for various pathogens, such as viruses, bacteria, and parasites. These vaccines can stop infection at the point of entry, preventing pathogens from spreading throughout the host and the population. They do this by focusing on mucosal immunity [1, 2].

Mucosal vaccinations have a role in preventive medicine that goes beyond their capacity to offer targeted protection. Secretory IgA antibodies, which are essential for neutralizing toxins and preventing pathogen adherence to mucosal surfaces, can be induced by mucosal immunization. It has been demonstrated that mucosal vaccinations increase the host's capacity to fight invasive pathogens by inducing cellular immune responses, such as T lymphocyte activation. Because traditional vaccines may be less successful in preventing colonization and transmission in the context of mucosal infections, this multifaceted immune response is particularly advantageous [3, 4].

Mucosal vaccine development and production present substantial bioprocessing and scale-up challenges. To ensure stability and efficacy, mucosal vaccines need specialized formulation and delivery systems, unlike parenteral vaccines, which can be produced using tried-and-true methods. The optimization of antigen and adjuvant formulations for mucosal delivery, considering variables like mucosal adhesion properties, adjuvant toxicity, and antigen stability, presents bioprocessing challenges. Furthermore, producing mucosal vaccines poses special challenges because some formulations or delivery systems may not be compatible with conventional sterilization techniques. These include maintaining sterility and controlling contamination [5, 6].

Manufacturing process complexity increases with mucosal vaccine production scale-up, necessitating careful consideration of equipment needs, regulatory compliance, and process scalability. The development of affordable manufacturing processes that can fulfill the demands of large-scale vaccine production without sacrificing product quality or safety is imperative as the production moves from the laboratory to the industrial scale. Moreover, to guarantee the security, effectiveness, and uniformity of mucosal vaccinations commercially, regulatory bodies demand thorough documentation of manufacturing procedures and quality control methods. Mucosal vaccines can potentially transform mucosal infection prevention and enhance public health outcomes globally if these obstacles are overcome [7, 8].

TYPES OF MUCOSAL VACCINES

Mucosal vaccines are a broad category of vaccination approaches that aim to produce protective immune responses against pathogens by focusing on mucosal surfaces. Because of their simplicity of administration, capacity to elicit strong immune responses, and suitability for widespread vaccination campaigns, oral, nasal, and pulmonary vaccines stand out among the various types of mucosal vaccines as promising approaches, which are summarized in Fig. (**1**).

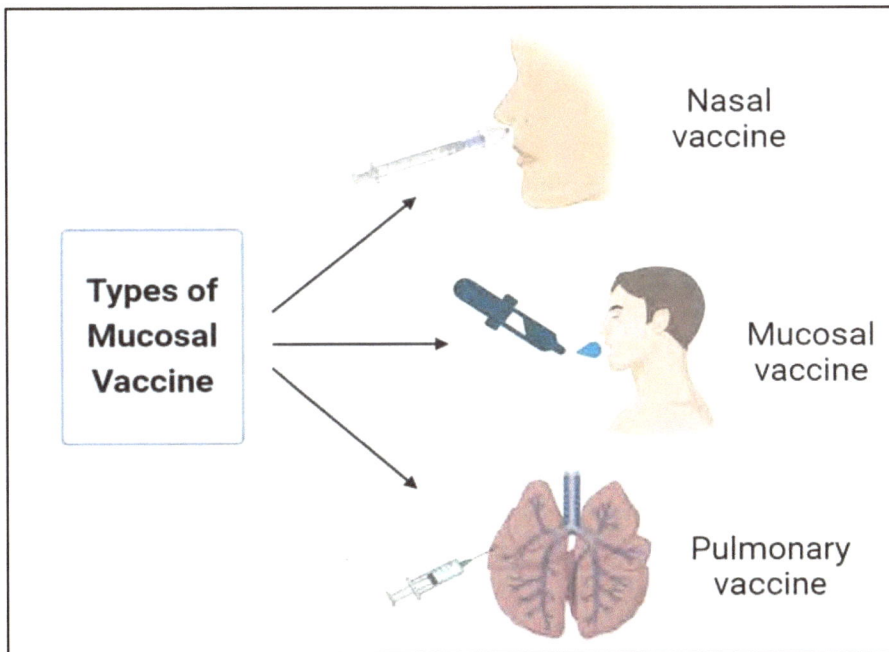

Fig. (1). Types of mucosal vaccines.

Oral Vaccines

One of the most well-known methods of immunizing the mucosa is oral vaccination. Because they are taken orally, usually as tablets, capsules, or liquid suspensions, they are easy to distribute and administer in large quantities, particularly in environments with limited resources. Oral vaccines can stimulate both systemic and mucosal immune responses by using the gut-associated lymphoid tissue (GALT), a network of tissues and lymphoid cells that runs the length of the gastrointestinal tract. Oral vaccinations against rotavirus, cholera, and poliovirus are notable examples. Live, attenuated, or inactivated pathogens, along with adjuvants or delivery mechanisms, are frequently included in these vaccines to improve immunogenicity and stability. Oral vaccinations have proven to be effective in preventing diarrheal illnesses, and they have played a significant role in international efforts to combat illnesses like rotavirus gastroenteritis and polio [9 - 11].

Nasal Vaccines

Another well-known class of mucosal vaccines that use the nasal mucosa as a delivery site for the vaccine is nasal vaccines. Nasal vaccination has several benefits, such as quick antigen absorption by mucosal-associated lymphoid tissue (MALT), no need for needle administration, and stimulation of systemic and local immune responses. Usually given as nasal sprays or droplets, nasal vaccines frequently contain live, attenuated, inactivated, or subunit antigens. Vaccines against respiratory syncytial virus (RSV), influenza, and measles are a few examples of nasal vaccinations. To increase vaccination efficacy, nasal vaccines can be made with adjuvants, mucosal adhesives, or delivery mechanisms like liposomes or nanoparticles. Nasal vaccination has the potential to replace needles in mass immunization campaigns and has demonstrated promise in eliciting protective immune responses against respiratory pathogens [12, 13].

Pulmonary Vaccines

A more recent development in mucosal vaccination is the pulmonary vaccine, which targets the respiratory mucosa for vaccine delivery. Some special benefits of pulmonary vaccination are needle-free administration, mucosal and systemic immune response induction, and direct access to immune cells in the lung-associated lymphoid tissue (LALT). Usually, aerosol sprays, dry powder inhalers, or nebulizers are used to administer pulmonary vaccines through inhalation. They could include subunit, live, or inactivated antigens; adjuvants and carrier systems are frequently used in their formulation to improve immunogenicity and stability. Vaccines against respiratory pathogens, influenza, and tuberculosis are a few examples of pulmonary vaccines. Pulmonary vaccination has attracted interest as a possible tactic for managing emerging respiratory viruses like SARS-CoV-2. It shows promise in the fight against respiratory infections, including those brought on by airborne pathogens [14, 15].

ADVANTAGES OF MUCOSAL VACCINATION

In contrast to conventional parenteral vaccination routes, mucosal vaccination provides several advantages that make it a potentially effective method of preventing infectious diseases. These benefits are provided by the distinct characteristics of mucosal surfaces and the specific immune responses they elicit. Fig. (**2**) shows the advantages of mucosal vaccination, which are described below.

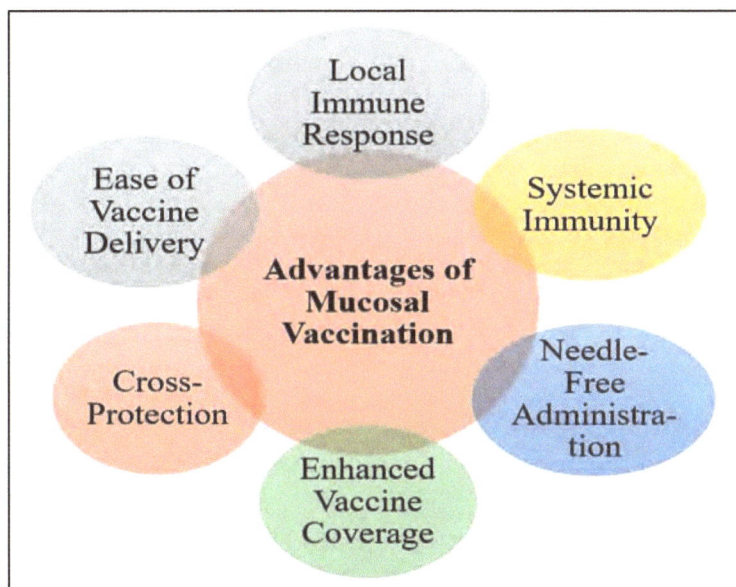

Fig. (2). Advantages of mucosal vaccination.

Local Immune Response

Mucosal vaccinations act as a first line of defense against infection by eliciting immune responses at the site of pathogen entry. Specialized immune cells, such as M, dendritic, and lymphocytes, are abundant on mucosal surfaces, such as those lining the gastrointestinal, respiratory, and genitourinary tracts. Mucosal vaccines work by stimulating the production of secretory IgA antibodies, which help neutralize pathogens and stop them from adhering to mucosal surfaces, by targeting these MALT. This local immune response can effectively prevent the establishment of infection and the spread of pathogens within the host [16, 17].

Systemic Immunity

Mucosal vaccination can produce systemic immunity in addition to local immune responses, protecting against the spread of infection and stopping the spread of disease. Activated immune cells from mucosal tissues migrate to systemic lymphoid organs in response to mucosal vaccines, where they can trigger systemic immune responses. When preventing infections brought on by pathogens like influenza virus and rotavirus, which target both the mucosal and systemic compartments, this dual mucosal and systemic immune response is especially helpful [18, 19].

Needle-Free Administration

The possibility of needle-free vaccination with mucosal vaccines can enhance vaccine acceptability, compliance, and accessibility, especially for those with needle phobia or restricted access to medical care. No needles or syringes are needed when administering oral, nasal, or pulmonary vaccines, thanks to non-invasive delivery techniques like inhalation, nasal sprays, and oral ingestion. Because of this, mucosal vaccination is particularly well-suited for widespread immunization campaigns, especially in areas with limited resources or during infectious disease outbreaks [20].

Enhanced Vaccine Coverage

Mucosal vaccination offers the potential to elicit broader and more comprehensive immune responses compared to conventional parenteral vaccination routes. Mucosal surfaces, with their wide surface area and various immune cells, constitute a vast immunological frontier. Mucosal vaccines can improve vaccine coverage and protection against various pathogens by simultaneously stimulating immune responses at several sites by targeting mucosal tissues. This is especially crucial for avoiding infections like respiratory and gastrointestinal illnesses that mostly affect mucosal surfaces [21].

Cross-Protection

Mucosal vaccination provides broader protection against antigenically diverse strains and variants by potentially eliciting cross-protective immune responses against related pathogens. Mucosal immune responses are characterized by high levels of cross-reactivity or the ability of immune cells triggered by a mucosal vaccination to recognize and react to related pathogens. This phenomenon, also referred to as cross-protection or heterotypic immunity, can offer partial or total protection against related pathogens within the same family or genus as well as antigenically distinct strains or variants of the same pathogen [22, 23].

Ease of Vaccine Delivery

Adjuvants or delivery systems that improve vaccine stability, immunogenicity, and mucosal adhesion are frequently used to formulate mucosal vaccines. These formulations can enhance immune cell activation and recruitment, facilitate antigen uptake by mucosal epithelial cells, and shield antigens from degradation in the harsh environment of the gastrointestinal tract. Furthermore, a range of delivery methods, including oral tablets, nasal sprays, and pulmonary inhalers, are available to administer mucosal vaccines, enabling accurate and convenient dosing [24].

Mucosal vaccination is a promising strategy for preventing infectious diseases because it provides several important benefits. Mucosal vaccines target mucosal surfaces, which can lead to local and systemic immune responses, enhance vaccine coverage, offer cross-protection against related pathogens, enable needle-free administration, and make vaccine delivery easier. To fully utilize this strategy and address the threats that infectious diseases pose to global health, mucosal vaccine development requires ongoing research and innovation.

BIOPROCESSING CHALLENGES

Antigen Selection and Design

Since the choice and design of antigens greatly influence vaccine efficacy and immunogenicity, antigen selection and design represent crucial bioprocessing challenges in mucosal vaccine development. The most appropriate antigens must be chosen for targeted pathogens to elicit strong and protective immune responses. While choosing antigens for mucosal vaccines, several factors need to be considered, such as immunogenicity, antigenicity, conservation across various strains or serotypes, and capacity to elicit both systemic and mucosal immune responses. To ensure optimal recognition and immune system interaction, antigens must also be designed to mimic the pathogen's native structure. A comprehensive comprehension of the pathogen's biology, virulence factors, and immune evasion mechanisms is necessary for this [25, 26].

Antigenicity, or an antigen's capacity to elicit an immune response, is one of the main factors considered during the antigen selection process. Immunogenic epitopes that trigger particular immune reactions, such as the generation of T cells, cytokines, and antibodies, must be present in antigens. It can be difficult to identify antigenic epitopes, especially in complex pathogens with several antigenic targets. Researchers can choose the most immunogenic antigens for vaccine development using methods like bioinformatics analysis, epitope mapping, and structural modeling to help identify and characterize antigenic epitopes [27, 28].

Antigens must be able to elicit robust and long-lasting immune responses, which makes immunogenicity another important factor in antigen selection. To achieve this, antigens that can trigger both innate and adaptive immune responses must be chosen carefully. Because they can stimulate pattern recognition receptors (PRRs) or interact with host immune cells, some antigens, like surface proteins or virulence factors, may be naturally immunogenic. For some antigens, additional adjuvants, conjugation to carrier proteins, or integration into cutting-edge delivery methods may be necessary to maximize their immunogenicity [29].

In order to create broadly protective mucosal vaccines that can offer cross-protection against antigenically diverse pathogens, antigen conservation across strains or serotypes is essential. A vaccine's coverage can be increased, and the likelihood of vaccine escape mutants arising decreases by choosing conserved antigens shared by several strains or serotypes. Nonetheless, a thorough examination of pathogen genomes, antigenic variability, and immune selection pressure is necessary to identify conserved antigens. Phylogenetic analysis, sequence alignment, and comparative genomics are a few techniques that can help find conserved antigenic targets for vaccine development [30, 31].

To offer the best defense against mucosal pathogens, antigens need to possess the qualities of immunogenicity, antigenicity, and conservation in addition to the ability to elicit both systemic and mucosal immune responses. Mucosal vaccines elicit systemic immune responses to thwart the spread and systemic infection and stimulate immune responses at mucosal surfaces, where pathogens usually enter the host. The key to the effectiveness of mucosal vaccines is the selection of antigens that can efficiently elicit mucosal immune responses, such as secretory IgA production, mucosal T cell activation, and mucosal cytokine secretion. To offer sustained defense against systemic infection, antigens must also elicit strong systemic immune responses, including neutralizing antibodies, memory T cells, and cytokine responses [32, 33].

Optimizing antigen recognition and immune system interaction requires designing antigens to resemble the pathogen's native structure. Because native conformational epitopes closely resemble the antigenic structures the immune system encounters during a natural infection, they are frequently more immunogenic than linear epitopes. The native conformation of recombinant antigens can be preserved through engineering by selecting suitable expression systems, purification procedures, and formulation techniques. The design of antigenic mimics for vaccine development can be guided by structural biology techniques such as cryo-electron microscopy, nuclear magnetic resonance (NMR) spectroscopy, and X-ray crystallography, which can offer insightful information about the three-dimensional structure of antigens [34, 35].

Developing effective mucosal vaccines requires selecting antigens that are highly immunogenic, conserved, highly antigenic, and capable of eliciting both mucosal and systemic immune responses. Researchers can find and create the best antigens for mucosal vaccine development by utilizing immunology, structural biology, bioinformatics, and vaccine design developments. This will lead to increased defense against infectious diseases [36].

Expression System Optimization

Expression system optimization is a crucial step in the bioprocessing of mucosal vaccine development. This step affects the antigenicity, immunogenicity, and production yield of vaccine antigens. The success of producing mucosal vaccines is mainly dependent on the expression system selected, and a number of factors influence this process. Scalability and production yield of the selected system are important factors in expression system optimization. Mucosal vaccines frequently require large amounts of antigen for testing and formulation, which calls for expression systems able to produce high-level recombinant proteins [37].

Bacterial expression systems, like Escherichia coli, are appealing for the production of mucosal vaccine antigens due to their high production yields and scalability. However, the antigenicity and immunogenicity of these antigens may be affected if bacterial expression systems fail to produce correctly folded or post-translationally modified antigens. In contrast, antigens that are correctly folded and post-translationally modified in eukaryotic expression systems like yeast, insect cells, or mammalian cells—can generate antigens that closely resemble the pathogen's original structure. Eukaryotic expression systems are preferred for producing complex antigens that require proper folding and glycosylation for optimal antigenicity and immunogenicity, even though they typically offer lower production yields than bacterial systems [38, 39].

The antigenicity and immunogenicity of the generated recombinant antigens are considered during the optimization of the expression system. To elicit strong and protective immune responses, mucosal vaccine antigens must closely resemble the pathogen's native structure. The antigenicity and immunogenicity of antigens produced by expression systems that generate them incorrectly folded or with post-translational modifications may be decreased, limiting the effectiveness of vaccines. Researchers use various techniques, such as codon optimization, signal peptide optimization, and fusion protein design, to maximize antigen expression and folding to overcome this difficulty [40, 41].

Redesigning the antigen gene's nucleotide sequence to improve translation efficiency and protein expression in the selected expression system is known as codon optimization. To ensure appropriate folding and post-translational modification, signal peptide optimization seeks to enhance recombinant protein secretion from the expression host. The process of designing fusion proteins entails combining the target antigen with tags or carrier proteins that facilitate appropriate folding, stability, and solubility, thereby enabling the purification and characterization of the antigen [42, 43].

Expression system optimization entails choosing the right promoters, vectors, and expression conditions to maximize protein production while reducing host cell toxicity and stress. Promoters have a major impact on protein expression levels and control how the antigen gene is transcribed. Robust promoters, like T7 or CMV promoters, can induce high-level expression of recombinant proteins. However, they may also place a metabolic strain on the host cell, resulting in decreased rates of growth or protein solubility [44].

Another important component of optimizing an expression system is vector design. Vectors contain vital components like the antigen gene expression cassette, antibiotic resistance genes, and the replication origin. Plasmid stability, copy number, and expression efficiency in the host cell can all be increased by optimizing vector design. Furthermore, optimizing expression conditions can improve protein expression and folding while reducing host cell stress and proteolytic degradation. These conditions include culture media composition, temperature, pH, and induction techniques [45, 46].

Expression system optimization heavily depends on downstream processing considerations; purification techniques affect antigen purity, yield, and stability. To ensure vaccine safety and efficacy and to meet regulatory requirements, mucosal vaccine antigens must be highly pure. Common purification methods for recombinant proteins include hydrophobic interaction chromatography, size exclusion chromatography, ion exchange chromatography, and affinity chromatography [47].

His-tag and GST-tag purification are two examples of tag-based purification techniques that can streamline antigen purification and ease downstream processing. Tag removal procedures might be necessary to remove any potential immunogenicity or interference with vaccine formulation. To achieve high purity and yield of recombinant antigens, optimizing purification methods entails choosing suitable chromatography resins, buffer conditions, and elution strategies [48].

Purification Methods for Mucosal Antigens

The creation of pure and stable antigens appropriate for vaccine formulation and testing is ensured by purification techniques for mucosal antigens, which are essential to developing successful mucosal vaccines. Whether isolated from pathogens or derived from recombinant expression systems, mucosal antigens frequently need to be purified to retain their immunogenicity and antigenicity while removing pollutants and impurities [49]. When developing mucosal vaccines, various purification methods are frequently used, each with its own benefits and drawbacks. Purification methods used for mucosal antigens are described below and summarized in Fig. (**3**).

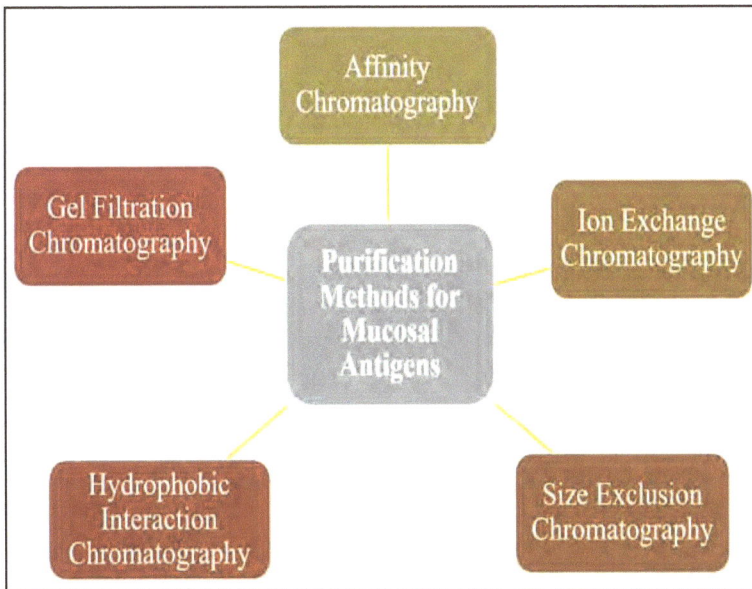

Fig. (3). Purification methods used for mucosal antigens.

Affinity chromatography is a popular technique for the purification of mucosal antigens, especially those generated in recombinant expression systems. The specific interaction between a target antigen or tag on the antigen of interest and a ligand immobilized on a chromatography resin is the basis for affinity chromatography. Maltose-binding protein (MBP-tag), glutathione S-transferase (GST-tag), and polyhistidine (His-tag) are common affinity tags used for antigen purification. High specificity and yield provided by affinity chromatography enable quick and effective purification of recombinant antigens. Removing the tag from the purified antigen using affinity chromatography, however, might involve extra steps because tags can obstruct the creation of vaccines or trigger unintended immune reactions [50, 51].

Ion exchange chromatography is another popular technique for purifying mucosal antigens, especially those obtained from complicated biological materials or pathogens. Proteins are separated by their net charge using ion exchange chromatography, whereby positively charged proteins bind to negatively charged ion exchange resins and vice versa. Based on their charge characteristics, proteins can be selectively eluted from the resin by varying the chromatography buffer's pH and ionic strength. Several mucosal antigens with different charge characteristics can be purified thanks to ion exchange chromatography's high resolution and adaptability. However, to obtain high purity and yield of the target antigen, ion exchange chromatography may need numerous purification steps and extensive optimization [52, 53].

Mucosal antigens are frequently purified using size exclusion chromatography, also called gel filtration chromatography, according to the molecular size and shape of the antigens. Larger proteins are excluded and elute first in size exclusion chromatography, which separates proteins by permitting smaller proteins to enter the porous matrix of the chromatography resin. Larger proteins elute earlier than smaller proteins, separating proteins based on their hydrodynamic radius. As a mild and non-denaturing purification technique, size exclusion chromatography is appropriate for maintaining mucosal antigens' natural structure and antigenicity. Size exclusion chromatography might not be able to fully purify mucosal antigens on a large scale or with sufficient resolution [54, 55].

One purification technique that is frequently used for mucosal antigens with hydrophobic characteristics is hydrophobic interaction chromatography (HIC). More hydrophobic proteins bind to the hydrophobic ligands on the chromatography resin, separating proteins according to their hydrophobicity *via* hydrophobic interaction chromatography. Based on their hydrophobic characteristics, proteins can be selectively eluted from the resin by varying the pH and salt concentration of the chromatography buffer. High selectivity and resolution are provided by hydrophobic interaction chromatography, which makes it possible to purify mucosal antigens with different levels of hydrophobicity. To attain high purity and yield of the target antigen, hydrophobic interaction chromatography may necessitate optimizing buffer conditions and resin selection [56, 57].

Tag-based purification techniques are frequently employed when producing mucosal antigens through recombinant expression systems. To aid in the target antigen's purification, tags like polyhistidine (His-tag), glutathione S-transferase (GST-tag), and maltose-binding protein (MBP-tag) can be fused to it. The specific interaction between a corresponding ligand immobilized on a chromatography resin and the tag is the basis for tag-based purification techniques. Mucosal antigens can be quickly and effectively purified using tag-based purification techniques, which bind the tagged antigen selectively to the resin and eliminate leftover contaminants. To avoid any potential interference with vaccine formulation or unwanted immune responses, tag removal procedures might be necessary [58, 59].

Formulation and Stability Considerations

Mucosal vaccine development requires careful attention to formulation and stability issues to guarantee that antigens retain their potency, safety, and effectiveness during production, storage, and administration. Regarding vaccinations, mucosal vaccines are not like other parenteral vaccinations because of the harsh conditions at mucosal surfaces and the requirement to stimulate both systemic and mucosal immune responses. Therefore, formulation strategies must be carefully thought out to maximize immune responses after administration, protect antigens from degradation, and improve their stability [60, 61].

Antigen stabilization is a crucial formulation component, especially for mucosal antigens vulnerable to protease degradation, pH extremes, or temperature changes. Encasing antigens in biocompatible forms, like liposomes, nanoparticles, or microparticles, can improve antigen stability and shield it from enzymatic degradation. These carriers preserve the structural integrity of antigens, protect them from proteolytic enzymes, and enable controlled release at mucosal sites. Moreover, stabilizers like sugars, polyols, or surfactants can be added to vaccine formulations to stop protein adsorption to container surfaces, denaturation, or aggregation while being stored and transported [62].

Adjuvants are essential for improving antigen immunogenicity and fostering strong immune responses in the formulation of mucosal vaccines. Adjuvants for mucosal surfaces activate innate immune cells, facilitating the uptake, presentation, and secretion of antigens and the release of cytokines. Bacterial toxins, such as heat-labile enterotoxin (LT) or cholera toxin (CT), as well as artificial derivatives or nanoparticles made to resemble pathogen-associated molecular patterns (PAMPs) and activate pattern recognition receptors (PRRs), are frequently used as mucosal adjuvants. Adjuvants must be chosen with caution, though, to balance immunostimulatory effects with possible safety issues like toxicity, inflammation, or unwanted immune activation [63, 64].

Mucosal surfaces are where pathogens usually enter the host, so mucosal vaccine formulations must be specifically designed to maximize antigen uptake and immune responses. The effectiveness of vaccines can be increased by employing techniques like particulate carriers, mucoadhesive polymers, and absorption enhancers to increase antigen absorption and retention across mucosal epithelia. Mucoadhesive polymers, like alginate or chitosan, stick to mucosal surfaces to increase antigen uptake by mucosal immune cells and prolong the duration of antigen residence. Surfactants and bile salts are absorption enhancers that break down the mucosal barrier to increase paracellular transport and absorption of antigens. Particulate carriers, like liposomes or nanoparticles, help deliver antigens to MALT (mucosal-associated lymphoid tissues), which triggers the immune response [65, 66].

Mucosal vaccine formulations must take stability into account to guarantee vaccine efficacy and shelf life under a variety of storage and transportation circumstances. Vaccines must be stable when stored at various temperatures, humidity levels, and pH ranges to preserve antigen potency and vaccine integrity. To determine the stability and shelf-life of vaccine formulations, stability testing entails assessing them under conditions that accelerate aging, such as temperature stress, freeze-thaw cycles, and exposure to light or oxygen. To guarantee vaccination efficacy and stability after administration, compatibility with various delivery methods and routes must also be considered [67, 68].

SCALE-UP CHALLENGES IN MUCOSAL VACCINE PRODUCTION

The shift from laboratory to industrial scale is one of the challenges associated with mucosal vaccine production. To meet the rising demand while maintaining product quality and consistency, this shift necessitates optimizing production procedures, machinery, and facilities. Some of the difficulties are upscaling cell culture and fermentation, streamlining downstream processing and purification, creating manufacturing facilities that adhere to GMP standards, and managing regulatory constraints. Investing in infrastructure, technology, and research is necessary to overcome these obstacles and expedite the development and manufacturing of mucosal vaccines intended for broad administration and distribution.

The transition from Laboratory to Industrial Scale

A crucial stage in the transition from research and development to large-scale manufacturing and distribution is the shift in mucosal vaccine production from the laboratory to the industrial scale. Scaling up production to industrial levels introduces several challenges that must be addressed to ensure efficient and economical manufacturing processes, even though laboratory-scale processes offer insightful information and proof-of-concept data.

Production processes at the laboratory scale are usually carried out with manual or semi-automated procedures and small-scale equipment. Scientists can investigate different parameters and conditions to maximize antigen yield, purity, and quality because these processes are frequently highly controlled and optimized for research. However, large-scale production is not the intended use of laboratory-scale processes, and a significant amount of modification and optimization is needed to switch to industrial scale [69 - 71].

Upscaling production processes to meet rising demand while preserving product quality and consistency presents challenges in the laboratory-to-industrial scale transition. Because of their throughput, scalability, and efficiency limitations, laboratory-scale processes might not be appropriate for large-scale production. Thus, optimizing and redesigning production processes are crucial to guarantee product quality and consistency, maximize yield, reduce production costs, and boost productivity [72].

Large-scale bioreactors that can generate sizable amounts of vaccine antigens, automated systems, and high-throughput technologies are all necessary for upscaling production processes. Industrial-scale bioreactors are built to support higher cell densities and hold larger volumes of cell culture media, which allows for the production of larger amounts of vaccine antigens. Furthermore, to optimize cell growth, productivity, and product quality, process variables like temperature, agitation, and aeration must be closely monitored and adjusted [73].

The infrastructure and design of the facility also present major obstacles when moving from a laboratory to an industrial scale. Good Manufacturing Practice (GMP) guidelines must be followed in the design of industrial-scale manufacturing facilities to guarantee the production of high-quality, safe vaccinations for human use. To increase production efficiency, reduce the risk of cross-contamination, and make regulatory compliance easier, facility layout, equipment placement, and workflow design must be optimized. To support large-scale vaccine production while upholding environmental sustainability and regulatory compliance, facility infrastructure, including utilities, HVAC systems, and waste management, must also be reliable and scalable [74, 75].

Maximizing antigen yield, purity, and quality through upstream and downstream processing optimization presents another hurdle in the shift to an industrial scale. The scalability of laboratory-scale cell culture and fermentation processes to industrial volumes may be limited, necessitating the optimization of process parameters, feeding strategies, and media formulations. To handle large volumes of cell culture supernatant or lysate while achieving high purity and yield of vaccine antigens, purification and downstream processing techniques must also be optimized [76, 77].

Upstream Process Optimization

Enhancing the effectiveness, productivity, and consistency of procedures taking place before the purification stage, like cell culture, fermentation, and antigen expression, is known as upstream process optimization in the manufacture of mucosal vaccines. This optimization is required to achieve high antigenic material yields while preserving product quality and reducing production costs.

As distinct cell lines differ in their growth characteristics, productivity, and suitability for mucosal vaccine production, selecting the appropriate cell line is essential for optimizing antigen production. For instance, complex mucosal vaccine antigens that need appropriate folding and post-translational modifications are frequently produced using mammalian cell lines, such as Chinese hamster ovary (CHO) cells. Simpler antigens that don't require intricate glycosylation or protein folding are frequently produced using bacterial expression systems, such as Escherichia coli. When choosing a cell line, it is important to consider aspects like productivity, scalability, growth kinetics, and suitability for downstream processing techniques [78, 79].

Cell culture conditions must be optimized to maximize cell growth, viability, and productivity. To create the ideal environment for cell growth and antigen production, parameters like media composition, pH, temperature, agitation, and dissolved oxygen levels must be carefully controlled and optimized. The media optimization process entails choosing the right growth factors, supplements, and nutrient sources to promote cell proliferation and productivity while reducing the buildup of metabolic waste and cell death. Additionally, fed-batch or perfusion techniques can improve cell growth and productivity by consistently adding nutrients and eliminating waste from the culture medium [80, 81].

Antigen yield and productivity can only be maximized by optimizing fermentation processes. Choosing the right fermentation system batch, fed-batch or continuous, as well as maximizing process variables like agitation, aeration, temperature, and pH, are all part of fermentation optimization. These parameters need to be carefully controlled to minimize by-product formation and metabolic stress while maximizing cell growth, biomass accumulation, and antigen expression. Online monitoring and control systems can also monitor important fermentation parameters in real time and make timely adjustments to maximize process performance [82, 83].

Real-time upstream process monitoring, control, and optimization can be made possible by implementing advanced analytics and process analytical technologies (PAT). PAT uses analytical methods, sensors, and probes to track important process variables and product characteristics in real-time. Researchers can find process deviations, improve process conditions, and guarantee product quality and consistency throughout production by integrating PAT with process control systems. Furthermore, by applying advanced analytics like statistical modeling and multivariate data analysis, data-driven decision-making and process optimization based on past data and process trends can be made possible [84, 85].

Downstream Processing Scalability

To efficiently purify vaccine antigens from large volumes of cell culture supernatant or lysate while maintaining product quality and consistency, downstream processing scalability is essential in the production of mucosal vaccines. Following cell culture and fermentation, downstream processing includes purification, concentration, and formulation steps. In this context, scalability refers to the capacity to move from laboratory-scale procedures to industrial-scale manufacturing without sacrificing productivity, yield, or product quality [86].

Chromatography, filtration, centrifugation, and precipitation are common purification methods, each with its own benefits and drawbacks. For instance, chromatography provides excellent resolution and selectivity but may not be as scalable as other methods because of resin capacity and column size limitations. Conversely, filtration has the potential to achieve high throughput, but it might take several stages and optimization to get the right purity and yield. To guarantee reliable and repeatable outcomes at scale, purification technique optimization entails choosing the best procedures for the target antigen, fine-tuning process parameters, and implementing automation and control systems [87, 88].

To maximize antigen recovery, purity, and yield while minimizing production costs and cycle times, downstream processing scalability necessitates the optimization of process parameters such as buffer composition, pH, temperature, and flow rates. In particular, process parameters must be carefully controlled and monitored when scaling up production to industrial volumes to ensure consistency and reproducibility across batches. Implementing online monitoring and control systems, ensuring optimal performance and product quality throughout the purification process, is possible, which enables real-time process parameter adjustments based on analytical data [89].

The optimization of formulation and filling procedures is necessary for downstream processing scalability to guarantee the stability, effectiveness, and security of vaccine antigens throughout administration, storage, and transit. Formulation optimization entails the selection of suitable excipients, stabilizers, and preservatives to preserve antigen potency and stability under a range of storage conditions. Furthermore, vaccine stability and shelf-life can be improved while facilitating precise dosing and administration by optimizing filling processes like lyophilization or spray drying. By minimizing contamination risks and guaranteeing product integrity, automated filling and packaging systems enable high-throughput production of vaccine formulations [90, 91].

Ensuring the safety, efficacy, and consistency of mucosal vaccines intended for human use is contingent upon downstream processing scalability, which requires adherence to regulatory requirements and quality standards. For vaccine products to be safe, traceable, and high-quality, industrial-scale manufacturing facilities must abide by Good Manufacturing Practice (GMP) guidelines, Good Laboratory Practice (GLP) regulations, and other applicable regulatory requirements. Moreover, putting in place strong systems for quality control and assurance is crucial to ensuring regulatory compliance throughout the manufacturing lifecycle and monitoring and validating downstream processing activities, facilities, and equipment [92, 93].

Equipment and Facility Requirements

The downstream processing of mucosal vaccines depends heavily on the equipment and facilities needed to ensure effective vaccine antigen formulation, packaging, and purification while upholding regulatory compliance, product quality, and consistency. Scaling up production from laboratory to industrial scale requires specialized equipment and well-designed facilities to achieve these goals [94].

Detectors for tracking eluted fractions, pumps for delivering buffer, software for process control and data analysis, and columns filled with chromatography resins are the standard components of chromatography systems. Large volumes of feed material must be handled by industrial-scale chromatography systems, which also need to be dependable, strong, and able to produce high yields and purity of product. To achieve effective and economical purification of vaccine antigens at scale, large-scale columns with high-capacity resins, automated packing and unpacking systems, and sophisticated process control capabilities are necessary [95, 96].

In downstream processing, filtration systems are crucial for eliminating aggregates, particles, and other contaminants from vaccine antigens. Membrane filters, depth filters, and ultrafiltration/diafiltration (UF/DF) units are the most common components of filtration systems. These units clarify, concentrate, and exchange vaccine antigens with a buffer. Large volumes of feed material must be handled by industrial-scale filtration systems to achieve high throughput, product recovery, and purity. In particular, tangential flow filtration (TFF) systems with high productivity, scalability, and product quality are frequently used for vaccine antigen concentration and buffer exchange [97, 98].

The extraction and purification of vaccine antigens from cell culture supernatant or lysate is frequently accomplished using centrifugation systems. High-speed centrifuges, rotors, and control systems for process monitoring and control are the standard components of centrifugation systems. Large volumes of feed material must be handled by industrial-scale centrifugation systems to achieve high centrifugal forces, separation efficiency, and product recovery. Because they provide high throughput, scalability, and flexibility, continuous flow centrifugation systems like disc stack centrifuges are frequently used for the large-scale processing of vaccine antigens [99, 100].

To facilitate the production of vaccines on a large scale while upholding environmental sustainability and regulatory compliance, facility infrastructure, including utilities, HVAC systems, and waste management, needs to be reliable and expandable. To facilitate operations related to downstream processing, utilities like compressed air, steam, and water must be provided in the right amounts and at the right quality. To guarantee the safety and integrity of vaccine products, HVAC systems must provide controlled environmental conditions, such as temperature, humidity, and air quality. To handle and dispose of hazardous materials and byproducts and process waste according to environmental regulations, waste management systems must be put in place [101, 102].

To optimize production workflow, reduce manual handling, and maximize efficiency, facility design considerations include space requirements, material flow, and ergonomics. There must be enough room for material handling, staging, and storage in addition to the installation, upkeep, and operation of equipment. Material flow needs to be carefully planned to ensure that raw materials, intermediates, and finished products are moved throughout the facility smoothly and efficiently. Workstation design, equipment accessibility, and operator comfort are examples of ergonomic factors that need to be considered to support employee morale, productivity, and safety [103].

Regulatory Requirements for Scale-Up

Regulatory requirements for scale-up in mucosal vaccine production are essential to ensure the safety, efficacy, and quality of vaccine products for human use.

Table **1** outlines the regulatory requirements for scale-up in mucosal vaccine production.

Table 1. Regulatory requirements for scale-up in mucosal vaccine production

Regulatory Aspect	Description
Good Manufacturing Practice (GMP)	Adherence to GMP guidelines governing facility design, equipment qualification, personnel training, and quality control [104].
Preclinical Testing	Conduct preclinical studies in laboratory animals to evaluate safety, immunogenicity, and potential adverse effects [105].
Clinical Trials	Conduct clinical trials in human volunteers to assess safety, efficacy, dosage, and immune response [105].
Process Validation	Establish documented evidence that the manufacturing process consistently produces vaccines meeting quality standards [106].
Process Control	Implement measures to monitor, control, and ensure consistency of manufacturing processes [106].
Product Labeling and Packaging	Ensure accurate labeling and packaging of vaccine products with the necessary information and suitable materials [107].
Storage and Distribution	Adhere to GMP guidelines for proper storage, handling, and distribution of vaccine products [107].
Pharmacovigilance	Establish pharmacovigilance systems for monitoring, reporting, and investigating adverse events and safety issues [108].

STRATEGIES TO OVERCOME BIOPROCESSING AND SCALE-UP CHALLENGES

Strategies to overcome bioprocessing and scale-up challenges in mucosal vaccine production encompass a wide array of innovative approaches and technologies aimed at improving process efficiency, scalability, and product quality. These strategies leverage advanced bioprocessing technologies, high-throughput screening methods, cell line engineering techniques, continuous bioprocessing, process analytical technology (PAT) implementation, quality by design (QbD) principles, and collaborative approaches for knowledge sharing [109].

Advanced Bioprocessing Technologies

Advanced bioprocessing technologies represent a significant leap forward in the production of mucosal vaccines, offering solutions to traditional challenges such as scalability, productivity, and product quality. Among these advanced technologies are high-throughput screening methods, cell line engineering techniques, and continuous bioprocessing. Each of these plays a crucial role in streamlining vaccine development processes and ensuring the efficient production of high-quality mucosal vaccines [110].

High-Throughput Screening Methods

High-throughput screening (HTS) methods have revolutionized the field of vaccine development by allowing researchers to rapidly assess large numbers of vaccine candidates, adjuvants, and formulations. These methods enable the screening of thousands to millions of samples in a relatively short time, accelerating the identification of promising vaccine candidates and optimizing vaccine formulation parameters. HTS methods encompass a variety of techniques, including combinatorial libraries consisting of large collections of molecules (*e.g.*, peptides, proteins, or small molecules) with diverse structures and properties. These libraries are screened against target antigens to identify novel vaccine candidates with desired immunogenic properties [111, 112].

Microarray technology allows for the simultaneous screening of thousands of antigens or antibodies on a solid surface. Researchers can use microarrays to assess antigen-antibody interactions, epitope mapping, and immune responses in a high-throughput manner. NGS technologies enable the rapid sequencing and analysis of microbial genomes, transcriptomes, and metagenomes. Researchers can use NGS to identify antigenic targets, assess genetic diversity, and engineer expression hosts for vaccine production. Phage display technology involves the expression of peptide or protein libraries on the surface of bacteriophage particles. These libraries can be screened against target antigens to identify antigenic epitopes, protein-protein interactions, or neutralizing antibodies [113, 114].

HTS methods offer several advantages for mucosal vaccine development. For example, they allow for the rapid screening of large numbers of vaccine candidates, accelerating the vaccine discovery process. By automating the screening process, HTS methods reduce the time and resources required for vaccine development, making them cost-effective. HTS methods can be adapted to screen various types of molecules, including antigens, adjuvants, and formulations, making them versatile tools for vaccine research [115].

Cell Line Engineering Techniques

Cell line engineering techniques are crucial in optimizing host cell lines for vaccine antigen production. These techniques enable the development of high-producing cell lines with enhanced productivity, stability, and product quality. Cell line engineering encompasses a variety of strategies, such as gene editing technologies, such as CRISPR-Cas9, that allow for precise modification of the host cell genome to enhance protein expression, glycosylation patterns, and post-translational modifications. Researchers can use gene editing to knock out genes involved in host cell metabolism, reduce by-product formation, and improve antigen production [116].

Synthetic biology approaches enable the design and construction of synthetic pathways for producing complex molecules, such as antigens and adjuvants, in engineered host cells. Researchers can use synthetic biology to optimize metabolic pathways, increase flux through target pathways, and improve the yield and quality of vaccine antigens. Metabolic engineering strategies optimize cellular metabolism to enhance productivity, reduce by-product formation, and improve the yield and quality of vaccine antigens. Researchers can use metabolic engineering to manipulate enzyme expression, regulate metabolic flux, and increase precursor availability for antigen synthesis [117, 118].

Cell line engineering techniques have various benefits for mucosal vaccine production, such as engineered cell lines, which can produce higher levels of vaccine antigens, leading to increased process efficiency and reduced manufacturing costs. Engineered cell lines are often more stable and robust than their wild-type counterparts, reducing the risk of cell line instability and batch-t--batch variability. Engineered cell lines can produce vaccine antigens with improved glycosylation patterns, folding kinetics, and post-translational modifications, enhancing antigenicity and immunogenicity [119].

Continuous Bioprocessing

Continuous bioprocessing represents a paradigm shift in vaccine manufacturing, offering productivity, process control, and resource utilization advantages. Continuous bioprocessing involves the uninterrupted operation of bioreactor systems, downstream processing units, and formulation processes, leading to increased process efficiency and reduced manufacturing footprint. Continuous bioprocessing offers various benefits for mucosal vaccine production, such as continuous bioreactor systems enabling the continuous production of vaccine antigens, reducing downtime between batches, and increasing overall throughput [120, 121].

Continuous bioprocessing allows for real-time monitoring and control of key process parameters, such as cell density, nutrient concentration, and product titer, leading to enhanced process robustness and product quality. Compared to traditional batch processes, continuous bioprocessing systems require smaller manufacturing footprints, leading to reduced capital and operating costs [122].

Continuous bioprocessing encompasses a variety of unit operations, including continuous bioreactor systems, such as perfusion bioreactors and continuous stirred-tank bioreactors (CSTRs), which enable the continuous cultivation of mammalian, bacterial, or yeast cells for vaccine antigen production. These systems provide steady-state conditions, optimal nutrient supply, and waste removal, leading to increased cell density and productivity. Continuous downstream processing techniques, such as simulated moving bed chromatography and membrane filtration, enable the continuous purification of vaccine antigens from crude cell lysates [123, 124].

These techniques offer advantages in terms of process integration, yield, and purity, leading to reduced processing times and improved product quality. Integrated continuous manufacturing platforms streamline process development, scale-up, and technology transfer, accelerating the commercialization of mucosal vaccines. These platforms combine upstream and downstream unit operations into a single continuous process, reducing process complexity and improving overall process efficiency [125].

Process Analytical Technology (PAT) Implementation

The use of Process Analytical Technology (PAT) is a crucial development in bioprocessing, especially in the field of producing mucosal vaccines, where exact control and monitoring of crucial process parameters are necessary to guarantee the consistency and quality of the final product. PAT collects instruments, methods, and ideas to optimize, control, and monitor real-time bioprocessing activities. Researchers and manufacturers can improve process robustness, better understand process dynamics, and ultimately increase product quality and yield by incorporating PAT into vaccine manufacturing processes [126].

One important component of implementing PAT in the production of mucosal vaccines is using cutting-edge analytical technologies to monitor crucial process parameters in real-time. Thanks to methods like spectroscopy, chromatography, mass spectrometry, and flow cytometry, key process parameters, such as cell viability, nutrient concentrations, metabolite levels, and attributes related to product quality, can be continuously measured. These real-time data streams enable proactive intervention and adjustment to guarantee optimal process control by offering insightful information about the performance of the processes [127].

Another crucial part of implementing PAT is using multivariate data analysis (MVDA) and process modeling techniques to analyze complex bioprocess data and find correlations between process variables and product quality attributes. Researchers can instantly analyze large datasets to find trends, patterns, and departures from intended process targets. This enables prompt corrective action and process optimization. Furthermore, by optimizing process parameters and predicting process outcomes, process modeling techniques like empirical and mechanistic models can reduce the time and resources needed for experiments [128, 129].

To maintain process parameters within predetermined limits and guarantee product quality and consistency, PAT implementation entails developing and implementing advanced process control strategies. Closed-loop control systems, feedback control algorithms, and adaptive control strategies make real-time process parameter adjustments based on analytical measurements and predictive models possible. By tightly controlling key process parameters, manufacturers may reduce variability and guarantee constant product quality across several batches [130].

Quality by Design (QbD) Principles

The development and production of mucosal vaccines can be approached methodically and scientifically by applying the principles of Quality by Design (QbD), which emphasize the proactive design, optimization, and control of crucial process parameters to guarantee product quality and consistency. Establishing a comprehensive understanding of the interplay among formulation attributes, process parameters, and product performance is a key component of QbD principles. This understanding facilitates the identification of critical quality attributes (CQAs) and critical process parameters (CPPs) that affect the safety and efficacy of vaccines. Researchers and manufacturers can gain regulatory approval more quickly, improve product quality, and strengthen process robustness by incorporating QbD principles into vaccine development and manufacturing processes [131 - 133].

Establishing a quality target product profile (QTPP), which outlines the ideal characteristics of the finished vaccine product based on patient needs, legal requirements, and market expectations, is known as quality-based development (QbD). The QTPP acts as a guidebook throughout the vaccine development process, providing guidance on formulation design, process development, and analytical testing techniques [134].

Critical quality attributes (CQAs) are those particular physical, chemical, biological, or microbiological features that dictate the safety, effectiveness, and caliber of the vaccine product. QbD entails identifying these CQAs. Examples of CQAs include antigen potency, purity, stability, and immunogenicity. By knowing how formulation and process parameters affect CQAs, researchers can prioritize efforts to optimize crucial aspects of vaccine development and manufacturing [135].

Critical process parameters (CPPs) are important variables that must be controlled within predetermined limits to guarantee product quality and consistency. They are identified and controlled as another important aspect of quality by design (QbD). Regarding cell culture, CPPs can include temperature, pH, agitation speed, and nutrient concentrations. They can include variables like chromatography conditions and filtration parameters for downstream processing. Manufacturers can reduce process variability and guarantee consistent product quality across batches by methodically identifying and managing critical process variables [136, 137].

QbD emphasizes applying risk-based methods to allocate funds and efforts to crucial vaccine development and production areas. Thanks to tools like process analytical technology (PAT), design of experiments (DoE), and failure mode and effects analysis (FMEA), researchers can methodically identify, evaluate, and reduce risks throughout the product lifecycle. By concentrating on critical risks and process parameters, manufacturers can minimize regulatory risks, improve product quality, and optimize process robustness [138].

Collaborative Approaches and Knowledge Sharing

Collaborative approaches and knowledge sharing are crucial to advancing the development and production of mucosal vaccines because they enable stakeholders to share best practices, resources, and expertise. Collaboration fosters innovation, speeds up scientific discovery, and expedites the translation of research findings into useful applications in the complex world of vaccine research and production. By leveraging collective knowledge and expertise, collaborative approaches drive progress in mucosal vaccine development and effectively address critical challenges [139].

Collaborative approaches include public-private partnerships (PPPs), consortia, and research networks that unite business, government, non-profit, and academic institutions. By combining resources, knowledge, and infrastructure, these collaborations generate synergies that address unmet needs in developing mucosal vaccines and jointly pursue common research objectives. PPPs allow stakeholders to work together toward common goals while utilizing their unique strengths by offering a platform for cooperative research, pre-competitive data sharing, and technology transfer [140].

When researchers, clinicians, policymakers, and business professionals get together to share ideas, present findings, and talk about new developments in mucosal vaccine research and development, collaborative approaches help to facilitate knowledge sharing through forums like conferences, workshops, and publications. These knowledge-sharing platforms facilitate cross-disciplinary interactions, networking, and collaboration initiation, cultivating a dynamic scientific community committed to advancing mucosal vaccine science [141].

Through collaborative approaches, resources such as reagents, cell lines, animal models, and research facilities that might be too costly or unavailable for individual researchers or organizations can be shared. By pooling their resources, collaborators can reduce entry barriers, advance research more quickly, and make the most of scarce resources. Additionally, shared resources encourage transparency, reproducibility, and standardization in research, raising scientific findings' validity and dependability [142].

Collaborative approaches facilitate capacity building and technology transfer in low- and middle-income countries (LMICs), where access to mucosal vaccine research infrastructure and expertise may be limited. LMIC researchers are empowered to address local health challenges and contribute to mucosal vaccine research through training, funding, and mentorship opportunities made possible by international collaborations and technology transfer initiatives. Collaborative approaches support equity, diversity, and inclusivity in mucosal vaccine research and aid in creating locally relevant solutions by promoting international partnerships and knowledge exchange [143, 144].

FUTURE DIRECTIONS AND INNOVATIONS

In the realm of mucosal vaccine development and production, future directions and innovations are poised to revolutionize the landscape, driven by advancements in next-generation vaccine platforms, the integration of artificial intelligence (AI) and machine learning (ML) in bioprocessing, and global initiatives aimed at accelerating vaccine development and production. Next-generation mucosal vaccine platforms, such as virus-like particles (VLPs), mRNA vaccines, and recombinant protein subunit vaccines, hold promise for eliciting robust mucosal and systemic immune responses, offering enhanced efficacy, safety, and delivery mechanisms. Additionally, integrating AI and ML technologies into bioprocessing workflows promises to optimize process efficiency, reduce costs, and accelerate development timelines. By analyzing large datasets generated during bioprocessing operations, AI and ML algorithms enable real-time monitoring, control, and optimization of critical process parameters, improving process robustness and product quality [145, 146].

Furthermore, global initiatives led by organizations like the Coalition for Epidemic Preparedness Innovations (CEPI), the World Health Organization (WHO), and the Global Alliance for Vaccines and Immunization (GAVI) are essential for fostering collaboration, resource-sharing, and capacity-building to accelerate mucosal vaccine development and production. These initiatives prioritize research and development efforts against emerging infectious diseases, aiming to strengthen global health security and ensure equitable access to vaccines worldwide. By leveraging next-generation vaccine platforms, harnessing the power of AI and ML in bioprocessing, and fostering international collaboration through global initiatives, the future of mucosal vaccine development holds the promise of safer, more effective, and globally accessible vaccines to combat a range of infectious threats and improve public health outcomes [147, 148].

CONCLUSION

There have been many bioprocessing and scale-up obstacles to producing an effective mucosal vaccine. These obstacles include the intricacies of mucosal delivery systems and the optimization of expression systems and purification techniques. These obstacles have hampered our capacity to respond to emerging infectious diseases and global health crises quickly, creating significant barriers to achieving efficient large-scale production. However, it is imperative to recognize the critical importance of overcoming these challenges for public health. Mucosal vaccines offer unique advantages in preventing infectious diseases by inducing robust mucosal and systemic immune responses, providing a first line of defense at the site of pathogen entry. By overcoming bioprocessing challenges and scaling up production, we can unlock the full potential of mucosal vaccines to combat a wide range of pathogens, including respiratory viruses, gastrointestinal pathogens, and sexually transmitted infections. Moreover, the successful development and deployment of mucosal vaccines have the potential to significantly reduce disease burden, hospitalization rates, and healthcare costs, ultimately saving lives and improving societal well-being. A call to action for continued research and collaboration in this field is essential as we look towards the future. By fostering interdisciplinary collaboration, sharing knowledge, and investing in innovative technologies, we can accelerate progress toward developing safe, productive, and globally accessible mucosal vaccines. Only through collective effort and unwavering dedication can we overcome the remaining challenges and harness the full potential of mucosal vaccination to protect public health on a global scale.

ACKNOWLEDGEMENTS

Authors are highly thankful to their Universities/Colleges for providing library facilities for the literature survey.

REFERENCES

[1] Anggraeni R, Ana ID, Wihadmadyatami H. Development of mucosal vaccine delivery: an overview on the mucosal vaccines and their adjuvants. Clin Exp Vaccine Res 2022; 11(3): 235-48.
[http://dx.doi.org/10.7774/cevr.2022.11.3.235] [PMID: 36451668]

[2]   Su F, Patel GB, Hu S, Chen W. Induction of mucosal immunity through systemic immunization: Phantom or reality? Hum Vaccin Immunother 2016; 12(4): 1070-9.
[http://dx.doi.org/10.1080/21645515.2015.1114195] [PMID: 26752023]

[3]   Correa VA, Portilho AI, De Gaspari E. Vaccines, adjuvants and key factors for mucosal immune response. Immunology 2022; 167(2): 124-38.
[http://dx.doi.org/10.1111/imm.13526] [PMID: 35751397]

[4]   Ogra PL, Faden H, Welliver RC. Vaccination strategies for mucosal immune responses. Clin Microbiol Rev 2001; 14(2): 430-45.
[http://dx.doi.org/10.1128/CMR.14.2.430-445.2001] [PMID: 11292646]

[5]   Meade E, Rowan N, Garvey M. Bioprocessing and the production of antiviral biologics in preventing and treating viral infectious disease. Vaccines (Basel) 2023; 11(5): 992.
[http://dx.doi.org/10.3390/vaccines11050992] [PMID: 37243096]

[6]   Madani F, Hsein H, Busignies V, Tchoreloff P. An overview on dosage forms and formulation strategies for vaccines and antibodies oral delivery. Pharm Dev Technol 2020; 25(2): 133-48.
[http://dx.doi.org/10.1080/10837450.2019.1689402] [PMID: 31690146]

[7]   Rosa SS, Prazeres DMF, Azevedo AM, Marques MPC. mRNA vaccines manufacturing: Challenges and bottlenecks. Vaccine 2021; 39(16): 2190-200.
[http://dx.doi.org/10.1016/j.vaccine.2021.03.038] [PMID: 33771389]

[8]   Hannas Z, Tan JS, Zhang Y, Lhermitte F, Cleuziat C, Motes-Kreimeyer L, Dhoms P, Bublot M. Manufacturing and Control of Viral Vectored Vaccines: Challenges. Viral Vectors in Veterinary Vaccine Development: A Textbook. 2021: 183-99.

[9]   Arora D. K Goyal A, R Paliwal S, Khurana B, P Vyas S. Oral mucosal immunization: Recent advancement and future prospects. Curr Immunol Rev 2010; 6(3): 234-59.
[http://dx.doi.org/10.2174/157339510791823637]

[10]   Bukhari A. B Cells in the Gut Associated Lymphoid Tissue (Galt) (Doctoral dissertation, Loyola University Chicago).

[11]   Hudu SA, Shinkafi SH, Umar S. An overview of recombinant vaccine technology, adjuvants and vaccine delivery methods. Int J Pharm Pharm Sci 2016; 8(11): 19-24.
[http://dx.doi.org/10.22159/ijpps.2016v8i11.14311]

[12]   Li M, Wang Y, Sun Y, Cui H, Zhu SJ, Qiu HJ. Mucosal vaccines: Strategies and challenges. Immunol Lett 2020; 217: 116-25.
[http://dx.doi.org/10.1016/j.imlet.2019.10.013] [PMID: 31669546]

[13]   Xu H, Cai L, Hufnagel S, Cui Z. Intranasal vaccine: Factors to consider in research and development. Int J Pharm 2021; 609: 121180.
[http://dx.doi.org/10.1016/j.ijpharm.2021.121180] [PMID: 34637935]

[14]   Tang J, Cai L, Xu C, *et al.* Nanotechnologies in Delivery of DNA and mRNA Vaccines to the Nasal and Pulmonary Mucosa. Nanomaterials (Basel) 2022; 12(2): 226.
[http://dx.doi.org/10.3390/nano12020226] [PMID: 35055244]

[15]   Heida R, Hinrichs WLJ, Frijlink HW. Inhaled vaccine delivery in the combat against respiratory viruses: a 2021 overview of recent developments and implications for COVID-19. Expert Rev Vaccines 2022; 21(7): 957-74.
[http://dx.doi.org/10.1080/14760584.2021.1903878] [PMID: 33749491]

[16]   Eckmann L, Bamias G. Mucosal immune system. Yamada's Textbook of Gastroenterology. 2022: 242-70.
[http://dx.doi.org/10.1002/9781119600206.ch14]

[17]   Dewangan HK. Rational application of nanoadjuvant for mucosal vaccine delivery system. J Immunol Methods 2020; 481-482: 112791.

[http://dx.doi.org/10.1016/j.jim.2020.112791] [PMID: 32387695]

[18]   Lamichhane A, Azegami T, Kiyono H. The mucosal immune system for vaccine development. Vaccine 2014; 32(49): 6711-23.
[http://dx.doi.org/10.1016/j.vaccine.2014.08.089] [PMID: 25454857]

[19]   Govers C, Calder PC, Savelkoul HFJ, Albers R, van Neerven RJJ. Ingestion, immunity, and infection: nutrition and viral respiratory tract infections. Front Immunol 2022; 13: 841532.
[http://dx.doi.org/10.3389/fimmu.2022.841532] [PMID: 35296080]

[20]   Schulze K, Ebensen T, Riese P, Prochnow B, Lehr CM, Guzmán CA. New horizons in developing novel needle-free immunization strategies to increase vaccination efficacy. How to Overcome the Antibiotic Crisis: Facts, Challenges, Technologies and Future Perspectives. 2016: 207-34.

[21]   Groeger S, Meyle J. Oral mucosal epithelial cells. Front Immunol 2019; 10: 208.
[http://dx.doi.org/10.3389/fimmu.2019.00208] [PMID: 30837987]

[22]   Alturaiki W. The role of cross-reactive immunity to emerging coronaviruses. Saudi Med J 2023; 44(10): 965-72.
[http://dx.doi.org/10.15537/smj.2023.44.10.20230375] [PMID: 37777266]

[23]   Rose MA, Zielen S, Baumann U. Mucosal immunity and nasal influenza vaccination. Expert Rev Vaccines 2012; 11(5): 595-607.
[http://dx.doi.org/10.1586/erv.12.31] [PMID: 22827245]

[24]   Rhee JH. Current and new approaches for mucosal vaccine delivery. InMucosal vaccines 2020 pp. 325-356. Academic Press.
[http://dx.doi.org/10.1016/B978-0-12-811924-2.00019-5]

[25]   Burton DR. What are the most powerful immunogen design vaccine strategies? Reverse vaccinology 2.0 shows great promise. Cold Spring Harb Perspect Biol 2017; 9(11): a030262.
[http://dx.doi.org/10.1101/cshperspect.a030262] [PMID: 28159875]

[26]   Pavot V, Rochereau N, Genin C, Verrier B, Paul S. New insights in mucosal vaccine development. Vaccine 2012; 30(2): 142-54.
[http://dx.doi.org/10.1016/j.vaccine.2011.11.003] [PMID: 22085556]

[27]   Kotsias F, Cebrian I, Alloatti A. Antigen processing and presentation. Int Rev Cell Mol Biol 2019; 348: 69-121.
[http://dx.doi.org/10.1016/bs.ircmb.2019.07.005] [PMID: 31810556]

[28]   Vatti A, Monsalve DM, Pacheco Y, Chang C, Anaya JM, Gershwin ME. Original antigenic sin: A comprehensive review. J Autoimmun 2017; 83: 12-21.
[http://dx.doi.org/10.1016/j.jaut.2017.04.008] [PMID: 28479213]

[29]   Slifka MK, Amanna IJ. Role of multivalency and antigenic threshold in generating protective antibody responses. Front Immunol 2019; 10: 956.
[http://dx.doi.org/10.3389/fimmu.2019.00956] [PMID: 31118935]

[30]   Masomian M, Ahmad Z, Ti Gew L, Poh CL. Development of next generation Streptococcus pneumoniae vaccines conferring broad protection. Vaccines (Basel) 2020; 8(1): 132.
[http://dx.doi.org/10.3390/vaccines8010132] [PMID: 32192117]

[31]   Kangabam R, Sahoo S, Ghosh A, *et al.* Next-generation computational tools and resources for coronavirus research: From detection to vaccine discovery. Comput Biol Med 2021; 128: 104158.
[http://dx.doi.org/10.1016/j.compbiomed.2020.104158] [PMID: 33301953]

[32]   Raya Tonetti F, Arce L, Salva S, *et al.* Immunomodulatory properties of bacterium-like particles obtained from immunobiotic lactobacilli: Prospects for their use as mucosal adjuvants. Front Immunol 2020; 11: 15.
[http://dx.doi.org/10.3389/fimmu.2020.00015] [PMID: 32038659]

[33]   Karczmarzyk K, Kęsik-Brodacka M. Attacking the intruder at the gate: Prospects of mucosal anti

SARS-CoV-2 vaccines. Pathogens 2022; 11(2): 117.
[http://dx.doi.org/10.3390/pathogens11020117] [PMID: 35215061]

[34] Guarra F, Colombo G. Computational Methods in Immunology and Vaccinology: Design and Development of Antibodies and Immunogens. J Chem Theory Comput 2023; 19(16): 5315-33.
[http://dx.doi.org/10.1021/acs.jctc.3c00513] [PMID: 37527403]

[35] Thomas S, Abraham A. Progress in the development of structure-based vaccines. Vaccine Design: Methods and Protocols, Resources for Vaccine Development. 2022; 3: 15-33.
[http://dx.doi.org/10.1007/978-1-0716-1892-9_2]

[36] Baker JR Jr, Farazuddin M, Wong PT, O'Konek JJ. The unfulfilled potential of mucosal immunization. J Allergy Clin Immunol 2022; 150(1): 1-11.
[http://dx.doi.org/10.1016/j.jaci.2022.05.002] [PMID: 35569567]

[37] Chauhan S, Khasa YP. Challenges and Opportunities in the Process Development of Chimeric Vaccines. Vaccines (Basel) 2023; 11(12): 1828.
[http://dx.doi.org/10.3390/vaccines11121828] [PMID: 38140232]

[38] Burnett MJB, Burnett AC. Therapeutic recombinant protein production in plants: Challenges and opportunities. Plants People Planet 2020; 2(2): 121-32.
[http://dx.doi.org/10.1002/ppp3.10073]

[39] Bagno FF, Godói LC, Figueiredo MM, *et al.* Chikungunya E2 protein produced in E. coli and HEK293-T cells—comparison of their performances in ELISA. Viruses 2020; 12(9): 939.
[http://dx.doi.org/10.3390/v12090939] [PMID: 32858804]

[40] Salem R, El-Kholy AA, Waly FR, Ayman D, Sakr A, Hussein M. Generation and utility of a single-chain fragment variable monoclonal antibody platform against a baculovirus expressed recombinant receptor binding domain of SARS-CoV-2 spike protein. Mol Immunol 2022; 141: 287-96.
[http://dx.doi.org/10.1016/j.molimm.2021.12.006] [PMID: 34915268]

[41] Song Y, Mehl F, Zeichner SL. Vaccine Strategies to Elicit Mucosal Immunity. Vaccines (Basel) 2024; 12(2): 191.
[http://dx.doi.org/10.3390/vaccines12020191] [PMID: 38400174]

[42] Komar AA. The art of gene redesign and recombinant protein production: approaches and perspectives. Protein therapeutics. 2017: 161-77.

[43] Gupta SK, Shukla P. Advanced technologies for improved expression of recombinant proteins in bacteria: perspectives and applications. Crit Rev Biotechnol 2016; 36(6): 1089-98.
[http://dx.doi.org/10.3109/07388551.2015.1084264] [PMID: 26384140]

[44] Kesidis A, Depping P, Lodé A, *et al.* Expression of eukaryotic membrane proteins in eukaryotic and prokaryotic hosts. Methods 2020; 180: 3-18.
[http://dx.doi.org/10.1016/j.ymeth.2020.06.006] [PMID: 32534131]

[45] Baghban R, Farajnia S, Rajabibazl M, *et al.* Yeast expression systems: overview and recent advances. Mol Biotechnol 2019; 61(5): 365-84.
[http://dx.doi.org/10.1007/s12033-019-00164-8] [PMID: 30805909]

[46] Rouches MV, Xu Y, Cortes LBG, Lambert G. A plasmid system with tunable copy number. Nat Commun 2022; 13(1): 3908.
[http://dx.doi.org/10.1038/s41467-022-31422-0] [PMID: 35798738]

[47] Kilgore R, Minzoni A, Shastry S, *et al.* The downstream bioprocess toolbox for therapeutic viral vectors. J Chromatogr A 2023; 1709: 464337.
[http://dx.doi.org/10.1016/j.chroma.2023.464337] [PMID: 37722177]

[48] Chiocchini C, Vattem K, Liss M, *et al.* From electronic sequence to purified protein using automated gene synthesis and *in vitro* transcription/translation. ACS Synth Biol 2020; 9(7): 1714-24.
[http://dx.doi.org/10.1021/acssynbio.0c00060] [PMID: 32502345]

[49]   Holley CK, Dobrovolskaia MA. Innate immunity modulating impurities and the immunotoxicity of nanobiotechnology-based drug products. Molecules 2021; 26(23): 7308.
[http://dx.doi.org/10.3390/molecules26237308] [PMID: 34885886]

[50]   Dutta S, Bose K. Protein Purification by Affinity Chromatography. InTextbook on Cloning, Expression and Purification of Recombinant Proteins. Singapore: Springer Nature Singapore, 2022; pp. 141-171.
[http://dx.doi.org/10.1007/978-981-16-4987-5_6]

[51]   Mishra V. Affinity tags for protein purification. Curr Protein Pept Sci 2020; 21(8): 821-30.
[http://dx.doi.org/10.2174/1389203721666200606220109] [PMID: 32504500]

[52]   Li Z, Huang X, Tang Q, Ma M, Jin Y, Sheng L. Functional properties and extraction techniques of chicken egg white proteins. Foods 2022; 11(16): 2434.
[http://dx.doi.org/10.3390/foods11162434] [PMID: 36010434]

[53]   Briskot T. Science and Risk-Based Development of Ion Exchange Chromatography.

[54]   Temporini C, Colombo R, Calleri E, Tengattini S, Rinaldi F, Massolini G. Chromatographic tools for plant-derived recombinant antibodies purification and characterization. J Pharm Biomed Anal 2020; 179: 112920.
[http://dx.doi.org/10.1016/j.jpba.2019.112920] [PMID: 31706629]

[55]   Beck J, Hochdaninger G, Carta G, Hahn R. Resin structure impacts two-component protein adsorption and separation in anion exchange chromatography. J Chromatogr A 2023; 1705: 464208.
[http://dx.doi.org/10.1016/j.chroma.2023.464208] [PMID: 37453173]

[56]   Saadi S, Makhlouf C, Nacer NE, *et al.* Whey proteins as multifunctional food materials: Recent advancements in hydrolysis, separation, and peptidomimetic approaches. Compr Rev Food Sci Food Saf 2024; 23(1): e13288.
[http://dx.doi.org/10.1111/1541-4337.13288] [PMID: 38284584]

[57]   Lietta E, Pieri A, Cardillo AG, Vanni M, Pisano R, Barresi AA. An Experimental and Modeling Combined Approach in Preparative Hydrophobic Interaction Chromatography. Processes (Basel) 2022; 10(5): 1027.
[http://dx.doi.org/10.3390/pr10051027]

[58]   Hirschi S, Ward TR, Meier WP, Müller DJ, Fotiadis D. Synthetic biology: Bottom-up assembly of molecular systems. Chem Rev 2022; 122(21): 16294-328.
[http://dx.doi.org/10.1021/acs.chemrev.2c00339] [PMID: 36179355]

[59]   Xu Z, Walker S, Wise MC, *et al.* Induction of tier-2 neutralizing antibodies in mice with a DNA-encoded HIV envelope native like trimer. Nat Commun 2022; 13(1): 695.
[http://dx.doi.org/10.1038/s41467-022-28363-z] [PMID: 35121758]

[60]   Eshaghi B, Schudel A, Sadeghi I, *et al.* The role of engineered materials in mucosal vaccination strategies. Nat Rev Mater 2023; 9(1): 29-45.
[http://dx.doi.org/10.1038/s41578-023-00625-2]

[61]   Venu G, Dutta S, Panwar K, *et al.* Mucosal vaccines: Strategies and challenges: A brief overview. Pharma Innov 2023; 12(6): 4980-90.

[62]   Xiao M, Tang Q, Zeng S, *et al.* Emerging biomaterials for tumor immunotherapy. Biomater Res 2023; 27(1): 47.
[http://dx.doi.org/10.1186/s40824-023-00369-8] [PMID: 37194085]

[63]   Tizard IR. Adjuvants and adjuvanticity. Vaccines for Veterinarians. 2021:75.

[64]   Stefanetti G, Borriello F, Richichi B, Zanoni I, Lay L. Immunobiology of carbohydrates: Implications for novel vaccine and adjuvant design against infectious diseases. Front Cell Infect Microbiol 2022; 11: 808005.
[http://dx.doi.org/10.3389/fcimb.2021.808005] [PMID: 35118012]

[65] Feng F, Wen Z, Chen J, Yuan Y, Wang C, Sun C. Strategies to develop a mucosa-targeting vaccine against emerging infectious diseases. Viruses 2022; 14(3): 520.
[http://dx.doi.org/10.3390/v14030520] [PMID: 35336927]

[66] Kumar R, Islam T, Nurunnabi M. Mucoadhesive carriers for oral drug delivery. J Control Release 2022; 351: 504-59.
[http://dx.doi.org/10.1016/j.jconrel.2022.09.024] [PMID: 36116580]

[67] Bajrovic I, Schafer SC, Romanovicz DK, Croyle MA. Novel technology for storage and distribution of live vaccines and other biological medicines at ambient temperature. Sci Adv 2020; 6(10): eaau4819.
[http://dx.doi.org/10.1126/sciadv.aau4819] [PMID: 32181330]

[68] Ghaemmaghamian Z, Zarghami R, Walker G, O'Reilly E, Ziaee A. Stabilizing vaccines *via* drying: Quality by design considerations. Adv Drug Deliv Rev 2022; 187: 114313.
[http://dx.doi.org/10.1016/j.addr.2022.114313] [PMID: 35597307]

[69] Sarkis M, Bernardi A, Shah N, Papathanasiou MM. Emerging challenges and opportunities in pharmaceutical manufacturing and distribution. Processes (Basel) 2021; 9(3): 457.
[http://dx.doi.org/10.3390/pr9030457]

[70] Neubauer P, Anane E, Junne S, Cruz Bournazou MN. Potential of integrating the model-based design of experiments approaches and process analytical technologies for bioprocess scale-down. Digital Twins: Applications to the Design and Optimization of Bioprocesses. 2021:1-28.

[71] Chopda V, Gyorgypal A, Yang O, *et al.* Recent advances in integrated process analytical techniques, modeling, and control strategies to enable continuous biomanufacturing of monoclonal antibodies. J Chem Technol Biotechnol 2022; 97(9): 2317-35.
[http://dx.doi.org/10.1002/jctb.6765]

[72] Bocker R, Silva EK. Pulsed electric field technology is a promising pre-treatment for enhancing the biorefinery of orange agro-industrial waste. RSC Advances 2024; 14(3): 2116-33.
[http://dx.doi.org/10.1039/D3RA07848E] [PMID: 38196909]

[73] Matanguihan C, Wu P. Upstream continuous processing: recent advances in production of biopharmaceuticals and challenges in manufacturing. Curr Opin Biotechnol 2022; 78: 102828.
[http://dx.doi.org/10.1016/j.copbio.2022.102828] [PMID: 36332340]

[74] Merikivi-Dahlqvist IA. Evaluation of release specifications for critical raw materials, drug substances, and drug products in the production process of recombinant adeno-associated virus vectors.

[75] Kulkarni N, DelRe N, Plumitallo T, Wong M. Improving Facility Layouts for Regulated Industries Using IE Techniques. InIIE Annual Conference. Proceedings. Institute of Industrial and Systems Engineers (IISE), 2020; pp. 1-6.

[76] Drobnjakovic M, Hart R, Kulvatunyou BS, Ivezic N, Srinivasan V. Current challenges and recent advances on the path towards continuous biomanufacturing. Biotechnol Prog 2023; 39(6): e3378.
[http://dx.doi.org/10.1002/btpr.3378] [PMID: 37493037]

[77] Ganeshan S, Kim SH, Vujanovic V. Scaling-up production of plant endophytes in bioreactors: concepts, challenges and perspectives. Bioresour Bioprocess 2021; 8(1): 63.
[http://dx.doi.org/10.1186/s40643-021-00417-y] [PMID: 34760435]

[78] Cid R, Bolívar J. Platforms for production of protein-based vaccines: From classical to next-generation strategies. Biomolecules 2021; 11(8): 1072.
[http://dx.doi.org/10.3390/biom11081072] [PMID: 34439738]

[79] de Pinho Favaro MT, Atienza-Garriga J, Martínez-Torró C, *et al.* Recombinant vaccines in 2022: a perspective from the cell factory. Microb Cell Fact 2022; 21(1): 203.
[http://dx.doi.org/10.1186/s12934-022-01929-8] [PMID: 36199085]

[80] Reddy JV, Raudenbush K, Papoutsakis ET, Ierapetritou M. Cell-culture process optimization *via* model-based predictions of metabolism and protein glycosylation. Biotechnol Adv 2023; 67: 108179.

[http://dx.doi.org/10.1016/j.biotechadv.2023.108179] [PMID: 37257729]

[81]   Ge C, Selvaganapathy PR, Geng F. Advancing our understanding of bioreactors for industrial-sized cell culture: health care and cellular agriculture implications. Am J Physiol Cell Physiol 2023; 325(3): C580-91.
[http://dx.doi.org/10.1152/ajpcell.00408.2022] [PMID: 37486066]

[82]   Ezemba C, Ekwegbalu EA, Ezemba AS. Fermentation, types of fermenters, design & uses of fermenters, and optimization of the fermentation process.

[83]   De Brabander P, Uitterhaegen E, Delmulle T, De Winter K, Soetaert W. Challenges and progress towards industrial recombinant protein production in yeasts: A review. Biotechnol Adv 2023; 64: 108121.
[http://dx.doi.org/10.1016/j.biotechadv.2023.108121] [PMID: 36775001]

[84]   Wasalathanthri DP, Patel BA. The Role of Process Analytical Technology (PAT) in Biologics Development. InContinuous Pharmaceutical Processing and Process Analytical Technology, 2023; pp. 339-354.

[85]   Kim EJ, Kim JH, Kim MS, Jeong SH, Choi DH. Process analytical technology tools for monitoring pharmaceutical unit operations: a control strategy for continuous process verification. Pharmaceutics 2021; 13(6): 919.
[http://dx.doi.org/10.3390/pharmaceutics13060919] [PMID: 34205797]

[86]   Gerstweiler L. Development of a continuous downstream process for microbial produced virus-like particle-based Group A Streptococcus vaccine (Doctoral dissertation).

[87]   São Pedro MN, Silva TC, Patil R, Ottens M. White paper on high-throughput process development for integrated continuous biomanufacturing. Biotechnol Bioeng 2021; 118(9): 3275-86.
[http://dx.doi.org/10.1002/bit.27757] [PMID: 33749840]

[88]   Soheilmoghaddam F, Rumble M, Cooper-White J. High-throughput routes to biomaterials discovery. Chem Rev 2021; 121(18): 10792-864.
[http://dx.doi.org/10.1021/acs.chemrev.0c01026] [PMID: 34213880]

[89]   Chahar DS, Ravindran S, Pisal SS. Monoclonal antibody purification and its progression to commercial scale. Biologicals 2020; 63: 1-13.
[http://dx.doi.org/10.1016/j.biologicals.2019.09.007] [PMID: 31558429]

[90]   Castro LS, Lobo GS, Pereira P, Freire MG, Neves MC, Pedro AQ. Interferon-based biopharmaceuticals: Overview on the production, purification, and formulation. Vaccines (Basel) 2021; 9(4): 328.
[http://dx.doi.org/10.3390/vaccines9040328] [PMID: 33915863]

[91]   Preston KB, Randolph TW. Stability of lyophilized and spray dried vaccine formulations. Adv Drug Deliv Rev 2021; 171: 50-61.
[http://dx.doi.org/10.1016/j.addr.2021.01.016] [PMID: 33484735]

[92]   Dodds D, Kindt Jr JW, da Costa C, Kazi N, Mahoney JT, Rupassara SI. Supply Chain Logistics and Business Ecosystems Needed to Develop Natural Vaccines with Novel, Safer, and Noninvasive Delivery Mechanisms.

[93]   Jayaraman P, Lim R, Ng J, Vemuri MC. Acceleration of translational mesenchymal stromal cell therapy through consistent quality GMP manufacturing. Front Cell Dev Biol 2021; 9: 648472.
[http://dx.doi.org/10.3389/fcell.2021.648472] [PMID: 33928083]

[94]   Mead MN, Seneff S, Wolfinger R, *et al.* COVID-19 mRNA Vaccines: Lessons Learned from the Registrational Trials and Global Vaccination Campaign. Cureus 2024; 16(1): e52876.
[PMID: 38274635]

[95]   Schmidt-Traub H, Susanto A. Chromatography Equipment: Engineering and Operation. Preparative Chromatography. 2020: 525-600.

[96]   Staubach S, Bauer FN, Tertel T, *et al.* Scaled preparation of extracellular vesicles from conditioned media. Adv Drug Deliv Rev 2021; 177: 113940.
[http://dx.doi.org/10.1016/j.addr.2021.113940] [PMID: 34419502]

[97]   Goodrich EM, Bohonak DM, Genest PW, Peterson E. Recent advances in ultrafiltration and virus filtration for production of antibodies and related biotherapeutics. Approaches to the Purification, Analysis, and Characterization of Antibody-Based Therapeutics. 2020: 137-66.
[http://dx.doi.org/10.1016/B978-0-08-103019-6.00007-2]

[98]   Müller D, Klein L, Lemke J, *et al.* Process intensification in the biopharma industry: Improving efficiency of protein manufacturing processes from development to production scale using synergistic approaches. Chem Eng Process 2022; 171: 108727.
[http://dx.doi.org/10.1016/j.cep.2021.108727]

[99]   Menesklou P, Sinn T, Nirschl H, Gleiss M. Scale-up of decanter centrifuges for the particle separation and mechanical dewatering in the minerals processing industry using a numerical process model. Minerals (Basel) 2021; 11(2): 229.
[http://dx.doi.org/10.3390/min11020229]

[100]   Göbel S, Pelz L, Reichl U, Genzel Y. Upstream processing for viral vaccines-Process intensification. InBioprocessing of viral vaccines 2022; pp. 137-173.
[http://dx.doi.org/10.1201/9781003229797-6]

[101]   Dolan SB. Transitioning from paper to digital vaccination records: integration into clinic workflows, time utilization following workflow modifications, and impact on the timeliness of vaccinations. University of Washington; 2020.

[102]   Permana I, Wang F. Performance improvement of a biotechnology vaccine cleanroom for contamination control. J Build Eng 2024; 82: 108248.
[http://dx.doi.org/10.1016/j.jobe.2023.108248]

[103]   Glock CH, Grosse EH, Neumann WP, Feldman A. Assistive devices for manual materials handling in warehouses: a systematic literature review. Int J Prod Res 2021; 59(11): 3446-69.
[http://dx.doi.org/10.1080/00207543.2020.1853845]

[104]   Roien R, Shrestha R, Yadav K, *et al.* An assessment of adherence to the WHO-delineated good manufacturing practice by the pharmaceutical companies in Kabul, Afghanistan. Cost Eff Resour Alloc 2022; 20(1): 17.
[http://dx.doi.org/10.1186/s12962-022-00348-1] [PMID: 35366905]

[105]   Thakur A, Foged C. Nanoparticles for mucosal vaccine delivery. InNanoengineered biomaterials for advanced drug delivery 2020; pp. 603-646.
[http://dx.doi.org/10.1016/B978-0-08-102985-5.00025-5]

[106]   Moore LE, Vucen S, Moore AC. Trends in drug- and vaccine-based dissolvable microneedle materials and methods of fabrication. Eur J Pharm Biopharm 2022; 173: 54-72.
[http://dx.doi.org/10.1016/j.ejpb.2022.02.013] [PMID: 35219862]

[107]   Samad F, Burton SJ, Kwan D, *et al.* Strategies to reduce errors associated with 2-component vaccines. Pharmaceut Med 2021; 35(1): 1-9.
[http://dx.doi.org/10.1007/s40290-020-00362-9] [PMID: 33151497]

[108]   Sienkiewicz K, Burzyńska M, Rydlewska-Liszkowska I, Sienkiewicz J, Gaszyńska E. The importance of direct patient reporting of adverse drug reactions in the safety monitoring process. Int J Environ Res Public Health 2021; 19(1): 413.
[http://dx.doi.org/10.3390/ijerph19010413] [PMID: 35010673]

[109]   Puranik A, Dandekar P, Jain R. Exploring the potential of machine learning for more efficient development and production of biopharmaceuticals. Biotechnol Prog 2022; 38(6): e3291.
[http://dx.doi.org/10.1002/btpr.3291] [PMID: 35918873]

[110]   Ghattas M, Dwivedi G, Lavertu M, Alameh MG. Vaccine technologies and platforms for infectious

diseases: Current progress, challenges, and opportunities. Vaccines (Basel) 2021; 9(12): 1490.
[http://dx.doi.org/10.3390/vaccines9121490] [PMID: 34960236]

[111] Lee B, Nanishi E, Levy O, Dowling DJ. Precision Vaccinology Approaches for the Development of Adjuvanted Vaccines Targeted to Distinct Vulnerable Populations. Pharmaceutics 2023; 15(6): 1766.
[http://dx.doi.org/10.3390/pharmaceutics15061766] [PMID: 37376214]

[112] Tripathi NM, Bandyopadhyay A. High throughput virtual screening (HTVS) of peptide library: Technological advancement in ligand discovery. Eur J Med Chem 2022; 243: 114766.
[http://dx.doi.org/10.1016/j.ejmech.2022.114766] [PMID: 36122548]

[113] Plotnikova MA, Klotchenko SA, Lebedev KI, *et al.* Antibody microarray immunoassay for screening and differential diagnosis of upper respiratory tract viral pathogens. J Immunol Methods 2020; 478: 112712.
[http://dx.doi.org/10.1016/j.jim.2019.112712] [PMID: 31783022]

[114] Watts GS, Hurwitz BL. Metagenomic next-generation sequencing in clinical microbiology. Clin Microbiol Newsl 2020; 42(7): 53-9.
[http://dx.doi.org/10.1016/j.clinmicnews.2020.03.004]

[115] Singleton KL, Joffe A, Leitner WW. Review: Current trends, challenges, and success stories in adjuvant research. Front Immunol 2023; 14: 1105655.
[http://dx.doi.org/10.3389/fimmu.2023.1105655] [PMID: 36742311]

[116] Tihanyi B, Nyitray L. Recent advances in CHO cell line development for recombinant protein production. Drug Discov Today Technol 2020; 38: 25-34.
[http://dx.doi.org/10.1016/j.ddtec.2021.02.003] [PMID: 34895638]

[117] Yan X, Liu X, Zhao C, Chen GQ. Applications of synthetic biology in medical and pharmaceutical fields. Signal Transduct Target Ther 2023; 8(1): 199.
[http://dx.doi.org/10.1038/s41392-023-01440-5] [PMID: 37169742]

[118] Gotsmy M, Strobl F, Weiß F, *et al.* Sulfate limitation increases specific plasmid DNA yield and productivity in E. coli fed-batch processes. Microb Cell Fact 2023; 22(1): 242.
[http://dx.doi.org/10.1186/s12934-023-02248-2] [PMID: 38017439]

[119] Cid R, Bolívar J. Platforms for production of protein-based vaccines: From classical to next-generation strategies. Biomolecules 2021; 11(8): 1072.
[http://dx.doi.org/10.3390/biom11081072] [PMID: 34439738]

[120] Rathore AS, Zydney AL, Anupa A, Nikita S, Gangwar N. Enablers of continuous processing of biotherapeutic products. Trends Biotechnol 2022; 40(7): 804-15.
[http://dx.doi.org/10.1016/j.tibtech.2021.12.003] [PMID: 35034769]

[121] Khanal O, Lenhoff AM. Developments and opportunities in continuous biopharmaceutical manufacturing. InMAbs 2021; 13(1): p. 1903664.
[http://dx.doi.org/10.1080/19420862.2021.1903664]

[122] Wasalathanthri DP, Rehmann MS, Song Y, *et al.* Technology outlook for real-time quality attribute and process parameter monitoring in biopharmaceutical development—A review. Biotechnol Bioeng 2020; 117(10): 3182-98.
[http://dx.doi.org/10.1002/bit.27461] [PMID: 32946122]

[123] Mitra S, Murthy GS. Bioreactor control systems in the biopharmaceutical industry: a critical perspective. Syst Microbiol Biomanuf 2022; 2(1): 91-112.
[http://dx.doi.org/10.1007/s43393-021-00048-6] [PMID: 38624976]

[124] Keulen D, Geldhof G, Bussy OL, Pabst M, Ottens M. Recent advances to accelerate purification process development: A review with a focus on vaccines. J Chromatogr A 2022; 1676: 463195.
[http://dx.doi.org/10.1016/j.chroma.2022.463195] [PMID: 35749985]

[125] National Academies of Sciences, Engineering, and Medicine. Innovations in Manufacturing Drug Products. InInnovations in Pharmaceutical Manufacturing on the Horizon: Technical Challenges,

Regulatory Issues, and Recommendations. National Academies Press (US), 2021.

[126] Ralbovsky NM, Soukup RJ, Lomont JP, *et al.* *In situ* real time monitoring of emulsification and homogenization processes for vaccine adjuvants. Analyst (Lond) 2022; 147(3): 378-86.
[http://dx.doi.org/10.1039/D1AN01797G] [PMID: 34908043]

[127] Vora LK, Gholap AD, Jetha K, Thakur RRS, Solanki HK, Chavda VP. Artificial intelligence in pharmaceutical technology and drug delivery design. Pharmaceutics 2023; 15(7): 1916.
[http://dx.doi.org/10.3390/pharmaceutics15071916] [PMID: 37514102]

[128] Metze S. Scalability of single-use biopharmaceutical manufacturing processes using process analytical technology (PAT) tools.

[129] Goldrick S, Sandner V, Cheeks M, *et al.* Multivariate data analysis methodology to solve data challenges related to scale-up model validation and missing data on a micro-bioreactor system. Biotechnol J 2020; 15(3): 1800684.
[http://dx.doi.org/10.1002/biot.201800684] [PMID: 31617682]

[130] Kim EJ, Kim JH, Kim MS, Jeong SH, Choi DH. Process analytical technology tools for monitoring pharmaceutical unit operations: a control strategy for continuous process verification. Pharmaceutics 2021; 13(6): 919.
[http://dx.doi.org/10.3390/pharmaceutics13060919] [PMID: 34205797]

[131] Pradhan M, Parihar AK, Singh D, Singh MR. Quality by design and formulation optimization using statistical tools for safe and efficient bioactive loading. InAdvances and Avenues in Developing Novel Carriers for Bioactives and Biological Agents, 2020; pp. 555-594.
[http://dx.doi.org/10.1016/B978-0-12-819666-3.00019-5]

[132] Jagan BGVS, Murthy PN, Mahapatra AK, Patra RK. Quality by Design (QbD): Principles, underlying concepts, and regulatory prospects. Thaiphesatchasan 2021; 45(1): 54-69.
[http://dx.doi.org/10.56808/3027-7922.2473]

[133] van de Berg D, Kis Z, Behmer CF, *et al.* Quality by design modelling to support rapid RNA vaccine production against emerging infectious diseases. NPJ Vaccines 2021; 6(1): 65.
[http://dx.doi.org/10.1038/s41541-021-00322-7] [PMID: 33927197]

[134] Shirohiwala R, Shah C, Upadhyay U. Implementation of Qbd & AQbD approach in pharmaceutical formulation and analytical method development: A Comprehensive Research-Review.

[135] Schad M, Gautam S, Grein TA, Käß F. Process Analytical Technologies (PAT) and Quality by Design (QbD) for Bioprocessing of Virus-Based Therapeutics. InBioprocess and Analytics Development for Virus-based Advanced Therapeutics and Medicinal Products (ATMPs), Cham: Springer International Publishing, 2023; pp. 295-328.

[136] Khan A, Naquvi KJ, Haider MF, Khan MA. Quality by design-newer technique for pharmaceutical product development. Intelligent Pharmacy, 2023; 14.

[137] Wolf M, Bielser JM, Morbidelli M. Perfusion Cell Culture Processes for Biopharmaceuticals: Process Development, Design, and Scale-up. Cambridge University Press, 2020; 6.

[138] Musale P, Mankar SD. Quality by Design Approch Based in Analytical Method Validation. Asian Journal of Pharmaceutical Analysis 2023; 13(3): 190-6.
[http://dx.doi.org/10.52711/2231-5675.2023.00031]

[139] Daems R, Maes E. The race for COVID-19 vaccines: Accelerating innovation, fair allocation and distribution. Vaccines (Basel) 2022; 10(9): 1450.
[http://dx.doi.org/10.3390/vaccines10091450] [PMID: 36146528]

[140] Davis AM, Engkvist O, Fairclough RJ, Feierberg I, Freeman A, Iyer P. Public-private partnerships: Compound and data sharing in drug discovery and development. SLAS Discov 2021; 26(5): 604-19.
[http://dx.doi.org/10.1177/2472555220982268] [PMID: 33586501]

[141] Lawrence RS, Durch JS, Stratton KR, editors. Vaccines for the 21st century: a tool for

decisionmaking.

[142]　Boué S, Byrne M, Hayes AW, Hoeng J, Peitsch MC. Embracing transparency through data sharing. Int J Toxicol 2018; 37(6): 466-71.
[http://dx.doi.org/10.1177/1091581818803880] [PMID: 30282506]

[143]　Peacocke EF, Heupink LF, Frønsdal K, Dahl EH, Chola L. Global access to COVID-19 vaccines: a scoping review of factors that may influence equitable access for low and middle-income countries. BMJ Open 2021; 11(9): e049505.
[http://dx.doi.org/10.1136/bmjopen-2021-049505] [PMID: 34593496]

[144]　Nunes CM. The Role of Global Health Partnerships in Achieving Vaccine Equity: A case study of the COVAX Facility (Doctoral dissertation, London School of Hygiene & Tropical Medicine).

[145]　Pandey K, Pandey M, Kumar V, Aggarwal U, Singhal B. Bioprocessing 4.0 in biomanufacturing: paving the way for sustainable bioeconomy. Syst Microbiol Biomanuf 2023; 1-8.

[146]　Hameed SA, Paul S, Dellosa GKY, Jaraquemada D, Bello MB. Towards the future exploration of mucosal mRNA vaccines against emerging viral diseases; lessons from existing next-generation mucosal vaccine strategies. NPJ Vaccines 2022; 7(1): 71.
[http://dx.doi.org/10.1038/s41541-022-00485-x] [PMID: 35764661]

[147]　Mutasa R, Ramana G, Newmarch G, Seiter A, Schaeferhoff M, Sowers E, Schunk M, Gupta R, Slamet L, Guichard S, Harimurti P. ASEAN Regional Vaccine Manufacturing and Development: Regional Synthesis Report. 2023.

[148]　Nayak A. Recombinant Vaccines: The Revolution Ahead. Microbial Engineering for Therapeutics. Singapore: Springer Nature Singapore 2022; pp. 163-200.
[http://dx.doi.org/10.1007/978-981-19-3979-2_8]

CHAPTER 7

Mucosal Vaccines in Cancer Immunotherapy

Koushal Dhamija[1,*], Alok Bhardwaj[1], Sudhir Kumar[2], Shekhar Sharma[1] and **Rupali Sharma[3]**

[1] *Lloyd Institute of Management & Technology, Plot No.-11, Knowledge Park-II, Greater Noida, Uttar Pradesh-201306, India*

[2] *Faculty of Pharmaceutical Sciences, DAV University, Jalandhar, India*

[3] *Amity University Haryana, Manesar, Gurugram, India*

Abstract: Mucosal vaccines, which use the body's mucosal immune system to fight cancerous cells, represent a promising new avenue in cancer immunotherapy. This paper provides a thorough overview of the role of mucosal vaccines in cancer treatment, emphasizing their benefits, drawbacks, current research, and prospects for the future. There are many different kinds of vaccines for the mucosa, such as live attenuated, inactivated, subunit, DNA, and vector-based vaccines. They function by triggering a systemic immune response against particular cancer antigens by stimulating mucosal immunity at sites such as the respiratory, gastrointestinal, and genitourinary tracts. Enhanced mucosal immune response, needle-free administration, cost-effectiveness, and broad coverage against various cancer types are just a few benefits of this special mechanism. Mucosal vaccines have limitations despite their potential, including the requirement for adjuvants, immune responses specific to a given route, stability issues, and safety concerns. Promising outcomes are being shown by ongoing studies and clinical trials, some of which have assessed safety and efficacy in clinical settings and demonstrated efficacy in preclinical models. In cancer immunotherapy, mucosal vaccines have a wide range of uses, such as treating metastatic disease, preventing cancer from returning, and boosting the effectiveness of immunotherapeutic combinations. Moreover, customized treatment plans based on unique patient profiles may be possible by developing personalized vaccines. Mucosal vaccinations in cancer immunotherapy have a promising future. There is hope for better patient outcomes and worldwide cancer prevention strategies thanks to developments in vaccine technology, integration into standard treatment protocols, and personalized approaches. Finally, mucosal vaccines offer a novel strategy for cancer immunotherapy that has the power to alter patient survival rates and treatment paradigms drastically. Realizing the full potential of mucosal vaccines in the fight against cancer requires ongoing research and clinical development.

* **Corresponding author Koushal Dhamija:** Lloyd Institute of Management & Technology, Plot No.-11, Knowledge Park-II, Greater Noida, Uttar Pradesh-201306, India;
E-mail: drkoushaldhamija81@gmail.com

Keywords: Adoptive cell therapy, Cancer, Cancer antigens, Immunotherapy, Immunity, Mucosal vaccine, Mucosal-associated lymphoid tissues, Systemic immune response.

INTRODUCTION

With a significant impact on people, families, and societies, cancer continues to be one of the most common and difficult diseases in the world. Even with major advances in medicine, the disease's treatment is still complicated and frequently combines several different modalities, including radiation, chemotherapy, and surgery. These traditional methods have increased the survival rates of many cancer types. Still, they are frequently linked to severe side effects and poor results, especially in cases of advanced or metastatic disease [1].

Immunotherapy has changed the landscape of cancer treatment in recent years. In contrast to conventional therapies that target cancer cells directly, immunotherapy uses the body's immune system to identify, attack, and destroy cancerous cells. This creative approach has begun a new era in oncology, which offers the possibility of long-lasting effects, better survival rates, and improved quality of life for cancer patients [2].

Immunotherapy is a collective term for treatment modalities that aim to enhance the immune system's capacity to identify and eliminate cancer cells. Several of these have become important tactics in the fight against cancer, including adoptive cell transfer, immune checkpoint inhibitors, monoclonal antibodies, and cancer vaccines. By disabling the barriers that prevent immune responses, these treatments enable the body to develop a stronger anti-tumor defense or stimulate the immune system to target cancer cells [3, 4].

Immunotherapy's effectiveness varies among patients and tumor types despite its impressive success in treating some cancer types, such as melanoma, lung cancer, and hematologic malignancies. Immune evasion strategies, tumor heterogeneity, and the emergence of treatment resistance are just a few of the difficulties that make this area of study and innovation imperative [5].

Mucosal vaccines are a state-of-the-art cancer immunotherapy method that uses the body's mucosal immune system to fight cancer. Mucosal vaccines are delivered through mucosal surfaces, such as the respiratory, gastrointestinal, and genitourinary tracts, as opposed to traditional vaccines administered *via* injection. This novel mode of delivery presents several benefits, such as increased mucosal immune response, systemic immunity induction, and needle-free delivery, making it a compelling choice for cancer treatment and prevention [6, 7].

Different types of mucosal vaccines exist, each with a unique mechanism of action and possible uses in cancer immunotherapy. Live attenuated vaccines, which contain weakened versions of the pathogen, elicit a strong immune response without actually causing disease. Subunit vaccines, conversely, provoke particular immune responses against cancer cells by containing antigens specific to the pathogen. Additionally, versatile and potentially enabling personalized treatment approaches are other types of mucosal vaccines, including vector-based and DNA vaccines [8, 9].

The ability of mucosal vaccines to stimulate mucosal immunity, a vital part of the body's defense against infections and cancerous cells, holds promise for treating cancer. Immune cells such as T, B, and antigen-presenting cells are abundant on mucosal surfaces. These cells help coordinate immune responses and aid in removing malignant cells. Vaccines against mucosal surfaces can prime the immune system to recognize and eliminate cancer cells at primary and metastatic sites by inducing local and systemic immune responses. The advantage of needle-free administration that mucosal vaccines provide makes them more convenient and accessible for patients, especially in settings with limited resources. Immunotherapy may become more widely used as a standard cancer treatment modality due to its ease of administration, which could improve patient compliance [10, 11]. Mucosal vaccines differ from other cancer vaccine types, as shown in Table **1**.

Table 1. Difference between mucosal vaccines and other types of cancer vaccines.

Feature	Mucosal Vaccines	Other Types of Cancer Vaccines
Route of Administration	Oral, nasal, intranasal, or other mucosal routes.	Intramuscular, subcutaneous, or intradermal injection [12].
Target Tissues	Mucosal-associated lymphoid tissues (MALT).	Systemic lymphoid tissues [13].
Mechanism of Action	Induce mucosal and systemic immune responses.	Primarily stimulate systemic immune responses [14].
Immunogenicity	It may require potent adjuvants to overcome mucosal tolerance.	Often rely on adjuvants to enhance immune responses [15].
Antigen Stability	The formulation must protect antigens from degradation in the mucosal environment.	Stability is less of a concern due to systemic delivery [16].
Target Antigens	Tumor-specific or tumor-associated antigens.	Tumor-specific or tumor-associated antigens [17].
Delivery Considerations	Requires formulation optimization for mucosal adhesion and penetration.	Formulation optimization focused on antigen stability and immune response [18].

(Table 1) cont.....

Feature	Mucosal Vaccines	Other Types of Cancer Vaccines
Regulatory Approval	Specific regulatory considerations for mucosal vaccines may vary by region.	Adherence to general regulatory guidelines for vaccine development [19].
Potential Side Effects	Mucosal irritation, gastrointestinal symptoms, mucosal inflammation.	Injection site reactions, systemic immune activation, and rare adverse events [20].
Clinical Applications	Prevention, treatment, and adjuvant therapy for mucosal tumors; personalized vaccine approaches.	Treatment of systemic cancers, adjuvant therapy, personalized vaccine approaches [21].

Patients with advanced or refractory disease have new hope: cancer immunotherapy, which revolutionizes the approach to cancer treatment. The immune system's ability to combat cancer cells can be greatly enhanced by mucosal vaccines, which could lead to better treatment outcomes and a higher standard of living for patients. Mucosal vaccinations seem destined to become an essential part of the cancer treatment arsenal as this field's research progresses, opening up new possibilities for tailored and targeted therapy. However, to maximize their therapeutic efficacy and clinical benefit, more research is required to determine predictive biomarkers, optimize vaccine formulations, and clarify the best combination strategies [22, 23].

PRINCIPLES OF CANCER IMMUNOTHERAPY

Cancer immunotherapy represents a groundbreaking approach in the fight against cancer, capitalizing on the inherent capabilities of the immune system to recognize and destroy malignant cells. At its core lies the principle of immune recognition, whereby the immune system identifies cancer cells as aberrant and mounts an attack against them. The key to this process is immune checkpoints, which are molecular pathways that regulate immune responses. Cancer cells often exploit these checkpoints to evade detection, but therapies targeting these checkpoints, such as PD-1/PD-L1 and CTLA-4 inhibitors, release the brakes on immune activity, enabling a robust anti-tumor response [24].

Activation of immune responses is another cornerstone, achieved through various means, including cytokine therapy, cancer vaccines, and adoptive cell transfer therapy. These strategies aim to bolster the immune system's ability to recognize and eliminate cancer cells, often with remarkable results. Moreover, personalized medicine has emerged as a guiding principle, recognizing the uniqueness of each patient's cancer and immune profile. Clinicians can optimize therapeutic outcomes while minimizing side effects by tailoring treatments to individual characteristics, such as tumor mutations and immune biomarkers. Combination therapies further enhance efficacy by targeting multiple pathways simultaneously or synergizing with conventional treatments like chemotherapy or radiation therapy [25, 26].

Managing immune-related adverse events (irAEs) has become increasingly important as immunotherapy evolves. While activating the immune system can be beneficial, it can also lead to unintended consequences such as autoimmune reactions. Close monitoring and timely intervention are crucial to mitigate these side effects and ensure patient safety. Furthermore, modulating the tumor microenvironment has emerged as a key strategy. The complex interplay between cancer cells and their surroundings influences immune responses, with some environments promoting tumor growth and immune evasion. Immunotherapies may seek to reshape this landscape, rendering it more conducive to immune cell infiltration and anti-tumor activity. Additionally, fostering long-term immune memory is essential for sustained therapeutic effects. Successful immunotherapy can generate memory T cells capable of recognizing and eliminating residual cancer cells, providing durable protection against recurrence [27, 28].

However, challenges remain, notably the development of resistance mechanisms. Cancer cells are highly adaptable and can evolve strategies to evade immune attack, limiting the effectiveness of immunotherapy over time. Understanding these resistance mechanisms is critical for devising strategies to overcome them, such as combination approaches targeting multiple vulnerabilities simultaneously. Clinical trials are pivotal in advancing the field, offering patients access to innovative therapies and generating data to inform future treatment strategies. By participating in clinical trials, patients contribute to the collective effort to unravel the complexities of cancer immunotherapy and bring new treatments to fruition [29, 30].

TYPES OF CANCER IMMUNOTHERAPY

Cancer immunotherapy encompasses a diverse array of treatment modalities designed to harness the power of the immune system to recognize and eliminate cancer cells. Types of cancer immunotherapy are described below and shown in Fig. (**1**).

Immune Checkpoint Inhibitors

Cancer immunotherapy has revolutionized the treatment of many different types of cancers with the advent of immune checkpoint inhibitors. These inhibitors specifically target molecules on immune cells known as checkpoints, which function as brakes on the immune system's response to cancer. Examples of these molecules include cytotoxic T-lymphocyte-associated protein 4 (CTLA-4), programmed cell death protein 1 (PD-1), and programmed death-ligand 1 (PD-L1) [31].

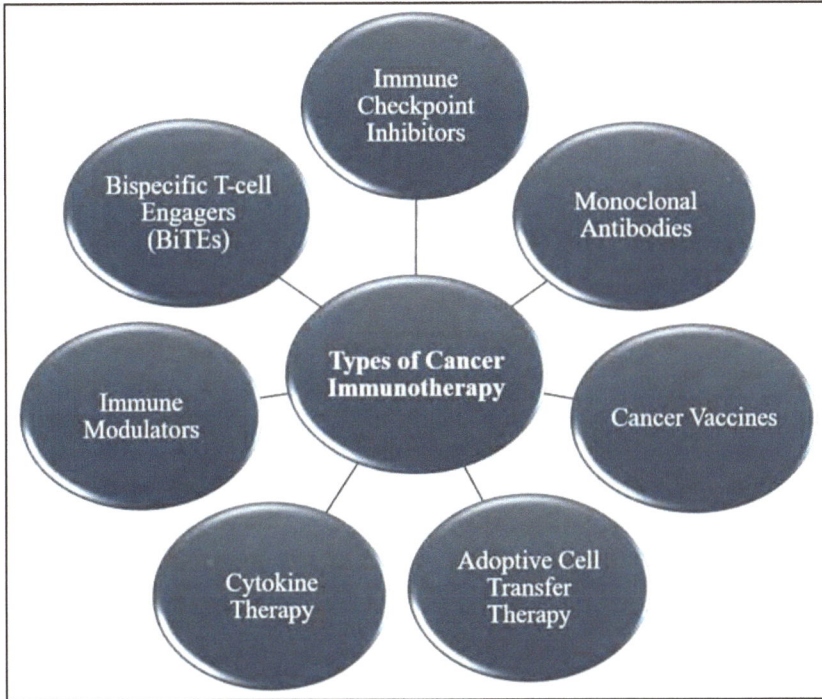

Fig. (1). Types of cancer immunotherapy.

Immune checkpoint inhibitors unlock the immune system's potential to identify and combat cancer cells more successfully by obstructing these checkpoints. Pembrolizumab and nivolumab are PD-1 inhibitors that stop cancer cells from using the PD-1 pathway to avoid immune surveillance. Similarly, to restore anti-tumor immune responses, PD-L1 inhibitors like durvalumab and atezolizumab target the connection between PD-L1 on tumor cells and PD-1 on immune cells. Furthermore, by inhibiting the inhibitory signals produced by CTLA-4, such as ipilimumab, CTLA-4 inhibitors improve T-cell activation and enable a stronger immune response against cancer cells [32].

Among the many cancer types for which these inhibitors have shown extraordinary efficacy are melanoma, lung cancer, renal cell carcinoma, bladder cancer, and Hodgkin's lymphoma. Even when conventional medicines have failed, they have considerably improved survival outcomes and given some patients permanent responses. However, because immune checkpoint inhibitors activate the immune system, they can potentially result in immune-related adverse events (irAEs). These unfavorable events can impact the body's systems and organs, such as the lungs, liver, gastrointestinal tract, skin, and endocrine glands. To protect patient safety and optimize therapeutic benefits, close observation and handling of irAEs are necessary [33, 34].

Immune checkpoint inhibitors have completely changed the way cancer is treated by utilizing the body's own immune system to combat it. Research is still being done to improve these treatments, find predictive biomarkers to help choose the right treatment, and create combination plans to increase their effectiveness in treating a wider range of cancer types and patient demographics.

Monoclonal Antibodies

Monoclonal antibodies (mAbs) have emerged as a cornerstone of cancer immunotherapy, revolutionizing the landscape of cancer treatment by leveraging the immune system's precision to target and attack cancer cells. Engineered in laboratories to mimic the body's natural immune response, these specialized molecules play a multifaceted role in combating cancer. Their mechanism of action is diverse and includes both direct and indirect approaches to eradicate cancer cells while sparing healthy tissue [35].

Mechanisms by which monoclonal antibodies exert their anti-cancer effects are through antibody-dependent cellular cytotoxicity (ADCC). In this process, monoclonal antibodies specifically recognize and bind to antigens on the surface of cancer cells, marking them for destruction by immune cells such as natural killer (NK) cells or macrophages. This immune-mediated killing mechanism enables the selective eradication of cancer cells while minimizing damage to surrounding healthy tissue [36].

Additionally, monoclonal antibodies can induce apoptosis, or programmed cell death, in cancer cells by interfering with critical signaling pathways necessary for survival. For example, trastuzumab, a monoclonal antibody approved for treating HER2-positive breast cancer, targets the HER2/neu receptor, disrupting downstream signaling pathways and inhibiting cancer cell proliferation and survival. Similarly, cetuximab and panitumumab target the epidermal growth factor receptor (EGFR) in colorectal and head and neck cancers, blocking receptor activation and downstream signaling cascades essential for tumor growth and progression [37, 38].

Moreover, monoclonal antibodies can be engineered to deliver cytotoxic agents directly to cancer cells, forming antibody-drug conjugates (ADCs). By conjugating cytotoxic payloads, such as toxins, radioisotopes, or chemotherapy drugs, to monoclonal antibodies, ADCs enable targeted delivery of potent anti-cancer agents specifically to tumor cells. This targeted approach minimizes systemic toxicity and enhances the therapeutic index of cytotoxic agents. Examples of ADCs include brentuximab vedotin, approved for the treatment of Hodgkin lymphoma and anaplastic large cell lymphoma, and trastuzumab emtansine (T-DM1), indicated for HER2-positive breast cancer [39].

Furthermore, monoclonal antibodies can modulate immune responses by targeting immune checkpoints, molecules that regulate the activity of immune cells. For instance, pembrolizumab and nivolumab are monoclonal antibodies that block the programmed cell death protein 1 (PD-1) receptor on T cells, unleashing the immune system's ability to recognize and attack cancer cells. By releasing the brakes on the immune response, these immune checkpoint inhibitors enhance anti-tumor immunity and promote durable responses in patients with various cancer types [24, 40].

Monoclonal antibodies have transformed cancer treatment paradigms, offering targeted precision and improved outcomes for patients across a spectrum of malignancies. They are often used as standalone therapies or combined with other treatment modalities, such as chemotherapy, radiation therapy, or other immunotherapies, to enhance efficacy and improve patient outcomes. However, like all therapeutic interventions, monoclonal antibodies may also be associated with adverse effects, including infusion reactions, immune-related adverse events, or toxicities related to the payload in ADCs [41].

Cancer Vaccines

Cancer vaccines represent an innovative approach to cancer immunotherapy, aiming to harness the immune system's ability to recognize and eliminate cancer cells. Unlike traditional vaccines that prevent infectious diseases by priming the immune system against specific pathogens, cancer vaccines stimulate immune responses against tumor-specific antigens to eradicate or control existing cancer cells. This emerging therapeutic strategy holds significant promise for the prevention, treatment, and potentially the cure of various types of cancer [2, 25, 42].

There are several types of cancer vaccines, each designed to target different aspects of the immune response to cancer. One approach involves using whole tumor cells or cell lysates as the vaccine antigen. These vaccines contain a broad range of tumor antigens, allowing for the activation of multiple immune pathways against cancer. Another strategy employs tumor-associated antigens (TAAs), proteins expressed by cancer cells but not by normal cells or expressed at higher levels in cancer cells. By targeting TAAs, cancer vaccines can specifically stimulate immune responses against cancer cells while sparing healthy tissues [17, 43].

Furthermore, cancer vaccines can comprise recombinant antigens, peptides, or nucleic acids encoding tumor-specific antigens. These vaccines deliver specific antigenic targets to the immune system, inducing targeted immune responses against cancer cells expressing those antigens. Additionally, genetic vaccines, such as DNA or RNA vaccines, deliver genetic material encoding tumor antigens directly into cells, expressing and processing them by the immune system, leading to the generation of immune responses against cancer cells [44].

Several cancer vaccines have shown promising results in clinical trials across various cancer types. Sipuleucel-T, an autologous cellular immunotherapy, was the first cancer vaccine approved by the FDA for the treatment of metastatic castration-resistant prostate cancer. It consists of autologous dendritic cells pulsed with a fusion protein containing prostatic acid phosphatase (PAP), a prostate cancer antigen. Sipuleucel-T stimulates the immune system to recognize and attack prostate cancer cells expressing PAP, improving overall survival in patients with advanced disease [45, 46].

Human papillomavirus (HPV) vaccine prevents infection with high-risk HPV types associated with cervical, anal, and oropharyngeal cancers. By targeting HPV-specific antigens, the vaccine induces robust immune responses that can prevent HPV infection and subsequent development of HPV-associated cancers. The HPV vaccine has demonstrated significant efficacy in reducing the incidence of cervical cancer and other HPV-related malignancies [47].

Additionally, the tumor microenvironment, characterized by immunosuppressive factors and immune evasion mechanisms, can hinder the effectiveness of cancer vaccines. Strategies to overcome these challenges include combination therapies with immune checkpoint inhibitors or other immunomodulatory agents and personalized vaccine approaches tailored to individual patients' tumor profiles. Cancer vaccines hold promise not only as therapeutic agents but also as preventive measures against cancer. Prophylactic vaccines targeting infectious agents linked to cancer, such as the HPV vaccine, have the potential to prevent a significant portion of cancer cases worldwide, highlighting the importance of vaccination in cancer prevention efforts [48, 49].

Adoptive Cell Transfer Therapy

Adoptive cell transfer (ACT) therapy is a promising approach in cancer treatment that involves harnessing the power of a patient's immune cells, typically T cells, to recognize and destroy cancer cells. This innovative immunotherapy has shown remarkable success in treating various types of cancer, including hematologic malignancies and solid tumors, by enhancing the immune system's ability to target and eradicate cancer cells [50].

ACT therapy begins with isolating immune cells, usually T cells, from a patient's blood or tumor tissue. These T cells are then selectively expanded and activated in the laboratory using various techniques, such as cytokine stimulation or genetic engineering, to enhance their anti-tumor activity. One of the most well-known forms of ACT therapy is chimeric antigen receptor (CAR) T-cell therapy. T cells are genetically modified to express synthetic receptors, known as CARs, that specifically recognize and bind to antigens present in cancer cells [51].

CAR T cell therapy has demonstrated remarkable efficacy in treating certain types of blood cancers, particularly B-cell malignancies such as acute lymphoblastic leukemia (ALL), chronic lymphocytic leukemia (CLL), and non-Hodgkin lymphoma (NHL). For example, tisagenlecleucel and axicabtagene ciloleucel, two CAR T cell therapies targeting CD19, have been approved by the FDA for the treatment of relapsed or refractory ALL and certain types of NHL, leading to high rates of complete remission in patients who have exhausted other treatment options [52, 53].

In addition to CAR T cell therapy, another form of ACT therapy is tumor-infiltrating lymphocyte (TIL) therapy. This therapy involves isolating and expanding T cells from tumor tissue that have naturally infiltrated the tumor microenvironment. These TILs are then infused back into the patient, where they can recognize and attack cancer cells more effectively. TIL therapy has shown promising results in melanoma, with durable responses observed in some patients, particularly those with metastatic disease [54].

While ACT therapy has demonstrated significant clinical benefits, challenges, and limitations need to be addressed to maximize its efficacy and applicability in cancer treatment. One disadvantage is the identification of suitable tumor antigens that can be targeted by T cells without causing off-target toxicity to healthy tissues. Advances in tumor antigen discovery and characterization are critical for developing more effective ACT therapies with improved specificity and safety profiles [55, 56].

Another challenge is the hostile tumor microenvironment, characterized by immunosuppressive factors and immune evasion mechanisms that can limit the effectiveness of ACT therapy. Strategies to overcome these challenges include combining ACT therapy with other immunomodulatory agents, such as immune checkpoint inhibitors or cytokines, to enhance the anti-tumor immune response and improve treatment outcomes. Furthermore, the manufacturing process of ACT therapy can be complex and time-consuming, requiring specialized infrastructure and expertise. Streamlining and standardizing the manufacturing process and reducing costs are essential for making ACT therapy more accessible to a broader range of patients [57, 58].

Cytokine Therapy

Cytokine therapy is a form of cancer immunotherapy that utilizes cytokines, small signaling proteins produced by immune cells, to modulate the immune system's response against cancer cells. These powerful molecules play a crucial role in regulating immune cell function, including the activation, proliferation, and differentiation of immune cells involved in anti-tumor immune responses. Cytokine therapy aims to harness the immunostimulatory properties of cytokines to enhance the body's natural ability to recognize and destroy cancer cells [59].

Interleukin-2 (IL-2) is one of the most extensively studied cytokines in cancer therapy and has been approved by the FDA for treating metastatic melanoma and metastatic renal cell carcinoma. IL-2 stimulates the proliferation and activation of T cells and natural killer (NK) cells, key immune system components involved in anti-tumor immunity. High-dose IL-2 therapy can induce durable responses in a subset of patients with advanced cancers, leading to long-term remission in some cases. However, IL-2 therapy is associated with significant toxicities, including capillary leak syndrome, hypotension, and organ dysfunction, limiting its widespread use [60, 61].

Another cytokine used in cancer therapy is interferon-alpha (IFN-α), which exhibits both immunomodulatory and anti-proliferative effects on cancer cells. IFN-α enhances the activity of immune cells, such as NK cells and T cells, and inhibits tumor cell proliferation and angiogenesis. IFN-α has been approved for the treatment of certain types of cancer, including melanoma, hairy cell leukemia, and renal cell carcinoma. However, its use is limited by side effects such as flu-like symptoms, fatigue, and depression [62].

While IL-2 and IFN-α have been the primary cytokines used in cancer therapy, other cytokines are also being investigated for their potential anti-cancer effects. For example, interleukin-12 (IL-12) is a potent immunostimulatory cytokine that promotes the activation and proliferation of T cells and NK cells and enhances the production of interferon-gamma (IFN-γ), a key mediator of anti-tumor immunity. Preclinical studies have shown promising results with IL-12 therapy in various cancer models, leading to ongoing clinical trials to evaluate its safety and efficacy in cancer patients [63, 64].

Cytokine-induced killer (CIK) cell therapy is a form of adoptive cell therapy that utilizes cytokine stimulation to expand and activate cytotoxic T cells with potent anti-tumor activity. CIK cells are generated by culturing peripheral blood mononuclear cells (PBMCs) with a combination of cytokines, such as IL-2, IFN-γ, and anti-CD3 antibodies, to enhance their cytotoxicity against cancer cells. CIK cell therapy has shown promising results in clinical trials for the treatment of solid tumors, including lung cancer, liver cancer, and gastric cancer, with manageable side effects [65].

Despite the promising potential of cytokine therapy in cancer treatment, several challenges and limitations need to be addressed to optimize its efficacy and safety. Strategies to minimize cytokine toxicity include the use of targeted delivery systems, such as liposomes or nanoparticles, to localize cytokine activity to the tumor microenvironment while sparing normal tissues. Another limitation is the development of resistance to cytokine therapy, which can occur due to tumor immune evasion mechanisms or the upregulation of immunosuppressive factors within the tumor microenvironment. Combination therapies with other immunomodulatory agents, such as immune checkpoint inhibitors or targeted therapies, may help overcome resistance and enhance the anti-tumor effects of cytokine therapy [66, 67].

Immune Modulators

Immune modulators are a diverse class of therapeutic agents that modulate the activity of the immune system, either by enhancing or suppressing immune responses, to achieve therapeutic effects in various diseases, including cancer. In cancer treatment, immune modulators enhance the body's natural ability to recognize and eliminate cancer cells while minimizing damage to healthy tissues [68].

Well-known immune modulators is interferon-alpha (IFN-α), a type I interferon that exhibits both immunostimulatory and antiproliferative effects on cancer cells. IFN-α enhances the activity of immune cells, such as natural killer (NK) and T cells, and inhibits tumor cell proliferation and angiogenesis. It has been approved for the treatment of certain types of cancer, including melanoma, hairy cell leukemia, and renal cell carcinoma. However, its use is limited by side effects such as flu-like symptoms, fatigue, and depression. Thalidomide inhibits the production of proinflammatory cytokines, such as tumor necrosis factor-alpha (TNF-α), and enhances the activity of immune cells, including T cells and NK cells. It has been approved for treating multiple myeloma and has shown efficacy in other hematologic malignancies, such as myelodysplastic syndromes and mantle cell lymphoma [69, 70].

Immune modulators can include agents that target immune checkpoint pathways and critical immune response regulators. Immune checkpoint inhibitors, such as antibodies targeting programmed cell death protein 1 (PD-1), programmed death-ligand 1 (PD-L1), and cytotoxic T-lymphocyte-associated protein 4 (CTLA-4), unleash the immune system's ability to recognize and attack cancer cells by blocking inhibitory signals that suppress T cell activity. Immune checkpoint inhibitors have revolutionized cancer treatment, with approvals across various cancer types, including melanoma, lung cancer, and renal cell carcinoma, leading to durable responses and improved survival outcomes in some patients [71, 72].

Toll-like receptor (TLR) agonists are another immune modulator class that stimulates innate immune responses and promotes antitumor immunity. TLR agonists activate immune cells, such as dendritic cells and macrophages, producing proinflammatory cytokines and priming adaptive immune responses against cancer cells. TLR agonists have shown promise in preclinical and clinical studies as monotherapy or in combination with other immunotherapies for the treatment of various cancers, including melanoma, breast cancer, and colorectal cancer [73].

Cytokines, such as interleukin-2 (IL-2) and interleukin-12 (IL-12), are potent immune modulators that stimulate immune cell activation and enhance antitumor immune responses. IL-2 activates T and NK cells, promoting their proliferation and cytotoxic activity against cancer cells. While IL-2 therapy has been approved for the treatment of metastatic melanoma and renal cell carcinoma, its use is limited by significant toxicities. IL-12 stimulates the production of interferon-gamma (IFN-γ) and enhances the cytotoxic activity of T cells and NK cells against cancer cells. Preclinical studies have shown promising results with IL-12 therapy in various cancer models, leading to ongoing clinical trials to evaluate its safety and efficacy in cancer patients [74].

Despite the promise of immune modulators in cancer therapy, challenges remain in optimizing their efficacy and minimizing toxicity. Strategies to overcome these challenges include the development of targeted delivery systems to localize immune modulator activity to the tumor microenvironment, the identification of predictive biomarkers to select patients who are most likely to benefit from treatment, and the exploration of combination therapies to enhance synergistic effects and overcome resistance mechanisms [75].

Bispecific T-cell Engagers (BiTEs)

Bispecific T-cell engagers (BiTEs) represent a groundbreaking class of immunotherapeutic agents designed to redirect a patient's immune cells, particularly T cells, to recognize and eliminate cancer cells. These engineered molecules can simultaneously bind to a T cell and a tumor cell, bringing them into close proximity and facilitating the formation of an immunological synapse, which triggers T cell activation and the subsequent destruction of cancer cells [76].

BiTEs comprise two single-chain antibody fragments, each targeting a distinct antigen: one binds to a surface protein expressed on T cells, typically CD3, while the other binds to an antigen specifically expressed on tumor cells. By bridging T cells and tumor cells, BiTEs activate T cells and induce their cytotoxic activity against cancer cells, releasing cytotoxic granules containing perforin and granzyme B, which mediate tumor cell lysis [77].

BiTEs is blinatumomab, which the FDA has approved for treating relapsed or refractory B-cell precursor Acute Lymphoblastic Leukemia (ALL) in adults and children. Blinatumomab targets CD19, a protein expressed on the surface of B-cell malignancies, and CD3, a component of the T-cell receptor complex. By engaging both CD19-positive B cells and CD3-positive T cells, blinatumomab activates T cells to selectively eliminate CD19-expressing leukemia cells, leading to high complete remission rates in patients with relapsed or refractory ALL [78, 79].

Blinatumomab and several other BiTEs targeting different antigens and cancers are under development and in clinical trials. For example, mosunetuzumab is a BiTE targeting CD3 and CD20, currently being investigated for treating non-Hodgkin lymphoma. Similarly, glofitamab is a BiTE targeting CD3 and CD20, showing promising results in relapsed or refractory B-cell non-Hodgkin lymphoma. BiTE therapy offers several advantages over traditional cancer treatments. Firstly, BiTEs have the potential to induce rapid and potent anti-tumor immune responses, leading to durable responses in some patients. BiTEs are highly specific for tumor cells, minimizing off-target toxicity to healthy tissues and reducing the risk of adverse effects associated with traditional chemotherapy [80, 81].

Additionally, BiTE therapy can overcome immune evasion mechanisms employed by cancer cells, such as downregulation of major histocompatibility complex (MHC) molecules or expression of immune checkpoint proteins, by directly engaging T cells and bypassing the need for antigen presentation by antigen-presenting cells. Despite these advantages, BiTE therapy has limitations and challenges that must be addressed. One challenge is the potential for cytokine release syndrome (CRS), a systemic inflammatory response resulting from the activation and proliferation of T cells, which can lead to symptoms ranging from fever and fatigue to life-threatening complications such as hypotension and multiorgan failure. Strategies to mitigate CRS include dose optimization, prophylactic treatment with corticosteroids, and close monitoring of patients during treatment [82, 83].

Another challenge is the development of resistance to BiTE therapy, which can occur due to various mechanisms, including antigen loss or downregulation, T cell exhaustion, or immune evasion by cancer cells. Combination therapies with other immunomodulatory agents, such as immune checkpoint inhibitors or cytokines, may help overcome resistance and enhance the efficacy of BiTE therapy [84].

MECHANISM OF ACTION OF MUCOSAL VACCINES IN CANCER IMMUNOTHERAPY

Mucosal vaccines represent a promising avenue in cancer immunotherapy, offering a unique mechanism of action that leverages the body's mucosal immune system to induce potent and durable anti-tumor responses. These vaccines are designed to be administered *via* mucosal routes, such as the oral, nasal, or intranasal routes, targeting mucosal-associated lymphoid tissues (MALT) and eliciting mucosal immune responses that can lead to systemic immunity against cancer [85].

The mechanism of action of mucosal vaccines in cancer immunotherapy involves various steps, which are shown in Fig. (2) and described below.

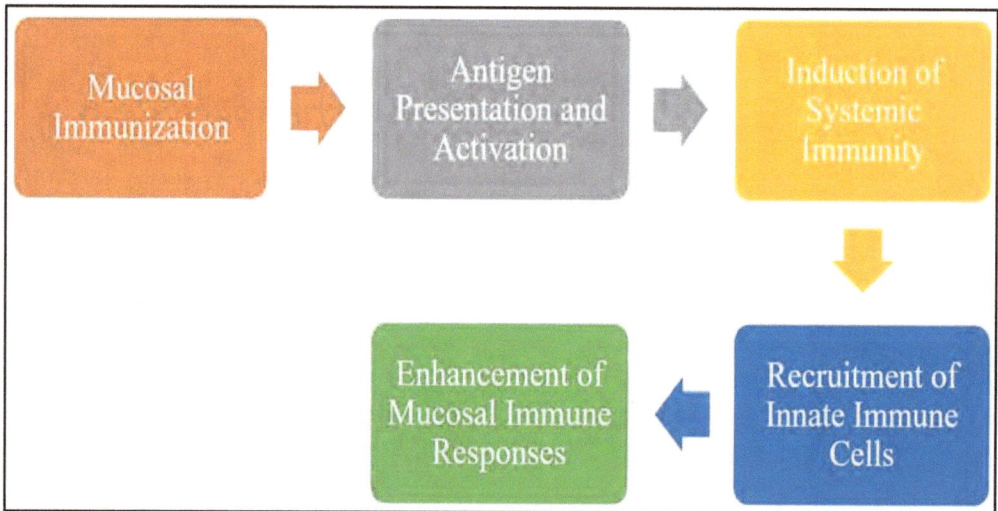

Fig. (2). Mechanism of action of mucosal vaccines in cancer immunotherapy.

Mucosal Immunization

Mucosal vaccines are administered *via* mucosal routes, allowing antigens to encounter specialized immune cells present in the mucosal-associated lymphoid tissues (MALT), such as Peyer's patches in the intestine or nasal-associated lymphoid tissue (NALT) in the nasal cavity. These immune cells, including dendritic cells, macrophages, and M cells, sample antigens and initiate immune responses locally [86].

Antigen Presentation and Activation

Antigen-presenting cells (APCs), such as dendritic cells, capture and process tumor antigens presented by mucosal vaccines. These APCs migrate to regional lymph nodes, presenting tumor antigens to T cells, which are then activated and differentiated into effector T cells, including cytotoxic T cells (CTLs) and helper T cells [87].

Induction of Systemic Immunity

Activated T cells traffic from the draining lymph nodes to systemic sites, where they recognize and eliminate cancer cells expressing the same antigens encountered at the mucosal site. This systemic immune response generates memory T cells capable of providing long-lasting protection against tumor recurrence or metastasis [88].

Recruitment of Innate Immune Cells

Mucosal vaccines can also recruit and activate innate immune cells, such as natural killer (NK) cells and macrophages, which play crucial roles in tumor surveillance and elimination. NK cells can directly kill cancer cells without prior sensitization and can be activated by cytokines produced in response to mucosal vaccination [89].

Enhancement of Mucosal Immune Responses

In addition to systemic immunity, mucosal vaccines can stimulate mucosal immune responses at the administration site, providing additional protection against tumor invasion at mucosal surfaces. These local immune responses may include the production of secretory IgA antibodies, which can neutralize tumor antigens and prevent tumor dissemination [90].

Overall, mucosal vaccines' mechanism of action in cancer immunotherapy involves the induction of both systemic and mucosal immune responses against tumor antigens, leading to the activation of effector T cells and the generation of long-lasting immune memory. By exploiting the body's mucosal immune system, mucosal vaccines offer a promising strategy for preventing and treating cancer, potentially providing broader protection against tumor recurrence and metastasis. Ongoing research aims to optimize mucosal vaccine formulations, delivery strategies, and antigen selection to enhance their efficacy and applicability in cancer immunotherapy.

ADVANTAGES OF MUCOSAL VACCINATION IN CANCER TREATMENT

Mucosal vaccination presents a multifaceted array of advantages that make it an intriguing and promising avenue for cancer treatment. By exploiting the unique properties of mucosal surfaces and the associated lymphoid tissues, mucosal vaccines offer a distinct mechanism of action that can effectively harness the body's immune system to combat cancer. The advantages of mucosal vaccination in cancer treatment are summarized in Fig. (**3**) and described below.

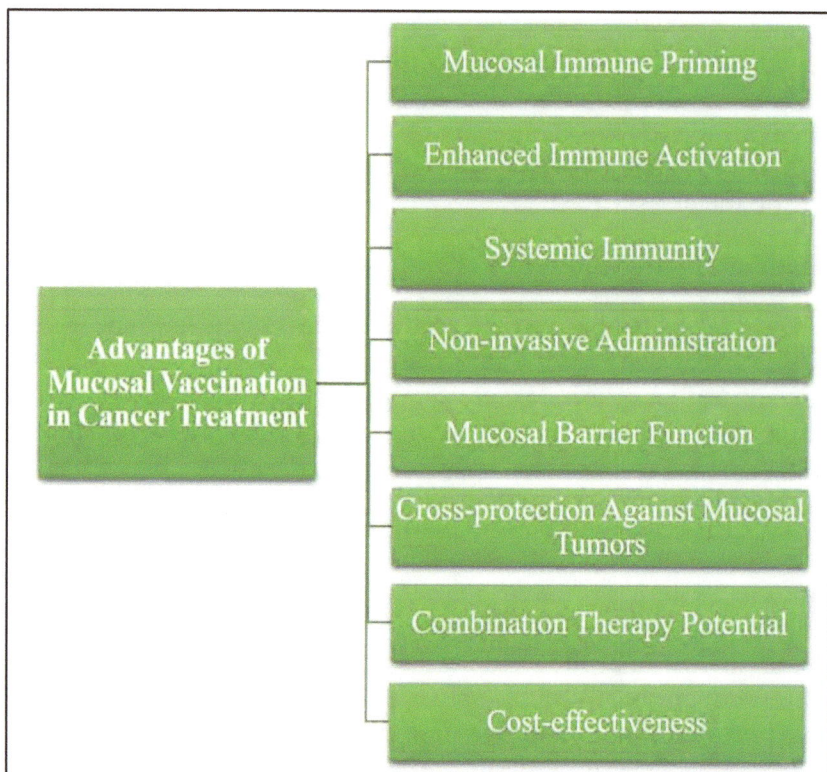

Fig. (3). Advantages of mucosal vaccination in cancer treatment.

Mucosal vaccination takes advantage of the proximity of mucosal-associated lymphoid tissues (MALT) to potential tumor development or metastasis sites. By delivering antigens directly to these mucosal sites, mucosal vaccines prime local immune responses against cancer cells, effectively establishing an initial line of defense against tumor invasion and dissemination. This localized immune priming may lead to faster and more efficient recognition and elimination of cancer cells [91].

The mucosal route of administration allows antigens to interact directly with specialized immune cells present in MALT, including dendritic cells, macrophages, and M cells. These cells efficiently capture, process, and present antigens to T cells, leading to robust immune activation and the generation of tumor-specific immune responses. Compared to systemic administration routes, mucosal vaccination can induce more potent and sustained immune responses due to the high density of immune cells in mucosal tissues [92].

In addition to local immune responses, mucosal vaccination can induce systemic immunity against cancer. Activated T cells, including cytotoxic T lymphocytes (CTLs), migrate from mucosal lymphoid tissues to systemic sites, infiltrating tumors and recognizing and eliminating cancer cells expressing the same antigens encountered at the mucosal site. This systemic immune response provides long-lasting protection against tumor recurrence or metastasis, extending the therapeutic benefit of mucosal vaccination beyond the initial site of administration [93, 94].

Mucosal vaccination offers a non-invasive and patient-friendly route of administration, which may improve patient compliance and acceptability compared to traditional injection-based vaccines. Oral, nasal, or intranasal delivery routes are generally well-tolerated and can be easily administered without needing needles or medical personnel. This ease of administration may enhance accessibility to cancer immunotherapy and reduce barriers to treatment initiation and adherence [95].

Mucosal surfaces serve as physical barriers against pathogens and toxins and play a crucial role in inducing mucosal immune responses. By delivering antigens directly to mucosal sites, mucosal vaccines can overcome mucosal tolerance mechanisms and enhance immune responses against cancer cells. The mucosal barrier function also helps retain antigens at the administration site, prolonging exposure to immune cells and enhancing vaccine efficacy [96].

Mucosal vaccination may provide cross-protection against mucosal tumors at different anatomical sites. For example, a mucosal vaccine targeting oral cancer antigens may induce immune responses that also confer protection against nasopharyngeal or esophageal cancers, which share common antigens or pathways. This broad-spectrum protection against mucosal tumors could significantly enhance the clinical utility of mucosal vaccines in cancer immunotherapy [97].

Mucosal vaccination can be easily combined with other cancer therapies, such as chemotherapy, radiation therapy, or immune checkpoint inhibitors, to enhance treatment outcomes. The localized immune activation induced by mucosal vaccines may synergize with systemic therapies, leading to improved anti-tumor effects and potentially reducing the risk of tumor recurrence. Furthermore, combining mucosal vaccines with other immunotherapeutic agents may overcome resistance mechanisms and enhance overall treatment efficacy [98].

Mucosal vaccination may offer cost advantages compared to traditional cancer treatments, particularly in resource-limited settings. The simplicity of administration and the potential for improved patient compliance may lead to reduced healthcare costs associated with cancer management. Additionally, mucosal vaccines can potentially reduce the need for invasive procedures and hospitalizations, further contributing to cost savings in cancer care [99].

Mucosal vaccination presents a comprehensive array of cancer treatment advantages, from enhanced immune activation and systemic immunity to non-invasive administration and cost-effectiveness. These advantages underscore the potential of mucosal vaccines as a promising approach in cancer immunotherapy, offering new opportunities for improving patient outcomes and reducing the burden of cancer worldwide. As research in this field advances, mucosal vaccination holds great promise for revolutionizing cancer treatment paradigms and improving the lives of patients affected by this devastating disease [100].

APPLICATIONS OF MUCOSAL VACCINATION IN CANCER TREATMENT

Mucosal vaccination, an innovative approach to cancer treatment, demonstrates versatile applications across various stages of cancer management. By leveraging the body's mucosal immune system, these vaccines offer unique advantages that hold promise in both prevention and treatment strategies against cancer. At the forefront of cancer prevention, mucosal vaccines have shown remarkable success in combating virally induced cancers, particularly those associated with human papillomavirus (HPV) and hepatitis B virus (HBV). Through oral or intranasal administration, mucosal vaccines induce robust immune responses at mucosal-associated lymphoid tissues (MALT), effectively preventing persistent viral infections and reducing the risk of HPV-related cervical, anal, and oropharyngeal cancers, as well as HBV-related liver cancer [101, 102].

Mucosal vaccination serves as a pivotal tool in therapeutic cancer vaccines, offering hope for the treatment of established cancers. These vaccines deliver tumor antigens directly to MALT, activating cytotoxic T lymphocytes (CTLs) and other effector cells to recognize and eliminate cancer cells. By targeting specific tumor antigens or tumor-associated antigens, mucosal vaccines stimulate mucosal and systemic immune responses against tumors, potentially leading to improved treatment outcomes. The localized immune activation induced by mucosal vaccines *via* intranasal or oral delivery routes enhances the induction of mucosal and systemic immune responses against tumors, thus holding promise for enhancing treatment efficacy [103, 104].

Mucosal vaccination presents a compelling adjunctive therapy option when combined with conventional cancer treatments, such as surgery, chemotherapy, or radiation therapy. By stimulating immune responses against residual tumor cells or micrometastases, mucosal vaccines may augment the efficacy of conventional therapies and mitigate the risk of tumor recurrence or metastasis. The synergistic effect between mucosal vaccines and systemic treatments can amplify anti-tumor effects, resulting in prolonged survival and improved clinical outcomes for cancer patients [105].

Mucosal vaccination holds particular relevance in treating mucosal tumors, which often present unique challenges due to their anatomical location and proximity to critical structures. Head, neck, lung, and gastrointestinal cancers are examples of malignancies arising from mucosal surfaces, making them suitable targets for mucosal vaccination strategies. By delivering vaccines directly to the tumor site, mucosal vaccines can elicit local immune responses against cancer cells, complementing standard treatments such as surgical resection or local radiotherapy. Additionally, the potential for cross-protection against mucosal tumors at different anatomical sites expands the therapeutic scope of mucosal vaccination, offering a promising avenue for addressing the heterogeneity of mucosal cancers [106, 107].

Mucosal vaccination holds potential as an immunotherapeutic approach for targeting minimal residual disease (MRD) in cancer patients. After primary treatment modalities, such as surgery or chemotherapy, residual tumor cells may persist in the body and contribute to disease relapse. Mucosal vaccines administered post-treatment can activate immune responses against MRD, effectively eliminating residual cancer cells and reducing the risk of disease recurrence. This proactive approach to immunotherapy may prove particularly beneficial in cancers with a high risk of relapse, such as breast cancer or melanoma [108].

Beyond active cancer treatment, mucosal vaccination plays a crucial role in cancer survivorship by enhancing long-term immune surveillance against cancer recurrence or secondary malignancies. Vaccines administered *via* mucosal routes bolster immune memory against tumor antigens, providing sustained protection against cancer relapse. Additionally, mucosal vaccines may mitigate the risk of secondary cancers associated with certain cancer treatments, such as radiation therapy or chemotherapy, by reinforcing immune responses against precancerous cells or residual tumor cells. This comprehensive approach to cancer survivorship underscores the potential of mucosal vaccination in promoting long-term health and well-being among cancer survivors [109, 110].

Mucosal vaccination represents a promising and versatile strategy in cancer treatment, offering multifaceted applications across the cancer care continuum. From prevention to adjuvant therapy, treatment of mucosal tumors, and immunotherapy for minimal residual disease, mucosal vaccination holds great potential for improving patient outcomes and reducing the burden of cancer worldwide. Continued research and development in this field are essential to unlock the full therapeutic potential of mucosal vaccination and advance the standard of care for patients with cancer [111].

CHALLENGES AND LIMITATIONS

Mucosal vaccination in cancer treatment faces several challenges and limitations that must be addressed to optimize immunogenicity, efficacy, and regulatory approval processes. One of the primary challenges is optimizing the immunogenicity of mucosal vaccines to induce robust and durable immune responses against cancer cells. Mucosal surfaces are inherently tolerogenic, making it challenging to stimulate strong immune responses without potent adjuvants or immunostimulatory agents. Additionally, the efficacy of mucosal vaccines may be compromised by factors such as antigen degradation, inefficient antigen uptake by mucosal immune cells, and the presence of immunosuppressive factors in the mucosal microenvironment. Strategies to enhance immunogenicity and efficacy include the incorporation of novel adjuvants, formulation optimization to improve antigen stability and delivery, and using antigen antigen-targeting strategies to enhance antigen presentation and immune activation [112].

A significant challenge in mucosal vaccination for cancer treatment is the selection of optimal target antigens. Identifying tumor-specific or tumor-associated antigens that are highly immunogenic and broadly expressed across different cancer types poses a significant hurdle. Furthermore, tumor heterogeneity and immune escape mechanisms may limit the effectiveness of vaccines targeting a single antigen. To overcome these challenges, researchers are exploring strategies such as the use of neoantigens derived from tumor-specific mutations, tumor-associated antigens with shared expression patterns across cancer types, and combinatorial approaches targeting multiple antigens or immune pathways to enhance vaccine efficacy and broaden the immune response [113].

Formulation and delivery considerations present additional challenges in developing mucosal vaccines for cancer treatment. Formulating vaccines for mucosal delivery requires consideration of factors such as antigen stability, mucosal adhesion, and mucosal penetration. Ensuring optimal vaccine formulation and delivery vehicles that protect antigens from degradation while promoting efficient uptake by mucosal immune cells is critical for vaccine efficacy. Furthermore, selecting appropriate delivery routes, such as oral, nasal, or intranasal administration, requires careful consideration of mucosal anatomy, immune physiology, and patient acceptability to maximize vaccine delivery and immune response induction [114].

Regulatory hurdles and approval processes present significant barriers to translating mucosal vaccines from preclinical studies to clinical use. Regulatory agencies require robust preclinical data demonstrating safety, efficacy, and immunogenicity before initiating clinical trials. Additionally, the unique challenges of mucosal vaccines, such as variability in mucosal immune responses and potential mucosal toxicity, require specific regulatory considerations. Navigating the regulatory landscape for mucosal vaccines in cancer treatment requires close collaboration between researchers, industry partners, and regulatory agencies to ensure compliance with regulatory standards and streamline the approval process [115].

FUTURE DIRECTIONS AND TRENDS

The future of mucosal vaccination in cancer treatment holds tremendous promise, with several exciting directions and emerging trends shaping the landscape of cancer immunotherapy. Next-generation mucosal vaccine platforms represent a key area of focus, with researchers exploring novel vaccine formulations and delivery systems to enhance the efficacy and versatility of mucosal vaccines. These platforms may include innovative adjuvants, nanoparticle-based carriers, and mucosal targeting strategies designed to optimize antigen presentation and immune activation at mucosal sites. By leveraging advancements in vaccine technology, next-generation mucosal vaccines hold the potential to overcome existing limitations and unlock new opportunities for cancer prevention and treatment [116].

Furthermore, combination therapies involving mucosal vaccines are emerging as a promising approach to enhance treatment outcomes in cancer patients. By integrating mucosal vaccines with other immunotherapeutic agents, such as immune checkpoint inhibitors, cytokines, or adoptive cell transfer therapies, researchers aim to synergize immune responses and overcome resistance mechanisms to achieve stronger and more durable anti-tumor effects. Combination therapies with mucosal vaccines may also involve the co-administration of conventional cancer treatments, such as chemotherapy or radiation therapy, to maximize the therapeutic benefit and improve patient outcomes [117].

Personalized vaccine approaches represent another important future direction in mucosal vaccination for cancer treatment. By tailoring vaccine formulations and target antigens to individual patients based on their unique tumor characteristics, genetic makeup, and immune profiles, personalized vaccines hold the potential to enhance treatment efficacy and minimize off-target effects. Advances in high-throughput sequencing, bioinformatics, and immunogenomics facilitate the identification of personalized vaccine targets and the development of customized vaccine regimens tailored to each patient's specific needs [118].

Integration with emerging technologies, such as nanotechnology, is poised to revolutionize the field of mucosal vaccination and further expand its therapeutic potential in cancer treatment. Nanoparticle-based vaccine carriers offer unique advantages, including enhanced antigen delivery, controlled release kinetics, and improved mucosal penetration, which can significantly enhance vaccine efficacy and immune responses. Additionally, nanotechnology enables the design of multifunctional vaccine platforms capable of incorporating adjuvants, targeting ligands, and imaging agents for real-time monitoring of vaccine distribution and immune responses. Integration with emerging technologies holds promise for overcoming existing challenges in mucosal vaccination and accelerating the translation of innovative vaccine concepts into clinical practice [119].

CONCLUSION

In conclusion, the future of mucosal vaccination in cancer treatment holds immense promise, driven by innovative approaches and emerging trends reshaping the landscape of cancer immunotherapy. Next-generation mucosal vaccine platforms, incorporating novel adjuvants, nanoparticle-based carriers, and mucosal targeting strategies, offer exciting opportunities to enhance vaccine efficacy and versatility. These advancements hold the potential to overcome existing limitations and unlock new avenues for cancer prevention and treatment. Furthermore, integrating mucosal vaccines with combination therapies, personalized vaccine approaches, and emerging technologies such as nanotechnology holds great potential to revolutionize cancer treatment by synergizing immune responses, tailoring treatments to individual patients, and leveraging cutting-edge delivery systems by capitalizing on these opportunities and addressing remaining challenges, including immunogenicity optimization, target antigen selection, formulation considerations, and regulatory hurdles, mucosal vaccination stands poised to play a transformative role in the prevention, treatment, and management of cancer. Ultimately, continued research efforts, multidisciplinary collaboration, and investment in mucosal vaccine development are essential to realize the full therapeutic potential of this innovative approach in cancer immunotherapy. With dedication and innovation, mucosal vaccination offers new hope for patients and clinicians in the ongoing fight against cancer, paving the way for a future where effective and personalized cancer treatments are within reach.

ACKNOWLEDGEMENTS

Authors are highly thankful to their Universities/Colleges for providing library facilities for the literature survey.

REFERENCES

[1]   Ionna F, Bossi P, Guida A, *et al.* Recurrent/metastatic squamous cell carcinoma of the head and neck: a big and intriguing challenge which may be resolved by integrated treatments combining locoregional and systemic therapies. Cancers (Basel) 2021; 13(10): 2371.
[http://dx.doi.org/10.3390/cancers13102371] [PMID: 34069092]

[2]   Gao S, Yang X, Xu J, Qiu N, Zhai G. Nanotechnology for boosting cancer immunotherapy and remodeling tumor microenvironment: the horizons in cancer treatment. ACS Nano 2021; 15(8): 12567-603.
[http://dx.doi.org/10.1021/acsnano.1c02103] [PMID: 34339170]

[3]   Bondhopadhyay B, Sisodiya S, Chikara A, *et al.* Cancer immunotherapy: a promising dawn in cancer research. Am J Blood Res 2020; 10(6): 375-85.
[PMID: 33489447]

[4]   Dhar R, Seethy A, Singh S, *et al.* Cancer immunotherapy. J Cancer Res Ther 2021; 17(4): 834-44.
[http://dx.doi.org/10.4103/jcrt.JCRT_1241_20] [PMID: 34528529]

[5]   Zhang Y, Zhang Z. The history and advances in cancer immunotherapy: understanding the characteristics of tumor-infiltrating immune cells and their therapeutic implications. Cell Mol Immunol 2020; 17(8): 807-21.
[http://dx.doi.org/10.1038/s41423-020-0488-6] [PMID: 32612154]

[6]   Wu Z, Li S, Zhu X. The mechanism of stimulating and mobilizing the immune system enhances anti-tumor immunity. Front Immunol 2021; 12: 682435.
[http://dx.doi.org/10.3389/fimmu.2021.682435] [PMID: 34194437]

[7]   Lavelle EC, Ward RW. Mucosal vaccines — fortifying the frontiers. Nat Rev Immunol 2022; 22(4): 236-50.
[http://dx.doi.org/10.1038/s41577-021-00583-2] [PMID: 34312520]

[8]   Yadav DK, Yadav N, Khurana SM. Vaccines: present status and applications. In Animal

biotechnology, 2020; pp. 523-542.
[http://dx.doi.org/10.1016/B978-0-12-811710-1.00024-0]

[9]   Bashiri S, Koirala P, Toth I, Skwarczynski M. Carbohydrate immune adjuvants in subunit vaccines. Pharmaceutics 2020; 12(10): 965.
[http://dx.doi.org/10.3390/pharmaceutics12100965] [PMID: 33066594]

[10]   Mempel TR, Lill JK, Altenburger LM. How chemokines organize the tumour microenvironment. Nat Rev Cancer 2024; 24(1): 28-50.
[http://dx.doi.org/10.1038/s41568-023-00635-w] [PMID: 38066335]

[11]   Kumar AR, Devan AR, Nair B, Vinod BS, Nath LR. Harnessing the immune system against cancer: current immunotherapy approaches and therapeutic targets. Mol Biol Rep 2021; 48(12): 8075-95.
[http://dx.doi.org/10.1007/s11033-021-06752-9] [PMID: 34671902]

[12]   Hedaya MA. Routes of Drug Administration. InPharmaceutics. 2024; pp. 537-554.
[http://dx.doi.org/10.1016/B978-0-323-99796-6.00006-0]

[13]   Rubel MZU, Ichii O, Namba T, *et al.* Systemic autoimmune abnormalities alter the morphology of mucosa-associated lymphoid tissues in the rectum of MRL/MpJ-*Fas^{lpr/lpr}* mice. Exp Anim 2024; 73(3): 270-85.
[http://dx.doi.org/10.1538/expanim.23-0129] [PMID: 38311397]

[14]   Li M, Wang Y, Sun Y, Cui H, Zhu SJ, Qiu HJ. Mucosal vaccines: Strategies and challenges. Immunol Lett 2020; 217: 116-25.
[http://dx.doi.org/10.1016/j.imlet.2019.10.013] [PMID: 31669546]

[15]   Correa VA, Portilho AI, De Gaspari E. Vaccines, adjuvants and key factors for mucosal immune response. Immunology 2022; 167(2): 124-38.
[http://dx.doi.org/10.1111/imm.13526] [PMID: 35751397]

[16]   Dewangan HK. Rational application of nanoadjuvant for mucosal vaccine delivery system. J Immunol Methods 2020; 481-482: 112791.
[http://dx.doi.org/10.1016/j.jim.2020.112791] [PMID: 32387695]

[17]   Wang QT, Nie Y, Sun SN, *et al.* Tumor-associated antigen-based personalized dendritic cell vaccine in solid tumor patients. Cancer Immunol Immunother 2020; 69(7): 1375-87.
[http://dx.doi.org/10.1007/s00262-020-02496-w] [PMID: 32078016]

[18]   Teng Z, Meng LY, Yang JK, He Z, Chen XG, Liu Y. Bridging nanoplatform and vaccine delivery, a landscape of strategy to enhance nasal immunity. J Control Release 2022; 351: 456-75.
[http://dx.doi.org/10.1016/j.jconrel.2022.09.044] [PMID: 36174803]

[19]   Tsai CJY, Loh JMS, Fujihashi K, Kiyono H. Mucosal vaccination: onward and upward. Expert Rev Vaccines 2023; 22(1): 885-99.
[http://dx.doi.org/10.1080/14760584.2023.2268724] [PMID: 37817433]

[20]   Mudgal R, Nehul S, Tomar S. Prospects for mucosal vaccine: shutting the door on SARS-CoV-2. Hum Vaccin Immunother 2020; 16(12): 2921-31.
[http://dx.doi.org/10.1080/21645515.2020.1805992] [PMID: 32931361]

[21]   Niemi JVL, Sokolov AV, Schiöth HB. Neoantigen vaccines; clinical trials, classes, indications, adjuvants, and combinatorial treatments. Cancers (Basel) 2022; 14(20): 5163.
[http://dx.doi.org/10.3390/cancers14205163] [PMID: 36291947]

[22]   Heuler J, Chandra H, Sun X. Mucosal Vaccination Strategies against *Clostridioides difficile* Infection. Vaccines (Basel) 2023; 11(5): 887.
[http://dx.doi.org/10.3390/vaccines11050887] [PMID: 37242991]

[23]   Vermaelen K. Vaccine strategies to improve anti-cancer cellular immune responses. Front Immunol 2019; 10: 8.
[http://dx.doi.org/10.3389/fimmu.2019.00008] [PMID: 30723469]

[24]   Parvez A, Choudhary F, Mudgal P, *et al.* PD-1 and PD-L1: architects of immune symphony and immunotherapy breakthroughs in cancer treatment. Front Immunol 2023; 14: 1296341.
[http://dx.doi.org/10.3389/fimmu.2023.1296341] [PMID: 38106415]

[25]   Le I, Dhandayuthapani S, Chacon J, Eiring AM, Gadad SS. Harnessing the immune system with cancer vaccines: From prevention to therapeutics. Vaccines (Basel) 2022; 10(5): 816.
[http://dx.doi.org/10.3390/vaccines10050816] [PMID: 35632572]

[26]   Wang RC, Wang Z. Precision medicine: Disease subtyping and tailored treatment. Cancers (Basel) 2023; 15(15): 3837.
[http://dx.doi.org/10.3390/cancers15153837] [PMID: 37568653]

[27]   Ramos-Casals M, Brahmer JR, Callahan MK, *et al.* Immune-related adverse events of checkpoint inhibitors. Nat Rev Dis Primers 2020; 6(1): 38.
[http://dx.doi.org/10.1038/s41572-020-0160-6] [PMID: 32382051]

[28]   Liu L, Liu Z, Gao J, *et al.* CD8+ T cell trajectory subtypes decode tumor heterogeneity and provide treatment recommendations for hepatocellular carcinoma. Front Immunol 2022; 13: 964190.
[http://dx.doi.org/10.3389/fimmu.2022.964190] [PMID: 35967384]

[29]   Gondhowiardjo SA, Handoko , Jayalie VF, *et al.* Tackling Resistance to Cancer Immunotherapy: What Do We Know? Molecules 2020; 25(18): 4096.
[http://dx.doi.org/10.3390/molecules25184096] [PMID: 32911646]

[30]   Mateo J, Steuten L, Aftimos P, *et al.* Delivering precision oncology to patients with cancer. Nat Med 2022; 28(4): 658-65.
[http://dx.doi.org/10.1038/s41591-022-01717-2] [PMID: 35440717]

[31]   Shiravand Y, Khodadadi F, Kashani SMA, *et al.* Immune checkpoint inhibitors in cancer therapy. Curr Oncol 2022; 29(5): 3044-60.
[http://dx.doi.org/10.3390/curroncol29050247] [PMID: 35621637]

[32]   Goleva E, Lyubchenko T, Kraehenbuehl L, Lacouture ME, Leung DYM, Kern JA. Our current understanding of checkpoint inhibitor therapy in cancer immunotherapy. Ann Allergy Asthma Immunol 2021; 126(6): 630-8.
[http://dx.doi.org/10.1016/j.anai.2021.03.003] [PMID: 33716146]

[33]   Zam W, Ali L. Immune checkpoint inhibitors in the treatment of cancer. Curr Rev Clin Exp Pharmacol 2022; 17(2): 103-13.
[http://dx.doi.org/10.2174/27724336MTE1eMDQh5] [PMID: 33823768]

[34]   Gupta PK, Gupta PK. Target organ toxicity. Problem-Solving Questions in Toxicology: A Study Guide for the Board and Other Examinations. 2020:83-117.

[35]   Brito JS. Cancer immunotherapy (doctoral dissertation, universidade de Coimbra).

[36]   Raskov H, Orhan A, Salanti A, Gaggar S, Gögenur I. Natural killer cells in cancer and cancer immunotherapy. Cancer Lett 2021; 520: 233-42.
[http://dx.doi.org/10.1016/j.canlet.2021.07.032] [PMID: 34302920]

[37]   Han Y, Liu D, Li L. PD-1/PD-L1 pathway: current researches in cancer. Am J Cancer Res 2020; 10(3): 727-42.
[PMID: 32266087]

[38]   Swain SM, Shastry M, Hamilton E. Targeting HER2-positive breast cancer: advances and future directions. Nat Rev Drug Discov 2023; 22(2): 101-26.
[http://dx.doi.org/10.1038/s41573-022-00579-0] [PMID: 36344672]

[39]   Marei HE, Cenciarelli C, Hasan A. Potential of antibody–drug conjugates (ADCs) for cancer therapy. Cancer Cell Int 2022; 22(1): 255.
[http://dx.doi.org/10.1186/s12935-022-02679-8] [PMID: 35964048]

[40]   Ishida Y. PD-1: its discovery, involvement in cancer immunotherapy, and beyond. Cells 2020; 9(6):

1376.
[http://dx.doi.org/10.3390/cells9061376] [PMID: 32492969]

[41]   Barbari C, Fontaine T, Parajuli P, *et al.* Immunotherapies and combination strategies for immuno-oncology. Int J Mol Sci 2020; 21(14): 5009.
[http://dx.doi.org/10.3390/ijms21145009] [PMID: 32679922]

[42]   Liu D, Che X, Wang X, Ma C, Wu G. tumor vaccines: Unleashing the power of the immune system to fight cancer. Pharmaceuticals (Basel) 2023; 16(10): 1384.
[http://dx.doi.org/10.3390/ph16101384] [PMID: 37895855]

[43]   Srivastava AK, Guadagnin G, Cappello P, Novelli F. Post-translational modifications in tumor-associated antigens as a platform for novel immuno-oncology therapies. Cancers (Basel) 2022; 15(1): 138.
[http://dx.doi.org/10.3390/cancers15010138] [PMID: 36612133]

[44]   Saxena M, van der Burg SH, Melief CJM, Bhardwaj N. Therapeutic cancer vaccines. Nat Rev Cancer 2021; 21(6): 360-78.
[http://dx.doi.org/10.1038/s41568-021-00346-0] [PMID: 33907315]

[45]   Sutherland SIM, Ju X, Horvath LG, Clark GJ. Moving on from sipuleucel-T: new dendritic cell vaccine strategies for prostate cancer. Front Immunol 2021; 12: 641307.
[http://dx.doi.org/10.3389/fimmu.2021.641307] [PMID: 33854509]

[46]   Wang I, Song L, Wang BY, Rezazadeh Kalebasty A, Uchio E, Zi X. Prostate cancer immunotherapy: a review of recent advancements with novel treatment methods and efficacy. Am J Clin Exp Urol 2022; 10(4): 210-33.
[PMID: 36051616]

[47]   Medeiros R, Vaz S, Rebelo T, Figueiredo-Dias M. Prevention of human papillomavirus infection. Beyond cervical cancer: a brief review. Acta Med Port 2020; 33(3): 198-201.
[http://dx.doi.org/10.20344/amp.12259] [PMID: 32130098]

[48]   Kim SK, Cho SW. The evasion mechanisms of cancer immunity and drug intervention in the tumor microenvironment. Front Pharmacol 2022; 13: 868695.
[http://dx.doi.org/10.3389/fphar.2022.868695] [PMID: 35685630]

[49]   Garbuglia AR, Lapa D, Sias C, Capobianchi MR, Del Porto P. The use of both therapeutic and prophylactic vaccines in the therapy of papillomavirus disease. Front Immunol 2020; 11: 188.
[http://dx.doi.org/10.3389/fimmu.2020.00188] [PMID: 32133000]

[50]   Yadav RK, Kumari B, Singh P, Ali A, Sharma S, Hajela K. Advances in Adoptive Cellular Therapy (ACT). Advances in Precision Medicine Oncology. 2021: 119.

[51]   Abdalla AME, Xiao L, Miao Y, *et al.* Nanotechnology promotes genetic and functional modifications of therapeutic T cells against cancer. Adv Sci (Weinh) 2020; 7(10): 1903164.
[http://dx.doi.org/10.1002/advs.201903164] [PMID: 32440473]

[52]   Sheykhhasan M, Manoochehri H, Dama P. Use of CAR T-cell for acute lymphoblastic leukemia (ALL) treatment: a review study. Cancer Gene Ther 2022; 29(8-9): 1080-96.
[http://dx.doi.org/10.1038/s41417-021-00418-1] [PMID: 34987176]

[53]   Locke FL, Go WY, Neelapu SS. Development and use of the anti-CD19 chimeric antigen receptor T-cell therapy axicabtagene ciloleucel in large B-cell lymphoma: a review. JAMA Oncol 2020; 6(2): 281-90.
[http://dx.doi.org/10.1001/jamaoncol.2019.3869] [PMID: 31697310]

[54]   Hulen TM, Chamberlain CA, Svane IM, Met Ö. ACT up TIL now: the evolution of tumor-infiltrating lymphocytes in adoptive cell therapy to treat solid tumors. Immuno 2021; 1(3): 194-211.
[http://dx.doi.org/10.3390/immuno1030012]

[55]   Fernández-Rodríguez C, González-Fernández S, Coto-Lesmes R, Pedrosa I. Behavioral activation and acceptance and commitment therapy in the treatment of anxiety and depression in cancer survivors: a

randomized clinical trial. Behav Modif 2021; 45(5): 822-59.
[http://dx.doi.org/10.1177/0145445520916441] [PMID: 32316765]

[56]   Jin S, Sun Y, Liang X, *et al.* Emerging new therapeutic antibody derivatives for cancer treatment. Signal Transduct Target Ther 2022; 7(1): 39.
[http://dx.doi.org/10.1038/s41392-021-00868-x] [PMID: 35132063]

[57]   Sun Y, Li F, Sonnemann H, *et al.* Evolution of CD8+ T cell receptor (TCR) engineered therapies for the treatment of cancer. Cells 2021; 10(9): 2379.
[http://dx.doi.org/10.3390/cells10092379] [PMID: 34572028]

[58]   Kuske M, Haist M, Jung T, Grabbe S, Bros M. Immunomodulatory properties of immune checkpoint inhibitors—more than boosting T-cell responses? Cancers (Basel) 2022; 14(7): 1710.
[http://dx.doi.org/10.3390/cancers14071710] [PMID: 35406483]

[59]   Chulpanova DS, Kitaeva KV, Green AR, Rizvanov AA, Solovyeva VV. Molecular aspects and future perspectives of cytokine-based anti-cancer immunotherapy. Front Cell Dev Biol 2020; 8: 402.
[http://dx.doi.org/10.3389/fcell.2020.00402] [PMID: 32582698]

[60]   Ko B, Takebe N, Andrews O, Makena MR, Chen AP. Rethinking oncologic treatment strategies with interleukin-2. Cells 2023; 12(9): 1316.
[http://dx.doi.org/10.3390/cells12091316] [PMID: 37174716]

[61]   Demaria O, Gauthier L, Vetizou M, *et al.* Antitumor immunity induced by antibody-based natural killer cell engager therapeutics armed with not-alpha IL-2 variant. Cell Rep Med 2022; 3(10): 100783.
[http://dx.doi.org/10.1016/j.xcrm.2022.100783] [PMID: 36260981]

[62]   Zhang Z, Zhu Y, Xu D, *et al.* IFN-α facilitates the effect of sorafenib *via* shifting the M2-like polarization of TAM in hepatocellular carcinoma. Am J Transl Res 2021; 13(1): 301-13.
[PMID: 33527025]

[63]   Lan T, Chen L, Wei X. Inflammatory cytokines in cancer: comprehensive understanding and clinical progress in gene therapy. Cells 2021; 10(1): 100.
[http://dx.doi.org/10.3390/cells10010100] [PMID: 33429846]

[64]   Nguyen KG, Vrabel MR, Mantooth SM, *et al.* Localized interleukin-12 for cancer immunotherapy. Front Immunol 2020; 11: 575597.
[http://dx.doi.org/10.3389/fimmu.2020.575597] [PMID: 33178203]

[65]   Ventura A. Combinatory therapeutic approaches for haematological and solid tumors with Cytokine-Induced Killer (CIK) cells.

[66]   Manzari MT, Shamay Y, Kiguchi H, Rosen N, Scaltriti M, Heller DA. Targeted drug delivery strategies for precision medicines. Nat Rev Mater 2021; 6(4): 351-70.
[http://dx.doi.org/10.1038/s41578-020-00269-6] [PMID: 34950512]

[67]   Vafaei S, Zekiy AO, Khanamir RA, *et al.* Combination therapy with immune checkpoint inhibitors (ICIs); a new frontier. Cancer Cell Int 2022; 22(1): 2.
[http://dx.doi.org/10.1186/s12935-021-02407-8] [PMID: 34980128]

[68]   Federico S, Pozzetti L, Papa A, *et al.* Modulating the innate immune response by targeting toll-like receptors: a perspective on their agonists and antagonists. J Med Chem 2020; 63(22): 13466-513.
[http://dx.doi.org/10.1021/acs.jmedchem.0c01049] [PMID: 32845153]

[69]   Malik AE, Issekutz TB, Derfalvi B. The role of type III interferons in human disease. Clin Invest Med 2021; 44(2): E5-E18.
[http://dx.doi.org/10.25011/cim.v44i2.36622] [PMID: 34152702]

[70]   Domingo S, Solé C, Moliné T, Ferrer B, Ordi-Ros J, Cortés-Hernández J. Efficacy of thalidomide in discoid lupus erythematosus: insights into the molecular mechanisms. Dermatology 2020; 236(5): 467-76.
[http://dx.doi.org/10.1159/000508672] [PMID: 32659758]

[71] Pandey P, Khan F, Qari HA, Upadhyay TK, Alkhateeb AF, Oves M. Revolutionization in cancer therapeutics *via* targeting major immune checkpoints PD-1, PD-L1 and CTLA-4. Pharmaceuticals (Basel) 2022; 15(3): 335.
[http://dx.doi.org/10.3390/ph15030335] [PMID: 35337133]

[72] Miller M, Hanna N. Advances in systemic therapy for non-small cell lung cancer. BMJ 2021; 375: n2363.
[http://dx.doi.org/10.1136/bmj.n2363] [PMID: 34753715]

[73] Dongye Z, Li J, Wu Y. Toll-like receptor 9 agonists and combination therapies: strategies to modulate the tumour immune microenvironment for systemic anti-tumour immunity. Br J Cancer 2022; 127(9): 1584-94.
[http://dx.doi.org/10.1038/s41416-022-01876-6] [PMID: 35902641]

[74] Nguyen HM, Guz-Montgomery K, Saha D. Oncolytic virus encoding a master pro-inflammatory cytokine interleukin 12 in cancer immunotherapy. Cells 2020; 9(2): 400.
[http://dx.doi.org/10.3390/cells9020400] [PMID: 32050597]

[75] Pérez-Romero K, Rodríguez RM, Amedei A, Barceló-Coblijn G, Lopez DH. Immune landscape in tumor microenvironment: Implications for biomarker development and immunotherapy. Int J Mol Sci 2020; 21(15): 5521.
[http://dx.doi.org/10.3390/ijms21155521] [PMID: 32752264]

[76] Raghani NR, Chorawala MR, Mahadik M, Patel RB, Prajapati BG, Parekh PS. Revolutionizing cancer treatment: comprehensive insights into immunotherapeutic strategies. Med Oncol 2024; 41(2): 51.
[http://dx.doi.org/10.1007/s12032-023-02280-7] [PMID: 38195781]

[77] Goebeler ME, Bargou RC. T cell-engaging therapies — BiTEs and beyond. Nat Rev Clin Oncol 2020; 17(7): 418-34.
[http://dx.doi.org/10.1038/s41571-020-0347-5] [PMID: 32242094]

[78] Lussana F, Gritti G, Rambaldi A. Immunotherapy of acute lymphoblastic leukemia and lymphoma with T cell–redirected bispecific antibodies. J Clin Oncol 2021; 39(5): 444-55.
[http://dx.doi.org/10.1200/JCO.20.01564] [PMID: 33434063]

[79] Meckler JF, Levis DJ, Vang DP, Tuscano JM. A Novel bispecific T-cell engager (BiTE) targeting CD22 and CD3 has both *in vitro* and *in vivo* activity and synergizes with blinatumomab in an acute lymphoblastic leukemia (ALL) tumor model. Cancer Immunol Immunother 2023; 72(9): 2939-48.
[http://dx.doi.org/10.1007/s00262-023-03444-0] [PMID: 37247022]

[80] Mocquot P, Mossazadeh Y, Lapierre L, Pineau F, Despas F. The pharmacology of blinatumomab: state of the art on pharmacodynamics, pharmacokinetics, adverse drug reactions and evaluation in clinical trials. J Clin Pharm Ther 2022; 47(9): 1337-51.
[http://dx.doi.org/10.1111/jcpt.13741] [PMID: 35906791]

[81] Bock AM, Nowakowski GS, Wang Y. Bispecific antibodies for non-Hodgkin lymphoma treatment. Curr Treat Options Oncol 2022; 23(2): 155-70.
[http://dx.doi.org/10.1007/s11864-021-00925-1] [PMID: 35182296]

[82] Dutta S, Ganguly A, Chatterjee K, Spada S, Mukherjee S. Targets of immune escape mechanisms in cancer: basis for developing and evolving cancer immune checkpoint inhibitors. Biology (Basel) 2023; 12(2): 218.
[http://dx.doi.org/10.3390/biology12020218] [PMID: 36829496]

[83] Jin XI. ZHANG HF, Hua-Chun LI, Xin-Hong PA, RENKE D. Cytokine release assessment: a good de-risk approach to bi-specific T-cell engagers in non-clinical development. Zhongguo Yaolixue Yu Dulixue Zazhi 2021; 522-30.

[84] Ruella M, Korell F, Porazzi P, Maus MV. Mechanisms of resistance to chimeric antigen receptor-T cells in haematological malignancies. Nat Rev Drug Discov 2023; 22(12): 976-95.
[http://dx.doi.org/10.1038/s41573-023-00807-1] [PMID: 37907724]

[85]   Wang B, Pei J, Xu S, Liu J, Yu J. Recent advances in mRNA cancer vaccines: meeting challenges and embracing opportunities. Front Immunol 2023; 14: 1246682.
[http://dx.doi.org/10.3389/fimmu.2023.1246682] [PMID: 37744371]

[86]   Hameed SA, Paul S, Dellosa GKY, Jaraquemada D, Bello MB. Towards the future exploration of mucosal mRNA vaccines against emerging viral diseases; lessons from existing next-generation mucosal vaccine strategies. NPJ Vaccines 2022; 7(1): 71.
[http://dx.doi.org/10.1038/s41541-022-00485-x] [PMID: 35764661]

[87]   Wang F, Ullah A, Fan X, *et al.* Delivery of nanoparticle antigens to antigen-presenting cells: from extracellular specific targeting to intracellular responsive presentation. J Control Release 2021; 333: 107-28.
[http://dx.doi.org/10.1016/j.jconrel.2021.03.027] [PMID: 33774119]

[88]   Kawasaki T, Ikegawa M, Kawai T. Antigen presentation in the lung. Front Immunol 2022; 13: 860915.
[http://dx.doi.org/10.3389/fimmu.2022.860915] [PMID: 35615351]

[89]   Ben-Shmuel A, Biber G, Barda-Saad M. Unleashing natural killer cells in the tumor microenvironment–the next generation of immunotherapy? Front Immunol 2020; 11: 275.
[http://dx.doi.org/10.3389/fimmu.2020.00275] [PMID: 32153582]

[90]   Anggraeni R, Ana ID, Wihadmadyatami H. Development of mucosal vaccine delivery: an overview on the mucosal vaccines and their adjuvants. Clin Exp Vaccine Res 2022; 11(3): 235-48.
[http://dx.doi.org/10.7774/cevr.2022.11.3.235] [PMID: 36451668]

[91]   Rhee JH. Current and new approaches for mucosal vaccine delivery. InMucosal vaccines, 2020; pp. 325-356.
[http://dx.doi.org/10.1016/B978-0-12-811924-2.00019-5]

[92]   Czerkinsky C, Holmgren J. Immunomodulation at Mucosal Surfaces: Prospects for Developing Antiinfectious and Antiinflammatory Vaccines. InImmune Modulating Agents, 2020; pp. 529-537.

[93]   Ferber S, Gonzalez RJ, Cryer AM, von Andrian UH, Artzi N. Immunology guided biomaterial design for mucosal cancer vaccines. Adv Mater 2020; 32(13): 1903847.
[http://dx.doi.org/10.1002/adma.201903847] [PMID: 31833592]

[94]   Ou BS, Saouaf OM, Baillet J, Appel EA. Sustained delivery approaches to improving adaptive immune responses. Adv Drug Deliv Rev 2022; 187: 114401.
[http://dx.doi.org/10.1016/j.addr.2022.114401] [PMID: 35750115]

[95]   Ahmed T, Freitas D, Huang X, Rui Simon Qu Q, Traverso G, Kirtane A. Physical methods to overcome tissue barriers in vaccine delivery. Vaccine Insights 2023; 2(10): 363-80.
[http://dx.doi.org/10.18609/vac/2023.050]

[96]   Zhang Y, Li M, Du G, Chen X, Sun X. Advanced oral vaccine delivery strategies for improving the immunity. Adv Drug Deliv Rev 2021; 177: 113928.
[http://dx.doi.org/10.1016/j.addr.2021.113928] [PMID: 34411689]

[97]   Beyaert S, Machiels JP, Schmitz S. Vaccine-based immunotherapy for head and neck cancers. Cancers (Basel) 2021; 13(23): 6041.
[http://dx.doi.org/10.3390/cancers13236041] [PMID: 34885150]

[98]   Chitsike L, Duerksen-Hughes P. The potential of immune checkpoint blockade in cervical cancer: Can combinatorial regimens maximize response? A review of the literature. Curr Treat Options Oncol 2020; 21(12): 95.
[http://dx.doi.org/10.1007/s11864-020-00790-4] [PMID: 33025260]

[99]   Kazi N, Kindt Jr JW, Kahanda I, da Costa C, Carnahan R, Mason H, Wilson BA, Rupassara SI. Perspective Chapter: Natural Adjuvants for Mucosal Vaccines—The Promise of Tomatine as an Inherent Adjuvant in Tomatoes.

[100] Lin Y, Wang C, He X, Yao Q, Chen J. Comparative cost-effectiveness of first-line pembrolizumab plus chemotherapy vs. chemotherapy alone in persistent, recurrent, or metastatic cervical cancer. Front Immunol 2024; 14: 1345942.
[http://dx.doi.org/10.3389/fimmu.2023.1345942] [PMID: 38274823]

[101] Boilesen DR, Nielsen KN, Holst PJ. Novel antigenic targets of HPV therapeutic vaccines. Vaccines (Basel) 2021; 9(11): 1262.
[http://dx.doi.org/10.3390/vaccines9111262] [PMID: 34835193]

[102] Kannampuzha S, Gopalakrishnan AV, Padinharayil H, *et al.* Onco-Pathogen mediated cancer progression and associated signaling pathways in cancer development. Pathogens 2023; 12(6): 770.
[http://dx.doi.org/10.3390/pathogens12060770] [PMID: 37375460]

[103] Xie X, Song T, Feng Y, *et al.* Nanotechnology-based multifunctional vaccines for cancer immunotherapy. Chem Eng J 2022; 437: 135505.
[http://dx.doi.org/10.1016/j.cej.2022.135505]

[104] Trincado V, Gala RP, Morales JO. Buccal and sublingual vaccines: A review on oral mucosal immunization and delivery systems. Vaccines (Basel) 2021; 9(10): 1177.
[http://dx.doi.org/10.3390/vaccines9101177] [PMID: 34696284]

[105] Zheng K, Feng Y, Li L, Kong F, Gao J, Kong X. Engineered bacterial outer membrane vesicles: a versatile bacteria-based weapon against gastrointestinal tumors. Theranostics 2024; 14(2): 761-87.
[http://dx.doi.org/10.7150/thno.85917] [PMID: 38169585]

[106] Gambirasi M, Safa A, Vruzhaj I, Giacomin A, Sartor F, Toffoli G. Oral Administration of Cancer Vaccines: Challenges and Future Perspectives. Vaccines (Basel) 2023; 12(1): 26.
[http://dx.doi.org/10.3390/vaccines12010026] [PMID: 38250839]

[107] Nizard M, Diniz MO, Roussel H, *et al.* Mucosal vaccines. Hum Vaccin Immunother 2014; 10(8): 2175-87.
[http://dx.doi.org/10.4161/hv.29269] [PMID: 25424921]

[108] Lin G, Li J. Circulating HPV DNA in HPV-associated cancers. Clin Chim Acta 2023; 542: 117269.
[http://dx.doi.org/10.1016/j.cca.2023.117269] [PMID: 36841427]

[109] Qin L, Zhang H, Zhou Y, Umeshappa CS, Gao H. Nanovaccine□based strategies to overcome challenges in the whole vaccination cascade for tumor immunotherapy. Small 2021; 17(28): 2006000.
[http://dx.doi.org/10.1002/smll.202006000] [PMID: 33768693]

[110] Fridman WH, Zitvogel L, Sautès-Fridman C, Kroemer G. The immune contexture in cancer prognosis and treatment. Nat Rev Clin Oncol 2017; 14(12): 717-34.
[http://dx.doi.org/10.1038/nrclinonc.2017.101] [PMID: 28741618]

[111] Finn OJ. Cancer vaccines: between the idea and the reality. Nat Rev Immunol 2003; 3(8): 630-41.
[http://dx.doi.org/10.1038/nri1150] [PMID: 12974478]

[112] Freytag LC, Clements JD. Mucosal adjuvants: new developments and challenges. In Mucosal immunology, 2015; pp. 1183-1199.

[113] Lischer C. Computational Methods to Find and Rank MHC-I Restricted Tumor-Associated Antigens to Improve Therapeutic Efficacy and Tolerability of Antigen-based Cancer Immunotherapy (Doctoral dissertation, Dissertation, Erlangen, Friedrich-Alexander-Universität Erlangen-Nürnberg (FAU), 2023).

[114] Sharma R, Agrawal U, Mody N, Vyas SP. Polymer nanotechnology based approaches in mucosal vaccine delivery: Challenges and opportunities. Biotechnol Adv 2015; 33(1): 64-79.
[http://dx.doi.org/10.1016/j.biotechadv.2014.12.004] [PMID: 25499178]

[115] Salalli R, Dange JR, Dhiman S, Sharma T. Vaccines development in India: advances, regulation, and challenges. Clin Exp Vaccine Res 2023; 12(3): 193-208.
[http://dx.doi.org/10.7774/cevr.2023.12.3.193] [PMID: 37599804]

[116] Sadozai H, Gruber T, Hunger RE, Schenk M. Recent successes and future directions in immunotherapy of cutaneous melanoma. Front Immunol 2017; 8: 1617.
[http://dx.doi.org/10.3389/fimmu.2017.01617] [PMID: 29276510]

[117] Mougel A, Terme M, Tanchot C. Therapeutic cancer vaccine and combinations with antiangiogenic therapies and immune checkpoint blockade. Front Immunol 2019; 10: 467.
[http://dx.doi.org/10.3389/fimmu.2019.00467] [PMID: 30923527]

[118] Bolhassani A, Safaiyan S, Rafati S. Improvement of different vaccine delivery systems for cancer therapy. Mol Cancer 2011; 10(1): 3.
[http://dx.doi.org/10.1186/1476-4598-10-3] [PMID: 21211062]

[119] Jin Z, Gao S, Cui X, Sun D, Zhao K. Adjuvants and delivery systems based on polymeric nanoparticles for mucosal vaccines. Int J Pharm 2019; 572: 118731.
[http://dx.doi.org/10.1016/j.ijpharm.2019.118731] [PMID: 31669213]

SUBJECT INDEX

A

B

C

D

Bovine